Single-Case Designs for Applied Research

To Thomas G. Haring (1953–1993), mentor and friend

Single-Case Designs for Applied Research

Craig H. Kennedy

University of Connecticut

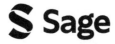

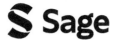

FOR INFORMATION:

2455 Teller Road
Thousand Oaks, California 91320
E-mail: order@sagepub.com

1 Oliver's Yard
55 City Road
London, EC1Y 1SP
United Kingdom

Unit No 323-333, Third Floor, F-Block
International Trade Tower Nehru Place
New Delhi 110 019
India

18 Cross Street #10-10/11/12
China Square Central
Singapore 048423

Printed in the United States of America

Library of Congress Control Number: 2024038455

ISBN: 978-1-0719-1598-1

This book is printed on acid-free paper.

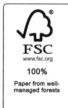

FSC
www.fsc.org
100%
Paper from well-managed forests

Acquisitions Editor: Leah Fargotstein

Editorial Assistant: Jennifer Milewski

Production Editor: Vijayakumar

Copy Editor: Melinda Masson

Typesetter: TNQ Tech Pvt. Ltd.

Indexer: TNQ Tech Pvt. Ltd.

Cover Designer: Scott Van Atta

Marketing Manager: Victoria Velasquez

24 25 26 27 28 10 9 8 7 6 5 4 3 2 1

BRIEF CONTENTS

DETAILED CONTENTS

PREFACE

Successful researchers practice innovation, not imitation. Research methods and the procedures that define their use are tools to be used in the pursuit of answering questions. It is the experimental question that drives the experimental method an investigator uses for any particular study. Experimental method is always subservient to the larger pursuit of more effective interventions, more precise assessments, or resolution to some long-standing problems.

I have thoroughly revised this research methods book as a starting place to explore behavioral, emotional, and cognitive phenomena with a focus on answering salient questions and solving problems in need of resolution. This book focuses on one type of research methodology: single-case designs. This design type is not the only meaningful approach to experimentation; there are many useful methodological tools that exist. However, single-case designs offer a unique set of characteristics that over the past 70+ years have proven to be reliably effective experimental tools.

The strengths of $N = 1$ designs are their unique capacity for establishing experimental control (i.e., internal validity) while providing a similarly unique ability for the experimental design to be altered as an experiment progresses. These strengths are closely associated, and probably unique to single-case designs. However, such a focus minimizes the utility of single-case designs in providing compelling information about the external validity of an experimental outcome. These are the trade-offs an investigator accepts when using single-case design methodology: an emphasis on rigorous experimental control, but limits on what can be claimed regarding external validity. Again, researchers use $N = 1$ designs when they are the correct methodological tool for the problem being studied.

This book is written for students interested in learning how to use single-case designs as a research tool in practical settings. The book is not about codifying a set of rules that must be stringently followed. Such a perspective on experimentation is antithetical to the idea of research and scientific progress—although, I am afraid, it is the way many students learn about experimental design, irrespective of disciplinary boundaries. Therefore, my goal in writing this book is to teach future researchers how to *think* about the use and logic of single-case designs.

The book is intended as a graduate-level text, perhaps at the advanced level of study. One of the complexities of writing a methodology text on single-case designs is that this approach to research is inextricably linked to behavior analysis. The two have developed contemporaneously and have contributed to the success of each other. Single-case designs were originally developed as tools to analyze behavioral mechanisms in the experimental analysis of behavior. It was not until the development of applied behavior analysis that people considered the use of single-case designs for more utilitarian purposes. This makes teaching students about the basic elements of single-case designs, such as measurement and multiple-baseline designs, relatively easy because there is no need for content knowledge relating to behavioral mechanisms. However, when the more advanced design concepts are encountered, their discussion is often based on the analysis of behavioral processes. Therefore, to grasp the more complex single-case design issues, a strong working knowledge of behavior analysis is helpful. This makes writing a broadly accessible textbook on single-case designs a difficult balance. I have tried, and hopefully succeeded, in striking a balance between the two.

Three books in particular have shaped my own understanding of single-case designs: Sidman's *Tactics of Scientific Research*, Johnston et al.'s *Strategies and Tactics of Behavioral Research*, and Campbell and Stanley's *Experimental and Quasi-Experimental Designs for Research*. The former two books have influenced my understanding of what $N=1$ designs are, and the latter has helped me understand what they are not. The influence of these books on my understanding of experimental design will be obvious to anyone who is familiar with them.

This book is structured in five parts. Part I establishes the background for using single-case designs by discussing why people conduct experiments and reviewing the history of single-case designs. Part II discusses strategic issues in conducting single-case experiments, focusing on establishing functional relations, types of replication, the development of experimental questions, and how one assesses whether a particular practice is evidence based. Part III presents issues key to collecting useful information—quantifying behaviors, recording their occurrences, and establishing consistent data collection and intervention protocols. Specific design tactics are presented in Part IV. Some of these designs have appeared in previous textbooks; others are more recent innovations from the research literature including repeated-acquisition designs and brief experimental analyses. Finally, Part V explores issues related to understanding the data emerging from single-case research. These areas include the visual analysis of data, the quantitative analysis of data, and the estimation of social validity. My goal is for these chapters, as a collection, to provide a foundation in the essential elements of single-case design that will allow the reader to learn more about this unique approach to experimentation.

Throughout the book I use "classic" or "high-impact" studies that are often the first instances of a particular experimental technique. By doing so, I hope to note when a particular design type emerged in the research literature and provide the opportunity for readers to assess how much has changed (or stayed the same) with the types of designs used in single-case research. This strikes me as a reasonable pedagogical technique. A second characteristic of this book is an emphasis on single-case designs as idiographic research methods. While single-case designs can incorporate multiple participants into a single experimental design, the underlying logic of these designs is always idiographic. Thus, I frequently make use of the term "$N = 1$" as a synonym for single-case designs. With the rapidly increasing interest in single-case designs across a range of research disciplines, the emphasis on its idiographic foundations seems apropos.

A few qualifications are in order. First, I must apologize for an overreliance on my own research to illustrate certain ideas and concepts. This citation frequency in no way reflects the importance of my own work. Instead, it is a reflection of the fact that an investigator is most familiar with their own research. Therefore, this is the source material most readily accessible to me as an author. Also, Chapter 2 of this book presents an abbreviated history of single-case designs, behavior analysis, and education. Its contents likely reflect my own professional training in behavior analysis and education, and my personal interest in the history of these fields.

Undoubtedly, I have made omission and commission errors because of my poorly developed historiography skills.

Leah Fargotstein and Jennifer Milewski at Sage have been invaluable in bringing this text to publication. In addition, I would like to thank the prepublication reviewers whose feedback substantively improved the book:

Judah B. Axe, *Simmons University*

Bridget Sweeney Blakely, *Drexel University*

Susan R. Copeland, *University of New Mexico*

Kyle De Young, *University of Wyoming*

Cynthia DiCarlo, *Louisiana State University*

Caroline DiPipi-Hoy, *East Stroudsburg University*

Nicole Gravina, *University of Florida*

Megan Griffin, *Whitworth University*

Brittany L. Hott, *University of Oklahoma*

Sara Jozwik, *University of Wisconsin–Milwaukee*

Molly E. Milam, *York College of Pennsylvania*

Reem Muharib, *Texas State University*

Jennifer Ninci, *University of Hawaii–Manoa*

Corey Peltier, *University of Oklahoma*

Robert Pennington, *University of North Carolina–Charlotte*

Sudha Ramaswamy, *Mercy College*

Samantha Riggleman, *Saint Joseph's University*

Emily Shumate, *University of Massachusetts–Lowell*

Scott Spaulding, *University of Washington*

Shane T. Spiker, *Arizona State University*

Joanna B. Thompson, *McNeese State University*

Benjamin N. Witts, *St. Cloud State University*

I would also like to thank my many colleagues over the decades who have provided me with interesting ideas and outstanding critical feedback that has helped shape my own understanding of single-case designs. Finally, I would like to note that I have dedicated the second edition of this book to my late advisor Thomas G. Haring. Tom died far too early in his life, but he had already become a significant researcher and deep thinker who influenced several generations of scholars. He was also a lot of fun. In the 10 years we worked together, he taught me a great deal about being a researcher, but also about how to live a meaningful life.

Craig H. Kennedy
New Haven, CT
February 2024

ABOUT THE AUTHOR

Craig H. Kennedy is a professor of educational psychology and pediatrics at the University of Connecticut. He received his terminal degree from the University of California, Santa Barbara (education), master's degree from the University of Oregon (special education), and bachelor's degree from the University of California, Santa Barbara (experimental psychology). He spent much of his academic career at Vanderbilt University where he was a professor of special education and pediatrics and served as department chair and senior associate dean. He has also served as provost and executive vice president of academic affairs at the University of Connecticut and dean of education at the University of Georgia.

He is a board-certified behavior analyst whose research focuses on health conditions and challenging behavior in people with autism and other neurodevelopmental disabilities. His early research focused on establishing and developing video modeling and peer support strategies as evidence-based practices. He is currently editor-in-chief of *Research and Practice for Persons With Severe Disabilities* and is a former associate editor of the *Journal of Applied Behavior Analysis* and *Journal of Behavioral Education*. He is a longtime member of the American Psychological Association (APA), Association for Behavior Analysis International, and TASH. He is also the inaugural recipient of the B. F. Skinner Foundation New Researcher Award from the APA and Alice H. Hayden Emerging Leader Award from TASH. During his career he has published over 180 scholarly papers and secured over $17 million in extramural support for his teaching, research, and service.

THE APPLIED IMPORTANCE OF RESEARCH

1 WHY CONDUCT EXPERIMENTS?

LEARNING OBJECTIVES

After reading this chapter, you will be able to

1.1 Articulate the elements of a systematic experimental inquiry.

1.2 Describe the hallmark characteristics of experimental progress.

1.3 Summarize the assumptions and beliefs that guide researchers in conducting their experiments.

Most gains made in educational practice have resulted from researchers conducting experiments. Whether those gains have been made by group-comparison methods, ethnography, epidemiology, econometrics, or single-case designs, the mechanism by which progress has occurred is *experimentation*. The use of experimental methods to better understand educational practices was championed by a diverse group of scholars in the early 20th century, including John Dewey (1958), George Herbert Mead (see Baldwin, 1987), B. F. Skinner (1954), and John B. Watson (1924). Each of these individuals noted that for systematic progress to occur, research was needed to allow education to rise above the politics, personal biases, and fads that dominate educational policymaking, then and now.

Although there is far to go in creating a universally effective and efficient educational system, the efforts of researchers have transformed educational practice in the last 50 years. What are now considered common practices in schools have emerged from the educational research of previous decades. Examples include peer-mediated instruction, data-based decision making, curriculum-based assessment, systematic instruction, positive behavior supports, token economies, inclusive education, phonics-based reading strategies, and accessing the general education curriculum, among many, many others.

These gains have been made by conducting experiments to answer questions to which there are no effective answers. By carefully crafting a question and then using a set of techniques to methodically study the phenomenon, a clearer idea of how different events interrelate can be revealed. In a sense, researchers ask specific questions regarding "How do things work?" If I want to know how a new teaching technique might improve student learning, my best bet is to conduct an experiment to answer that question. I could simply say "my way is obviously better" or "because we have always done things this way, it is the best way," *but I am more likely to improve student learning if I conduct experiments.*

WHAT IS AN EXPERIMENT?

An experiment is an approach to answering questions. By systematically studying a set of questions, researchers uncover answers that help guide them toward increasingly effective practices. However, there are important differences between how a layperson goes about answering a question and how a researcher answers a question. Humans have used at least three different ways of finding answers to questions.

The approach most familiar to people is the use of *common sense*. I mean to use *common sense* not in a derogatory way, but rather as a label for a set of strategies that are familiar to us. People arrive at assumptions about "how the world works" through everyday experience. For example, a child new to a school may notice that their classmates all raise their hands before answering the teacher's questions or asking for help. If students do not raise their hands, the teacher does not provide them with attention. The new child may quickly learn that they need to raise their hand to get the teacher's attention. If this occurs, they have used their everyday experiences to learn about how to behave in the new classroom and, perhaps, in other settings in the future. Not surprisingly, by and large, this approach works well for us in our daily lives.

However, there is a downside to answering questions through everyday experience. Although accumulated wisdom can often be effective in guiding our daily lives (your grandparents are, indeed, a source of important knowledge about how the world works), common sense also has its limitations. The primary limitation of common sense is that it is derived from correlated events and descriptions of situations. Simply the fact that two events tend to co-occur and there is a pattern to their co-occurrence does not mean that they are related. This places important constraints on how useful common sense is as a tool for understanding the world. For example, a person might observe that each day the sun rises in the east, crosses the sky, and sets in the west. For the majority of recorded history, people used this observation to infer that the sun circles the earth. Such an observation is confirmed by daily experience and makes sense if those experiences are the only basis for drawing conclusions. Although we like to think that as a modern, educated society we no longer believe the sun circles the earth, a recent survey of Americans found that 25% believed that *the sun circles the earth* (Allum et al., 2008; National Science Board, 2014).

Unfortunately, common sense stops at the level of correlation and does not pursue a more rigorous set of tests to verify or discount the nature of covariants. As the dictum taught in every introductory science class says, *"correlation does not imply causation."* Lest the reader think this is not a problem in the field of education, it may be instructive to note that the primary way educational policies are decided in a school district is the "school board." A school board's task is to make decisions about what is taught, who is taught where, how students are taught, and other related issues such as school discipline. However, despite the importance of these decisions, it has been noted that less than 10% of school board members have any type of degree relating to education and virtually none have training in research (Alsbury, 2008; Land, 2002).

Fortunately, people have developed other ways of answering questions that apply more rigorous tests about events before arriving at conclusions. An alternative to everyday experience as a means of understanding nature emerged in Ancient Greek and Persian cultures (Kantor, 1963). This approach, which we will call *logical analysis*, uses formal mathematical systems to test and arrive at conclusions. When conducting a logical analysis, a person needs to clearly define the question, use an established set of procedures to test possible answers to the question, and then arrive at a conclusion (Marr, 1986). For example, one could develop the following proposition: "All behavior occurs for a reason; reading is a form of behavior; therefore, the reasons why people read can be identified." A rule set could then be used to test the logical adequacy of the proposition and its conclusion: "The reasons why people read can be identified" (Cohen & Nagel, 1962). A number of individuals have attempted to show that such mathematical analyses are the basis of philosophical knowledge, sometimes referred to as "refined knowledge" (e.g., Whitehead & Russell, 1925).

However, there is a very important limitation to the logical approach. Although the system is clear and rigorous in what it does, the system is purely linguistic. That is, it never actually makes contact with natural phenomena and demonstrates the existence of the logical outcome. Although it presents hypotheses to test, the tests themselves are only verbal arguments. This has led to concerns that logical analysis is an inwardly defined system that is not tested in the real world. Harking back to our solar system question, one could formally propose that the sun circles the earth and develop a mathematical model of how it works (see Kuhn, 1957). Such a system, referred to as Ptolemaic astronomy, was the sine qua non of understanding our solar system for centuries. However, such a logical argument does not demonstrate the existence of the phenomenon; it demonstrates only that the phenomenon could exist as a logical outcome of a verbal argument. Such limitations to logical analysis set the occasion for the development of experimentation as an alternative way of learning about how the world works.

What makes experimentation different from common sense or logic is that it requires an individual to systematically test their assumptions (Bristow, 2010). Indeed, there are a set of characteristics that distinguish experimentation from other human endeavors that might not be immediately obvious to those not trained as researchers. First, a clear *experimental question* needs to be asked (see Chapter 5). Such questions are often referred to as "hypotheses" (see Box 1.1). However, there are different types of hypotheses, with some being more specific than others. For example, I might ask any of the following questions regarding a particular teaching technique:

1. "Does the use of time delay as a prompting technique lead to children acquiring addition and subtraction skills?"

2. "Does the use of time delay as a prompting technique result in faster acquisition of addition or subtraction skills than trial-and-error feedback?"

3. "Are parameters of the matching law, such as magnitude of reinforcement or latency of reinforcement, the reason that time delay is more effective than trial-and-error feedback in teaching basic mathematics skills?"

BOX 1.1: VARIOUS TYPES OF HYPOTHESES

An experimental question can be considered a type of hypothesis. However, in many areas of the social and health sciences, hypotheses have a more formal meaning and role in experimentation. This role can be traced to the early 20th century and the emergence of inferential statistics as a tool for agrarian research (Street, 1990). Tests using inferential statistics require the statement of a formal hypothesis (often referred to as a null hypothesis). In this sense, a hypothesis is not so much an experimental question as a statement about the anticipated results of the study. Once a formal hypothesis has been stated, the study can be conducted, the results statistically analyzed, and the statistical results used to either confirm the hypothesis or fail to reject the null hypothesis. However, with single-case designs such an arrangement is sometimes deemed unnecessary to competently conduct a study. Instead of creating formal hypotheses to confirm or reject, researchers focus on developing appropriate experimental questions and techniques to analyze them. The focus is not on the adequacy of an experimenter's prediction about the outcomes of their research (i.e., formal hypothesis testing), but on allowing the phenomenon to be revealed through careful experimentation. Researchers using single-case designs may use inferential statistics (see Chapter 17), but the emphasis is on experimental control and internal validity.

Hypothesis 1 is a general question about whether a particular teaching technique is effective. This is a very general type of hypothesis, but one that proposes a potentially important experimental question. Hypothesis 2 is more specific and asks whether one type of teaching technique is better than another. Hypothesis 3 asks a very specific question regarding what *mechanism* is responsible for the effectiveness of a particular teaching strategy. All of these are valid experimental questions that vary in specificity. Indeed, hypotheses can range from open-ended questions to very precise predictions about how things work. However, regardless of the level of specificity, *all hypotheses specify an experimental question in an objective manner that can be tested* (see Curry et al. [2020] and Mager [1962] for more on objective statements).

A second characteristic of research is that a clear plan is developed for objectively *measuring the events of interest*. That is, a researcher needs to identify what needs to be measured to adequately study the experimental question. For example, if I am studying the effects of a teaching technique on mathematics skill acquisition, one thing I need to measure is mathematics performance. In addition, based on the nature of my experimental question, I may also want to gather information on the types of errors that are made, the time that elapses between correct responses, performance on novel types of mathematics problems, and/or the occurrence of competing behaviors. Typically, *the events of interest are formalized into an observational code and a set of procedures outlined for when and how the events of interest will be measured* (see Part III of this book for more on *measurement*).

Another aspect of research that differs from other ways of exploring nature focuses on conducting an *experimental analysis*. The world is full of events that are constantly changing. This flux of activity is part of how our everyday lives function. However, it makes the systematic study of *causes* very difficult. If things are continually changing, it is hard to ascertain what are simply correlated events and what are causal relations among events. Therefore, researchers use experimental designs to distinguish between what is correlated from what is causal. To accomplish this, all events—also referred to as *variables*—are held constant except for one. This one variable—referred to as an *independent variable* (see Chapter 3)—is then allowed to operate, then withdrawn, then allowed to operate again, and so on. For example, if an investigator wants to study how teacher attention influences the challenging behavior of a child, adult attention could be selectively presented when challenging behavior occurs, then withdrawn for a period of time, and then re-presented. In addition, the researcher would need to hold all other potentially influential events constant (e.g., task type, task difficulty, and the presence of peers) while varying teacher attention so that there are no correlated events co-occurring with changes in teacher attention. If challenging behaviors (in this case the *dependent variable*) increase when attention is provided and decrease when attention is withdrawn, this pattern suggests that the behavior is related to teacher attention. By systematically presenting and withdrawing an independent variable while holding other variables constant and measuring changes in the dependent variable, experimental control can be demonstrated. By demonstrating experimental control through the use of research designs, an estimation of the degree to which a particular variable influences behavior can be established (see Part IV of this book for a discussion of types of experimental designs).

Once the experiment is conducted, a researcher needs to *analyze* the results. Typically, a series of exploratory analyses of the data are conducted to find out what types of patterns exist. These exploratory analyses seek to reveal how the independent variable influenced the dependent variable(s). Once the nature of the data patterns have been established, a researcher then seeks to summarize them for presentation to an audience. This is done so that the patterns that were found to occur as a result of the experiment can be clearly and concisely presented to other researchers. In essence, exploratory data analysis is a method for finding out "what the data have to say." These patterns are then summarized in tables and graphs so that information can be clearly communicated to a larger audience (see Part V of this book for a discussion of data analysis).

Finally, once a researcher has identified an experimental question, developed a measurement system, conducted an experimental analysis, and analyzed the results, one critical, final step needs to be completed. That is, *the results of the experiment need to be publicly reported and subjected to peer review.* A hallmark of experimentation is that the process is very transparent, meaning that any other person interested in what the researcher has done can obtain information about what occurred, where it was done, how it was done, when it was done, what resulted from those efforts, and how the researchers interpret their findings. A general rule of thumb is that the experiment is described in sufficient detail so that another person can read the paper reporting the study, replicate the procedures, and see if they obtain the same results. A manuscript reporting an experiment is then submitted to a *peer-reviewed journal* where experts evaluate the believability of the experiment and decide whether it was competently conducted and should be published. Finally, any experimental outcome is suspect until another group of researchers *replicate* the procedures and findings (see Chapter 4). This focus on public reporting, evaluation by experts, and replication by independent research groups makes the research process unlike most other human activities. There is no room in the process for vagueness, deceit, or false claims because everything is available for public scrutiny and rigorous evaluation (see the *Publication Manual* of the American Psychological Association [2020] for more information on the preparation and peer review of research papers). However, replication in its various instances is a challenging endeavor, and much attention is focused on the degree to which findings in the social sciences are replicable (see Box 1.2 and Chapter 4).

BOX 1.2: "THE REPLICATION CRISIS" AND SINGLE-CASE DESIGNS

Over the last decade there has been much discussion, some experimental analysis, and many emerging recommendations regarding the "replicability" of contemporary science. Much of that discussion has focused on the social sciences and particularly psychological research (Pashler & Wagenmakers, 2012; Simmons et al., 2011). A primary focus of these concerns has been the degree to which statistically significant findings from an initial experiment can be replicated by other researchers using similar procedures. From a single-case design perspective, it is important to frame this discussion about replicability in the context of experimental and quasi-experimental group design logic. The large majority of psychological research randomly assigns participants to an individual condition and then compares the central tendency and dispersion of the data from each of the groups. If the groups are shown to be statistically distinct, then an experimental effect is claimed. This is the core logic of most psychological experiments. However, note that there *is no requirement for replication to occur within an individual experiment*. Replication of findings in group-comparison studies requires additional experiments, and a concerning percentage of those follow-up studies fail to replicate the original findings. *The concern about replicability has not emerged as a strong concern in single-case design research.* Thus, not all psychological research seems to have a "replication crisis." The reasons for this are likely based on the strong emphasis on internal validity through replication used in single-case research. In any particular experiment, the effect of the independent variable is replicated at least once and is often replicated multiple times within an individual experiment (see Chapter 4). Single-case experiments that fail to replicate their findings are studies that fail to show experimental control, and the results are interpreted accordingly. Thus, the emphasis in single-case designs on internal validity likely reduces the risk of reporting false positive findings.

EXPERIMENTAL PROGRESS

Just as the process of conducting experiments differs substantially from everyday activities, so does the course of experimental progress. The stereotype most people have of research would suggest that it is an efficient, rigorous process that makes linear progress toward a particular goal. For instance, a researcher decides to solve a particular problem, devises an appropriate experimental question, and then conducts an experiment that solves the puzzle.

Such a streamlined process is rare. This is because research is a very messy, inefficient, and nonlinear process.

One of the most interesting aspects of experimental progress is the *unpredictability* of the endeavor. Rarely do experimental questions result in precisely what was hypothesized to occur. That is why strict hypothesis testing (Box 1.1) is not always employed in experiments. For example, a researcher may set out to study curricular issues relating to student misbehavior. The experimental question might focus on whether task difficulty is related to increased levels of student noncompliance—the harder the work, the less compliant the student. However, during the course of establishing a baseline, the researcher might notice variability from one day to the next in student behavior, even though task difficulty is being held constant from day to day. Upon further investigation the researcher might discover an unanticipated event covarying with noncompliance. For instance, the student may not have the opportunity to eat breakfast, and on days when they arrive late for school, the student misses the opportunity to have breakfast in the school cafeteria. This missing of a meal may be associated with noncompliance apart from, or in conjunction with, task difficulty. To adequately address this question a competent researcher would need to analyze not only task difficulty in relation to noncompliance, but also the role of missing breakfast in relation to these variables. Although this might seem unrelated to the original hypothesis, to adequately answer the question a somewhat different experimental question would need to be studied.

This aspect of the research process has led to the observation that "any experiment worth its salt will raise more questions than it answers" (Sidman, 1960, p. 8). Sometimes those new questions can be predicted before the experiment is conducted, and at other times, as in the breakfast example, those new questions will only be revealed once the experiment is in progress. This truism suggests that a wise researcher should stay vigilant during an experiment to a range of events that might influence behavior. B. F. Skinner (1983) once remarked that his most important scientific discoveries were due to serendipity and might have been missed had he not been willing to follow his data even though they did not fit his original hypothesis. For example, his discovery of the behavioral process we now call "superstitious behavior" (i.e., responding maintained by an adventitious reinforcement contingency) occurred because the apparatus he was using to condition behavior malfunctioned. The apparatus failure inadvertently produced a contingency that created response-independent reinforcement, thus demonstrating how superstitious behavior can be shaped and maintained (Skinner, 1948; Vyse, 2022).

Similarly, the course of a *program of research* rarely goes precisely in the direction a researcher anticipates. Consider the example of sleep deprivation and problem behavior. Several research groups in the 1990s identified correlations between sleep deprivation and increases in challenging behavior (Fisher et al., 2002; Horner et al., 1997; Kennedy & Itkonen, 1993; O'Reilly, 1995; Symons et al., 2000). This finding came about when researchers were attempting to account for day-to-day variability in challenging behavior that could not be understood from events being manipulated during functional behavioral assessments. If environmental events were held constant, challenging behavior still fluctuated from day to day. Upon further investigation, sleep deprivation emerged as an influential variable in its own right, although the researchers had not set out to study sleep (Kennedy, 2021).

In our own research (Kennedy et al., 2000; Kirby & Kennedy, 2003), this line of inquiry took an unexpected turn. Findings across researchers (Horner et al., 1997; Kennedy & Itkonen, 1993; O'Reilly, 1995) suggested that negatively reinforced behavior was being affected by sleep deprivation, but it was unclear whether positively reinforced behaviors were similarly affected. Two issues needed to be analyzed to answer this question. First, a range of variables might have been co-occurring with sleep deprivation that were influencing behavior. Second, the specific types of reinforcers maintaining behavior needed to be explicitly controlled. These concerns required complete control of the environment to isolate single reinforcer functions, while holding other variables constant, and the direct manipulation of sleep. Such requirements dictated that a model system be used to clarify questions regarding sleep deprivation. This led us to conduct a series of laboratory experiments with nonhumans that revealed that sleep deprivation increased negatively reinforced behaviors (e.g., Kennedy et al., 2000), but decreased or did not change positively reinforced behaviors (Kirby & Kennedy, 2003). Thus, given the questions that emerged from our initial research findings, the direction of subsequent research was adjusted accordingly, along with its implications for applied intervention.

This example illustrates that research is a highly inductive endeavor. Only by conducting experiments can we get clear answers to our questions, but at the same time the answers are often a surprise. Experimentation in many respects is like exploration. There are no signposts to guide a researcher; instead, they push forward into the unknown and create a road map for those who follow. This observation highlights the cumulative nature of experimental findings. Most "discoveries" are the result of dozens of experiments, often conducted by several different research groups (Simon, 1987, 2013). The reason for this can be described in a metaphor. Think of each experiment that people conduct as an individual piece of a large jigsaw puzzle. Each piece needs to be fit into place, but no single piece defines what the final product is. In the long term, the critical outcome is not the fitting of a single piece into the puzzle, but the completion of the entire puzzle.

Similarly, individual research studies replicate and build on each other. One research group may conduct an experiment demonstrating that students with learning disabilities can learn new skills, such as phonological decoding, in general education settings. They may then conduct a second study to extend this finding by comparing the rate of learning in special versus general education settings and find that they are similar. Another research group may conduct a related study asking a similar comparative question regarding the quantity and quality of social interactions in different settings and find that general education participation produces superior outcomes. Yet another research group may read all of these experimental findings and ask about the impact of academic and social development on students in general education settings who do not have disabilities. Other research groups may replicate these studies for students with moderate disabilities, another research group may focus on students with gifts and talents, and so on. The net result of these studies is a clearer picture of the strengths and limitations of educating students with and without disabilities in general education settings. No single study could answer all the relevant questions, but the conduct of a range of studies, each asking a slightly different question, both replicates the results of previous studies and extends those studies into new directions. The cumulative result of this process is improved knowledge about educational practices, but the development of such a knowledge base can take years and some-times decades (see Chapter 4).

Despite its nonlinear nature, however, experimentation does result in progress. It may be difficult to predict from one experiment to the next the particular course a line of research will take. However, the way the research process is oriented seems to ensure that progress is made. By requiring researchers to make public their procedures, findings, and interpretation of experimental results, the process is open to others for critique, debate, and replication. The accumulated result of this process is an improved understanding of an educational problem. The result at any single point in time may be more effective educational procedures, a better understanding of the complexity of the problem, or the realization that a particular line of research is not productive. Whatever the outcome, the process results in knowledge advancing beyond what could be known from common sense or logical analysis.

ASSUMPTIONS OF RESEARCHERS

Researchers approach experimentation with a different set of assumptions than most people use in their personal or professional lives. Often these assumptions are not explicitly recognized and, instead, are learned through the research apprenticeship process referred to as graduate training and postdoctoral study. Although most researchers do not spend a great deal of time contemplating *epistemological* assumptions relating to scientific inquiry (instead, they are likely engaged in the act of conducting research), there is a consistent set of beliefs that researchers hold. These assumptions tend to be very robust and occur across a broad range of disciplines and approaches to research (Lehr & Schauble, 2015; Linn, 1990; Underwood, 1957).

One assumption held by researchers was discussed at length in the previous section. *Everyday experience and even stringent logical analysis are not enough to understand the world.* Instead, *systematic inquiry* is needed to parse out correlation from causation. By engaging in carefully described and arranged procedures that others can replicate, researchers learn more about how the world works than by other approaches to acquiring knowledge.

A second assumption relates to the lawfulness of the world. Typically referred to as *determinism*, this belief postulates that events have identifiable causes. Apples fall from trees toward the ground, gasoline ignites at a certain temperature, and behaviors occur in certain patterns as a function of their consequences. If Behavior X occurs in a particular pattern, there must be a set of events related to Behavior X that cause it to occur in such a pattern. For example, if a child cries every time a parent drops them off at preschool, there must be something about the antecedent and consequent events that surround that episode that causes the child to cry. For nonresearchers, determinism is easier to accept and, perhaps, understand for the physical sciences than for educational or psychological phenomena (Goldenweiser, 1938; Pearl, 2009). Nevertheless, all events have a cause, and identifying those causes is the foundation of experimentation, whether a particular researcher articulates this assumption or not.

Closely related to the notion of determinism is the assumption of *material causes*. Hundreds of years ago, when asked why water turns from a liquid to a gas, most educated people would have invoked a metaphysical explanation—for example, that the essential spirits in the water had become excited and left for heaven. Or, a person acted the way they did because a "homunculus" in their head directed them to act that way. This type of explanation—still alive and well in our contemporary society—invokes causes that do not physically exist (Burgos, 2021; MacCorquodale & Meehl, 1948; Morey, 1991). To say the least, metaphysical causes are difficult to experimentally investigate.

By focusing on material causes, researchers are forced to deal with physical events as causal entities. Things that are being studied need to be operationally specified and accurately measured. In addition, to find the source of the occurrence of those events, some other event must be identified and tracked in relation to that which is the event of interest. If the occurrence of scolding by a parent tends to follow the yelling of a child and the nonoccurrence of scolding is related to the nonoccurrence of yelling, then scolding might be causally related to yelling. Additional manipulations of scolding as a consequence for yelling may suggest that the two events are so closely related, and in a particular pattern of occurrence, that we would say that yelling is caused by scolding. No appeal to forces that exist in some other place, time, or physical dimension is needed to explain the behavior (Skinner, 1950).

Earlier in this chapter I alluded to an aspect of experimentation that was different from most other ways of knowing—*replication*. In Chapter 4 we will discuss different types of replication in detail, but here I would like to present the idea that *independent replication* is one of the foundations of research. Any published report of research should explain why a study was conducted, exactly what was done, what the results were, and how those data might be interpreted. This allows other researchers to attempt to independently replicate the experiment to see if similar results can be obtained. In general, there is a consensus among researchers that any finding is suspect until it has been replicated (Haack, 2011; Maxwell et al., 2015). The infamous case of *"cold fusion"* is an exemplar of this issue (see Taubes, 1993). Briefly, a pair of physicists claimed to be able to initiate nuclear fission under low temperatures—something that was fundamentally inconsistent with what was known about this phenomenon through thousands and thousands of studies. Research groups from around the world attempted to replicate this finding, but even after many years and many experiments, no other research group could replicate the findings (indeed, the original researchers could not replicate their own findings!). Because no one could replicate the original results, researchers have come to regard the finding as an error in experimentation (i.e., poor experimental methods and/or inaccurate interpretation of results). The ability of others to replicate new findings is a critical component of the research process.

A belief in the *cumulative nature of research findings*, then, is an important assumption among researchers. As was previously discussed, each study is like an individual piece of a jigsaw puzzle, which is not complete until a range of experiments have been completed. This process (a) serves to check on the veracity of individual research findings, (b) is self-correcting in that errors will be found and alternative findings/interpretations publicly presented, and (c) results in an increased understanding of the phenomenon being investigated. In applied areas, such as educational research, there is also an implicit assumption that this whole process results in better educational practices (Chapter 6). The result is that students, teachers, and community members benefit from the work that we refer to as experimentation.

Along with a more complete understanding of a phenomenon, there is also an expectation that at some point a more *parsimonious* understanding of it will result. By parsimonious, what is meant is that a set of findings can be summarized in as simple a manner as does justice to the phenomenon. For example, when the initial finding emerged showing that *time delay* as a technique for transferring stimulus control (Touchette, 1971) could be extended to educational contexts (Halle et al., 1979), nobody knew exactly what would result. However, after many decades of research by multiple research groups, a great deal is known about when, where, how, and to what degree time delay is an effective teaching strategy. Not only are the general parameters of time delay well understood, but the techniques can be summarized as a handful of procedures for practitioners to use (Horn et al., 2023). In this case, parsimony resulted from a more complete knowledge of how the behavioral processes worked and how they could be organized. What resulted was not only a greater understanding of what comprised a certain area of research, but also an efficient way of organizing those findings.

CONCLUSION

Experimentation as an approach for answering educational questions emerged in the early 20th century (Tomlinson, 1997). Since then, experimentation has provided tremendous insight into processes that improve educational practices and outcomes for a wide variety of students. However, research itself is a difficult concept for most people to grasp, in part because the typical citizen has little knowledge of, and no direct experience with, the process. As a matter of course we propose questions and find answers to them in our everyday lives and, to the extent that things unfold as we anticipate, are psychologically satisfied with the results. There is no obvious need to pursue issues further, as long as things work as we expect. Despite the general success of common sense in our day-to-day experience, it often falls short when confronted with complex causes.

It is because of this limitation to common sense that people have developed a set of techniques for answering complex or nonintuitive problems that are referred to as experimentation. The research process is rigorous, not easily understood, and effortful. However, when done properly, it is an invaluable tool for knowledge generation. Experimentation is not a "thing" to be reified and kept at a distance, but a tool set for asking questions about the world. At its most utilitarian it is something to be used to solve people's problems.

In the remainder of this book we will explore one approach to experimentation, referred to as *single-case designs*. These designs embody the quintessential properties of experimental methods and are ideally suited for a range of questions relevant to educational contexts. They are an exciting set of tools that allow people to ask questions that can be answered using individual students, classrooms, or schools, with no need for "control" or "contrast" groups as comparisons. These designs have a rich history in educational, psychological, and health sciences research, as well as an exciting future for exploring currently unsolved questions relating to education.

1. What makes experimentation different from everyday experience?

2. Why is objective measurement a central focus of experimentation?

3. In what ways is a hypothesis an experimental question?

4. Why might there be so few failures to replicate when investigators use single-case designs for research?

5. Can you think of a systematic line of research in your area of interest and describe how it evolved over time?

2 TRANSLATIONAL FOUNDATIONS

LEARNING OBJECTIVES

After reading this chapter, you will be able to

2.1 Discuss the three key disciplines that are the historical antecedents to the single-case design research method.

2.2 Trace the emergence and development of the field of behavior analysis.

2.3 Explain how behavioral analysis and educational research have become interconnected fields of study.

*"The analysis of individual behavior is a problem in scientific demonstration, reasonably well understood (Skinner, 1953, Sec. 1), comprehensively described (Sidman, 1960), and quite thoroughly practiced (*Journal of the Experimental Analysis of Behavior, *1958–). That analysis has been pursued in many settings over many years. Despite variable precision, elegance, and power, it has resulted in general descriptive statements of mechanisms that can produce many of the forms that individual behavior may take"* (Baer et al., 1968, p. 91).

Donald M. Baer and his colleagues (1968) wrote that statement nearly 60 years ago regarding the status of the field of behavior analysis, from which single-case designs are derived. Most readers of this book were not yet born when this summary about the health and prosperity of behavior analysis was written. Since that time, research using single-case designs has provided tremendous insights into processes that improve educational practices and outcomes for a wide variety of students. For decades this approach to experimental design has yielded easier-to-implement and more effective interventions, a deeper understanding of *behavioral mechanisms*, more accurate and usable measurement systems, and greater benefits for students, families, and schools.

Single-case designs are used to demonstrate experimental control within a single participant. That, in a nutshell, is the definition of single-case designs. However, we need to unpack that deceptively simple definition to better understand what constitutes these designs. Single-case designs demonstrate experimental control using *one person as both the control and experimental participant*. For this reason, these designs are also referred to as *N* = 1 designs. Other names for this approach include single-case experimental designs, single-subject designs, and intrasubject replication designs. Unlike case histories, single-case designs demonstrate *a rigorous degree of experimental control*. Case histories are based on correlations among events, but single-case designs specifically hold all conditions constant except for the independent variable, which is systematically introduced and withdrawn to study its effects on behavior (see Chapter 3). In addition, single-case designs are not a single type of experimental design, but *an overarching approach to experimentation that has multiple variations*, all of which meet the defining characteristics of this approach to research (see Part IV).

Along with the characteristics just mentioned, there are some underlying assumptions in the use of single-case designs that should be explicitly noted. These assumptions constitute what is referred to as the *epistemological* basis of single-case designs, which is largely based on the field of behavior analysis (see Chiesa, 1994; Moore, 2008). First, this approach to research is *idiographic*. This type of research is used to approach subject matter by understanding how individuals behave, not by describing mathematical averages of groups (Molenaar & Campbell, 2009; Sidman, 1952). Stated differently, these designs are used to discover why a person does what they do and then test whether other people behave the same way under similar conditions. Proof is developed one participant at a time, under high degrees of experimental rigor. This can be contrasted with group-comparison research, which looks for general tendencies among large numbers of participants and differences among group averages (see Underwood [1957] and Box 2.1).

BOX 2.1: IDIOGRAPHIC VERSUS NOMOTHETIC APPROACHES TO EXPERIMENTATION

It has been observed that there are two "schools" of experimental design in applied psychology, and both emerged during the early 20th century from experimental psychology (Kazdin, 1978; Molenaar & Campbell, 2009). One approach is group-comparison designs, also referred to as experimental and quasi-experimental designs (Shadish et al., 2002). The second is single-case designs or N = 1 designs. These two approaches are not simply different ways of asking the same experimental question, but deeply distinct ways of framing experimental questions (Johnston et al., 2020). Group-comparison designs are based on *nomothetic* conceptualizations of experimentation derived from a *vaganotic* theory of measurement. Such efforts focus on sampling from a population in an effort to extrapolate experimental findings from the sample to the population as a whole. The goal is to describe populations of individuals and compare similarities and differences among them. In contrast, single-case designs are based on *idiographic* conceptualizations of experimentation derived from an *idemnotic* theory of measurement. The goal is to experimentally analyze individual cases in search of the mechanism of change. The goal is to experimentally describe processes acting at the individual level and build up evidence from subsequent replications. These are fundamentally distinct ways of framing an experimental question. An example might help illustrate this point. A nomothetic approach to test-taking performance would likely yield the finding that students who are fastest at taking tests produce higher scores when measured as a group. However, an idiographic approach would likely yield the finding that as an individual student increases their test-taking time, that person increases their error rate, and that effect occurs over and over again across students.[1] Neither approach is correct or incorrect. They are simply different ways of conceptualizing and conducting experiments.

---

[1] I would like to thank my colleague, Dr. Eric Loken at the University of Connecticut, for providing me with this example.

Another assumption has to do with the nature of the variables being studied. The only requirement that single-case designs impose on the variables used to study behavior is that they be physical events. This means that the events must have material existence. Another way of saying this is that everything measured as an effect or done as an intervention must be *operationalized*. To operationalize a variable, it needs to be described in objective terms that can be agreed upon as occurring, or not occurring, by anyone who understands the operational definition (see Chapters 7 and 8). This assumption means that some terms we use in everyday discourse are not amenable to being operationalized, even though we use them as if they have causal status. Examples of these *hypothetical constructs* include inferences about intentions ("I think they meant to do that"), mental states ("The student may have had a lapse in memory"), or emotions ("They acted that way because they were angry").

However, the need to operationalize experimental variables does not preclude the study of brain–behavior interactions. As long as internal events—also referred to as *private events*—can be operationalized and directly measured (i.e., they can be shown to exist), then they are permissible elements in single-case designs (Moore, 1984; see Box 2.2). Again, it is not the location of a variable but the ability to measure it, rather than infer it, that is at issue (see MacCorquodale & Meehl, 1948; Meehl, 2016).

BOX 2.2: CAN THE BRAIN BE PART OF THE ANALYSIS OF BEHAVIOR?

The answer to this question is an emphatic *yes*. However, if this question was posed 30 years ago, the answer would have been an equally emphatic *no*. A great deal has changed in neuroscience in recent years that allows direct measurement of events occurring in the brain. Examples of such data include events such as oxygen metabolism (measured via functional magnetic resonance imaging [fMRI]), binding of neurotransmitters to certain brain nuclei (measured via computed tomography [CT] scans), and neuronal firing patterns (measured via electrophysiological recording of event-related potentials [ERPs]). Because these are measurable events, not inferences or assumptions, they are variables that can be, and are being, used to analyze behavior. As neuroscience is advancing, increasing opportunities are occurring to expand the variables studied in single-case designs (Kennedy et al., 2001).

A third assumption is that an *inductive* approach to understanding human behavior is the most productive strategy. The overarching goal of conducting research is to explain something. Researchers who use single-case designs approach their subject matter with a great deal of respect for its complexity. Rather than developing a priori theories of why people learn and then conducting experiments to test the accuracy of the theory, single-case designs are typically used to explore the nature of mechanisms or causes from the data that are collected. This former approach is widely used in traditional psychological research and is referred to as "theory-driven research," "top-down theorizing," or "deductive research." This can be contrasted with a behavior-analytic approach that is often referred to as "grounded theory," "bottom-up theorizing," or "inductive research."

The general approach that single-case designs are used for is to directly study how human behavior functions and use that information to develop more robust explanations and interventions derived from these mechanisms. An example of this difference can be illustrated with research on choice making. In economics, *rational choice theory* has been used to explain consumer spending (Scott, 2000; von Neumann & Morgenstern, 1947). Rational choice theory states that consumers optimize their spending among available options (i.e., they spend rationally based on their expectations of value). This theory was developed independent of research data, and its adequacy was initially based on logical arguments (Thaler, 2016). When research was conducted, it was conducted to test the accuracy of the theory, not to ask open-ended questions about how consumers actually spend their money. This is an example of top-down theorizing.

A bottom-up approach can be illustrated by the work on concurrent operant schedules of reinforcement. Concurrent operants compare response allocation in situations where two different options are available for reinforcement. Or, put another way, this research focuses on experimentally analyzing *choice*. In concurrent reinforcement schedules, one experimental variable is altered at a time (e.g., delay or magnitude of reinforcement), its effect on choice is noted, and then another variable is analyzed, and so on. After many experiments were conducted, a general set of patterns became clear that described how choice making occurs. In this case, a quantitative formula was proposed, referred to as the *matching law*, that explained how organisms as simple as birds or organizations as complex as corporations make choices (Davison & McCarthy, 1987). For better or worse, we do not make choices rationally, but instead our behavior tends to be biased toward options with faster rather than larger payoffs. In this instance, the bottom-up approach produced a far more adequate explanation for this type of complex behavior (Herrnstein, 1990; Thaler & Ganser, 2015).

Using single-case designs, knowledge is developed incrementally, experiment by experiment. This is a very conservative approach to arriving at explanations but in the long term has proven to be the most productive strategy because of the high degree of direct contact researchers maintain with their subject matter (E. F. Keller, 2002). As the astronomer Sidney van den Bergh (1995) noted about the relation between theory and experimentation, *"Our job is to listen to what nature is telling us and not impose our own esthetics."* It is a naïve researcher who thinks they are more clever than nature.

All of these characteristics and assumptions associated with single-case designs are directly linkable to the historical antecedents of this approach. There are three historical precursors to what we refer to as single-case designs. They include *biology, medicine*, and *psychology*. Each of these disciplines—which are linked by the common theme of trying to understand animate life—developed research strategies that focused on idiographic, objective, and inductive approaches to arriving at explanations.

HISTORICAL ANTECEDENTS TO SINGLE-CASE DESIGNS

The concept of a new field, separate from physics or chemistry, focusing on understanding how living organisms develop and mature was not proposed until the early 19th century. The first proposal for a discipline that we now call *biology* came from Jean-Baptiste Lamarck's *Philosophical Zoology* (1809/2011). In this treatise, Lamarck called for a new scientific field to study how plants and animals come into existence, reproduce, and evolve. At this point in time, the term *philosophical* had a very different meaning from what we mean by the word in the 21st century. Emerging from the Age of Enlightenment (Brittan, 2015), philosophers were individuals who intensively studied a problem using systematic techniques that eventually evolved into what we call the *scientific method* (see Bacon, 1620/2000). Hallmarks of this new approach to acquiring knowledge were objective observation, manipulating one variable at a time, holding other variables constant, carefully recording findings, and replicating results. Today, this approach to gaining knowledge about the world is referred to as *empiricism* (Brittan, 2015).

The best-known scholar in biology during the mid-19th century was Charles Darwin. Both Darwin (1859) and Alfred R. Wallace (1875) developed the concept that individual organisms within a species vary slightly from one another and generation to generation and that environmental conditions can select some individuals to be more likely to reproduce, making the variations they exhibit more likely to occur in future generations. We now refer to these concepts as *evolutionary biology* (see Gould, 2002). Darwin and Wallace arrived at their conclusions simultaneously and by using similar research methods. That is, they studied individual cases (e.g., a particular bird species), looked for variations in individuals within the same species and across species, recorded their observations, noted the environmental conditions under which they lived, and used these data to draw conclusions about how nature is structured and functions.

The research of individuals such as Darwin and Wallace was largely *descriptive* in that they could not directly manipulate evolutionary processes, only describe patterns in these processes. During the last half of the 19th century, a more *experimental* approach was adopted, particularly in embryology (now referred to more generally as developmental biology). The goal of this area was to understand how organisms develop from a fertilized egg to a mature organism (E. F. Keller, 2002). Importantly, developmental biologists were eventually able to directly manipulate a variable of interest (e.g., a particular gene sequence) and observe its effects on the developing embryo. This allowed biologists to gather direct experimental evidence about how discrete events influence biological development and paved the way for the field of *genomics* that emerged a century later (Collins et al., 2003).

In a related and contemporaneous field of study, medicine also developed approaches for conducting experiments in the 19th century. Medicine has a long history of using *case histories* to inform physicians about new innovations in treating patients. For example, Ephraim McDowell was a surgeon practicing medicine in the early 19th century. At this time, internal surgery was largely an abstract concept, yet to be proactively practiced. If you had a tumor in your gut, for example, you would die a slow and painful death as the tumor grew and suppressed the functioning of various organs. McDowell (1817) developed a surgical technique for successfully removing ovarian cysts (a common, but deadly, type of tumor), which he replicated with other patients and then published so that other surgeons could use his technique with their patients. This was one of the first published case histories of a replicable technique for conducting successful internal surgery.

A significant limitation of case histories, as previously noted, is that they are based on an unfolding sequence of events that are not experimentally controlled, only systematically described. In addition, case histories rely on naturally occurring events, which limits what can be studied, as well as when. For example, a physician might be treating a patient, and along with the treatment they prescribed, the patient might also start a series of "self-prescribed" treatments without telling the doctor.

Combining the need for an experimental approach to medical issues and developments in experimental biology, Claude Bernard (1865/1927) introduced the idea of *experimental medicine*. A key component of Bernard's experimental medicine was the use of *model systems* to study questions relating to human physiology (Thompson, 1984). Model systems are experiments that use an analogous situation in a nonhuman species to analyze the effects and mechanisms influencing the phenomenon of interest in humans. For example, Bernard studied phenomena such as diabetes and blood oxygenation in animals to reveal how the pancreas and hemoglobin functioned in relation to disease processes seen in humans, respectively. This type of direct experimental approach using model systems has been the foundation for many of the medical innovations seen during the last 150 years (Cooter & Pickston, 2000). Again, this type of experimentation was based on idiographic, objective, and inductive research procedures. These were experimental precursors to single-case designs. (As an aside, the reader is also referred to the work of Charles S. Sherrington [1906/1989] for the use of model systems directly relating to neuroscience and behavior [Sherrington, 1975]).

A final area that has influenced single-case designs, and the one most familiar to readers of this book, is *experimental psychology*. Not surprisingly, the first researchers in experimental psychology at the beginning of the 20th century often emerged from medicine and biology. Two of the most prominent early researchers studying psychological topics were Ivan M. Sechenov and Ivan P. Pavlov. Sechenov (1965), often referred to as the "father of Russian physiology," was an international pioneer in neurophysiology. He had been trained in Europe in biology and medicine, and used these techniques to study human behavior via neural processes. His work was largely driven by the idea that all human action was a series of reflexes mediated by the nervous system. The experimental methods he used were based on his biological and medical training and reflected many of the characteristics previously discussed, including the use of model systems, idiographic techniques, and the inductive accumulation of experimental evidence. Like Pavlov, whom we will discuss next, Sechenov's focus was not on creating new experimental designs; instead, he applied what he had learned in biology and medicine to a new topic—psychology.

Pavlov (1897/1960) discovered the learning processes we now refer to as *respondent conditioning*. Pavlov was a physiologist studying digestive processes in mammals. Indeed, he won the Nobel Prize in Physiology or Medicine in 1904 for this work. However, his discovery of classical (respondent) conditioning was serendipitous. While studying salivary duct secretion in dogs using a model system, Pavlov and his colleagues noticed that saliva would begin flowing prior to the introduction of food to the dog's mouth. Typically, salivation is a reflexive event elicited by the presence of food in the mouth. However, Pavlov's subjects had learned to associate certain noises with the food and began salivating when they heard familiar noises (e.g., the footsteps of a laboratory technician). This meant that a physiological reflex could be conditioned to be psychologically associated with an arbitrary stimulus. This process—classical conditioning—is also referred to as *stimulus-response (S-R) psychology* (see Figure 2.1).

At the same time that Pavlov was conducting his work on classical conditioning, an American named Edward L. Thorndike (1898) was conducting his dissertation on another type of learning, which Thorndike labeled the "law of effect." Thorndike used a model system, much like a biologist, to analyze how learning occurred. His primary apparatus was a box that required some arbitrary response (e.g., pushing a lever) for the animal to escape and gain access to food. Access to the food was the driving force for the animal to learn a novel behavior. An example of the *learning curves* he obtained using this method is presented in Figure 2.2. The graph shows that over successive trials, the novel behavior was emitted faster and faster. This was the first time that the process of learning had been measured and analyzed using biologically derived methods. Thorndike used a variety of responses, including chaining behaviors into a sequence, and replicated his procedures from one animal to the next, even using different species to establish the generality of his learning curves. Interestingly, Thorndike, while a professor at Columbia University in the early 20th century, established one of the first programs in *educational psychology*, providing a bridge between experimental psychology and education (Joncich, 1968; Thorndike, 2011).

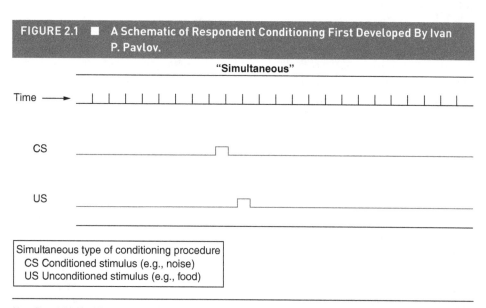

FIGURE 2.1 ■ A Schematic of Respondent Conditioning First Developed By Ivan P. Pavlov.

"Simultaneous"

Time

CS

US

Simultaneous type of conditioning procedure
CS Conditioned stimulus (e.g., noise)
US Unconditioned stimulus (e.g., food)

Note: By pairing the US with the CS, the CS comes to elicit the response previously occasioned by the US. (Figure 3, p. 22, from: Keller, F. S., & Schoenfeld, W. N. (1950). *Principles of psychology.* Copyright 1995 by the B. F. Skinner Foundation. Reproduced by permission.)

FIGURE 2.2 ■ A Learning Curve Demonstrating Edward L. Thorndike's Law of Effect.

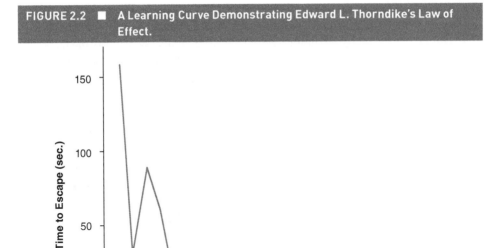

Note: The number of seconds required to escape from the puzzle box and obtain food is listed along the *y*-axis. The number of successive trials is presented along the *x*-axis. (From: Thorndike, E. L. (1898). Animal intelligence: An experimental study of the associative processes in animals. *Psychological Review Monograph Supplement 2*(4, Whole No. 8). Macmillan. In the public domain.)

Another influential figure in bringing a biologically based perspective to psychology was John B. Watson (1924). Watson is not so much known for his research as for his advocacy of an approach to psychology that was radically different from other psychologists of his time. Early in the 20th century, most psychologists focused on people's subjective experiences of events (e.g., describing the sensations experienced when seeing a particular color), often using group-comparison designs to contrast different experimental conditions (Boring, 1950). Watson's perspective was that only events that were observable by others (i.e., that could be objectively defined and observed) should be the subject matter of experimental psychology. This approach was quickly referred to as *behaviorism*. The focus of behaviorism was to make psychology as objective and precise as biology and other natural sciences. This perspective influenced an entire generation of young scholars who were looking to make psychology more scientific (Todd & Morris, 1994). (See Table 2.1 for a timeline of events relating to single-case designs and educational research from the 1800s to the early 1970s.)

Most notable among this next generation of behaviorists was B. F. Skinner. Skinner completed his doctorate at Harvard University approximately 35 years after Thorndike studied there. While conducting his dissertation, which would eventually be published as the *Behavior of Organisms* (1938), Skinner developed an approach to psychology that was heavily influenced by experimental biology (Boakes, 1984; Todd & Morris, 1995).

TABLE 2.1 ■ A Timeline of Critical Figures and Events in the History of Single-Case Designs[a]				
1800s	1900–1940s	1950s	1960s	1960–1970s
Precursors	Psychology	Experimental Analysis	Applied Behavior Analysis	Education
Biology	Thorndike (1898)	Fuller (1949)	Ferster & DeMyer (1961)	Hall et al. (1968)
Lamarck (1809/2011)	Sherrington (1906/1989)	Lindsley (1956)	Baer (1962)	Walker & Buckley (1968)
Darwin (1859)	Watson (1924)	Ferster & Skinner (1957)	Bijou (1963)	Lovitt & Curtis (1969)
Wallace (1875)	Skinner (1938)	*Journal of the Experimental Analysis of Behavior* (1958–present)	Lovaas et al. (1965)	Alper & White (1971)
			Journal of Applied Behavior Analysis (1968–present)	Haring & Phillips (1972)
		Ayllon & Michael (1959)		
Medicine				
Bernard (1865/1927)				
Pavlov (1897/1960)				

[a] See text for additional details.

In keeping with experimental biology, Skinner used less "complex" animals to model the behavior of people. This approach was based on the *continuity assumption*, derived from evolutionary biology, that is based on physiological, anatomical, and behavioral characteristics being genetically conserved across species, with subsequent species elaborating (and incorporating) features from which they had evolved. Hence, behavioral processes that are present in rodents or pigeons are likely to be conserved in primates, such as human beings. He also used highly simplified environments. The goal was to hold constant all possible environmental variables, except the variable of experimental interest (e.g., food presentation). By doing this, environmental processes influencing behavior can be individually identified, and the *functional relations* they enter into with behavior can be analyzed (see Chapter 3).

Along with these features, Skinner's approach also used biological practices in that it was idiographic, operational, and inductive. Skinner's experimental approach was to use a rodent or pigeon as the organism, select an arbitrary response that could be quickly emitted and repeated (i.e., a lever press), choose a biologically powerful stimulus (i.e., food), and study how reinforcement contingencies influence response patterns. This arrangement allowed for a single response to be measured continuously in time to study the effects of reinforcement on patterns of behavior. One such pattern is presented in Figure 2.3. This graph presents a *cumulative record* of behavior. Along the *x*-axis (horizontal line) is time. Along the *y*-axis (vertical line) each occurrence of behavior is recorded by a slight rise in the line. In this way, the *rate of responding* in real time can be recorded and visually analyzed (see Chapter 7). This general approach to studying behavior has become known as the *experimental analysis of behavior*, and a journal devoted to this approach to research was established in 1958 (*Journal of the Experimental Analysis of Behavior* [*JEAB*], 1958–present).

THE EMERGENCE OF BEHAVIOR ANALYSIS

Skinner's primary findings were that the *contingency* between a response and a reinforcing stimulus determines the probability of that response, and that intermittent *schedules of reinforcement* produce very distinct patterns of behavior (Ferster & Skinner, 1957; Skinner, 1938). For example, the contingent delivery of a reinforcer for a lever press on a fixed-interval schedule (i.e., reinforcement is only available for a response after a fixed amount of time has passed) produces a scalloped pattern of behavior increasing in probability as the end of the time interval nears (see Figure 2.3). This approach is referred to as *operant conditioning* or *response-stimulus (R-S)* psychology.

Skinner also conducted early experiments on topics such as behavioral pharmacology, superstition, anxiety, language use, and systematic instruction (see Skinner, 1983). However, there are two other reasons that Skinner is considered the most famous psychologist in history (Bjork, 1993). First, he extrapolated his laboratory findings from model systems to the everyday lives of people (Skinner, 1953). This allowed him tremendous insight into the causes of human behavior and created a great deal of resistance from laypersons and experts alike (reminiscent of the stormy reception that evolutionary biology received a century earlier).

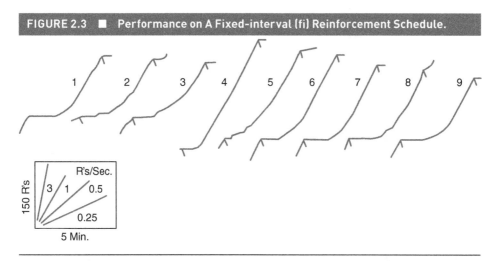

FIGURE 2.3 ■ Performance on A Fixed-interval (fi) Reinforcement Schedule.

Note: The cumulative record shows successive responses (R) as upward movement of the line along the *y*-axis or ordinate. Time is represented along the *x*-axis or abscissa. (Figure 156, p. 162, from: Ferster, C. B., & Skinner, B. F. (1957). *Schedules of reinforcement*. Copyright 1995 by the B. F. Skinner Foundation. Reproduced by permission.)

Second, he produced an entire generation of new researchers who went on to prominent scientific careers and who produced, themselves, subsequent generations of *behavior analysts*. Most of these individuals were trained by Skinner or his associates in the 1940s and 1950s at Harvard, Columbia, or Indiana University (Dinsmoor, 1990). A too brief mention of the most noteworthy of these individuals is given here. William K. Estes studied anxiety and learning (Healy et al., 1992a, 1992b). Peter B. Dews developed what became known as behavioral pharmacology (Dews, 1987). Joseph V. Brady co-developed behavioral pharmacology and integrated biomedical and behavior-analytic research (Hodos & Ator, 1994). Charles B. Ferster conducted the initial experiments on schedules of reinforcement and time out (Skinner, 1981). Murray Sidman worked on avoidance responding (Sidman, 1989). Richard J. Herrnstein developed the first analyses of choice making and the quantitative analysis of behavior (Baum, 2002). Many of these individuals are pictured in Figure 2.4, which was taken during the third conference on the experimental analysis of behavior in 1949.

FIGURE 2.4   ■   Group Photograph of People Attending the Third Conference on The Experimental Analysis of Behavior (1949).

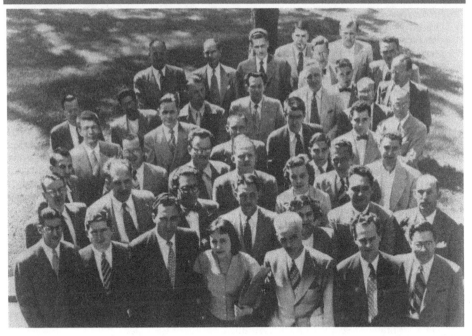

Note: Taken from the second floor of Schermerhorn Extension at Columbia University. Left to right, first row: Mike Kaplan, Donald Perlman, Nat Schoenfeld, Ruth (Morris) Bolman, Fred Keller, Fred Skinner, Phil Bersh. Second row: Harold Coppock, Ralph Hefferline, Helmut Adler, Fred Frick, Elaine (Hammer) Graham, Joe Notterman, Bill Jenkins. Third row: Ben Wyckofk, Joel Greenspoon, Bill Daniels, Van Lloyd, Dorothy Yates, unknown, Norm Guttman. Fourth row: Lloyd Homme, Joe Antonitis, Sam Cambell, Jim Dinsmoor, Charlie Ferster, George Collier. Fifth row: unknown, Burt Wolin, Doug Ellson, Fred Lit, Clancy Graham, Bill Verplanck, Bill Estes. Sixth row: Mac Parsons, Dave Anderson, Don Page, Murray Sidman, Phil Ratoosh, George Roth. Seventh row: Don Cook, Rod Funston. (Figure 5, p. 145, from: Dinsmoor, J. A. (1990). Academic roots: Columbia University, 1943–1951. *Journal of the Experimental Analysis of Behavior, 54,* 129–150. Copyright 1990 by the Society for the Experimental Analysis of Behavior. Reproduced by permission.)

Unlike the previous studies, Sidney W. Bijou in the late 1950s sought to study typical development from a behavior-analytic perspective. Bijou experimentally analyzed the behavior of young children in order to develop a behavioral theory of child development (Bijou, 1995). He also developed the first behavior-analytic conceptualization of intellectual disabilities (Bijou, 1963). Bijou's work laid the foundation for subsequent generations of psychologists and educators to study human development from a naturalistic, experimental perspective (Baer & LeBlanc, 1977).

In 1959, the first application of behavioral mechanisms from the laboratory occurred (Ayllon & Michael, 1959). The Ayllon and Michael (1959) study differed from previous experiments on human operant behavior in that it did not focus on establishing the generality of behavioral mechanisms from nonhumans to humans, but, instead, focused on using those behavioral mechanisms to solve a social problem. What Ayllon and Michael did was to use the concept of reinforcement contingencies to improve the living conditions of people with schizophrenia in an institutional setting. By arranging various contingencies for the delivery of salient events, Ayllon and Michael were able to improve the behavior not only of patients, but also of staff (whom the patients were dependent upon). In many respects, this was the first study in *applied behavior analysis* to be conducted, although it would be another decade before that term was introduced.

Charles B. Ferster was the first individual to take laboratory findings from behavior analysis and use them to improve the behavior of children with autism. Ferster and DeMyer (1961) conducted a series of experiments on how to shape and maintain behavior in children with autism. By using reinforcement contingencies, they were able to establish complex behaviors in children who were thought incapable of such performances. Their findings showed that even children with very complex disabilities could be taught through the use of systematic instruction.

A few years later, Wolf et al. (1964) published a study that showed how to alter the behavior of a child with autism in a therapeutic manner. Wolf et al. worked with a child with autism who engaged in self-injury and refused to wear eyeglasses. These authors worked with his staff and parents to implement a differential reinforcement program that included time out from positive reinforcement. The result was a dramatic decrease in self-injury and increased wearing of eyeglasses. In addition, there were generalized improvements in this boy's behavior across settings and tasks.

This work in autism was replicated and extended by Ivar O. Lovaas and his students. Lovaas, although he was not the first individual to work with children with autism, was the first to initiate a prolonged program of therapeutic research with this population. Lovaas was able to identify environmental causes for self-injury (Lovaas et al., 1965) and restrictions in the ability of children with autism to attend to complex stimuli (Lovaas et al., 1971), among other findings. In addition, many of the leaders in the field of autism collaborated with Lovaas in the 1960s and 1970s, including Edward G. Carr, Marjorie Charlop, Robert L. Koegel, Laura Schreibman, and Tristram Smith.

The advances of the early '60s in applying the experimental analysis of behavior to social problems rapidly spread to a range of topic areas. Donald M. Baer (1962) studied behavioral processes relating to typical and atypical child development and creativity. James A. Sherman

(1965) used reinforcement techniques to establish imitation and spoken language in adults with schizophrenia who were thought to be mute. Israel Goldiamond (1965) initiated the first studies of operant conditioning to reduce stuttering and increase fluent speech and coined the term *functional analysis*. Harlan Lane (1963) studied the development of language in people who were deaf. Murray Sidman began to study the receptive and expressive language of people with aphasia (Leicester et al., 1971). Arthur W. Staats studied the development of reading abilities (Staats et al., 1962).

At this time, behavior analysts were beginning their first forays into educational settings. Two early efforts are particularly noteworthy. B. F. Skinner (1961) developed the teaching machine. Skinner devised an electromechanical device that would present written questions to children, allow them to respond, and provide them feedback about the accuracy of their answers. This work was a forerunner of computer and web-based teaching strategies. In addition, Fred S. Keller (1968) developed the personalized system of instruction (PSI). Using PSI, students are taught curriculum content through a self-paced program that uses shaping of more and more complex question–answer pairings until the student meets a proficiency criterion. This approach has been widely adopted, particularly for adult learners at community colleges.

With all of this work occurring in the application of behavioral principles, the Society for the Experimental Analysis of Behavior (SEAB), publisher of *JEAB*, elected to create a new journal, the *Journal of Applied Behavior Analysis* (*JABA*, 1968–present). SEAB's goal was to establish a journal to publish applications of the experimental analysis of behavior to issues of social concern. Montrose M. Wolf was selected as the first editor of *JABA*, and the initial board of editors was comprised of many of the researchers previously mentioned (see Table 2.2).

A particularly influential paper by Baer et al. (1968) was published in the first volume of *JABA* that helped codify the dimensions of the new field of applied behavior analysis. Baer et al. outlined seven dimensions that characterized applied behavior analysis:

- The focus of this area is the *application* of behavioral principles to areas that are judged to be in need of improvement.

- The focus of change is on a person's *behavior* and requires objective and precise measurement.

- In order to demonstrate change in a person's behavior, single-case designs need to be used to *analytically* evaluate the effects of an intervention.

- The interventions that are used are specified in operational terms to clearly specify what is being done, so a replicable *technology* of behavior change can be created.

- The effects of interventions on behavior need to be understood in regard to known behavioral mechanisms to link these effects to a coherent *conceptual system*.

- The focus of analyses is on producing *effective* outcomes that show clear benefits to the recipients of the interventions.

- Interventions need to have *generalized* effects across relevant settings and behaviors.

TABLE 2.2 ■ The Founding Editorial Board for the *Journal of Applied Behavior Analysis*

Role	Personnel
Editor	Montrose M. Wolf, University of Kansas
Associate Editor	Donald M. Baer, University of Kansas
Executive Editor	Victor G. Laties, University of Rochester
Board of Editors	W. Stewart Agras, University of Vermont
	Teodoro Ayllon, Georgia State College
	Nathan H. Azrin, Anna State Hospital
	Albert Bandura, Stanford University
	Wesley C. Becker, University of Illinois Urbana-Champaign
	Jay S. Birnbrauer, University of North Carolina
	Charles B. Ferster, Georgetown University
	Israel Goldiamond, University of Chicago
	James G. Holland, University of Pittsburgh
	B. L. Hopkins, Southern Illinois University
	Fred S. Keller, Western Michigan University
	Peter J. Lang, University of Wisconsin
	Harold Leitenberg, University of Vermont
	Ogden R. Lindsley, University of Kansas
	O. Ivar Lovaas, University of California, Los Angeles
	Jack L. Michael, Western Michigan University
	Gerald R. Patterson, University of Oregon
	Todd R. Risley, University of Kansas
	James A. Sherman, University of Kansas
	Murray Sidman, Massachusetts General Hospital
	Gerald M. Siegel, University of Minnesota
	B. F. Skinner, Harvard University
	Howard N. Sloane, University of Utah
	Joseph E. Spradlin, Parsons Research Center
	Arthur W. Staats, University of Hawaii

Many of these dimensions are explicitly derived from the antecedents of applied behavior analysis in terms of scientific practices, such as being objective, analytical, and conceptual. The others are clearly tied to the applied nature of this endeavor. With a new journal and a clear view of what applied behavior analysis was, researchers from a range of disciplines began gravitating toward this new approach to solving social problems.

LINKING EDUCATIONAL RESEARCH AND BEHAVIOR ANALYSIS

One area that quickly adopted applied behavior analysis was educational research, particularly for students who were the most challenging to teach. Beginning in the 1950s and hitting a peak in the 1960s, universities throughout the United States started opening departments of special education to prepare teachers to effectively educate children and youth who were not adequately being served in the existing educational systems (Trent, 1994; Winzer, 2009). As a new approach to education, special education was being developed from scratch. The primary criterion for adopting a particular practice was not whether traditional educators thought it was the appropriate approach to use or consistent with existing theory, but whether the approach worked (Lagemann, 2002; see Chapter 6).

One of the first special educators to adopt applied behavior analysis was Norris G. Haring (Wolery, 2005). Haring's general approach was relatively straightforward: Special educators will be more effective teachers if they adopt a systematic approach to instruction based in the science of behavior (Haring, 2016; Haring & Phillips, 1972). This was a strategic decision that required a belief that the evidence supporting behavioral mechanisms at that time suggested that it could be applied to educational issues, such as special education.

In regard to the establishment of special education departments at universities, four departments stand out for having quickly adopted applied behavior analysis as an approach to educational issues. These departments were located at the University of Washington, the University of Kansas, the University of Oregon, and Peabody College (now part of Vanderbilt University). Interestingly, Haring was the founding chair of the first two departments. These departments, and others, quickly began producing new researchers who were linking behavior analysis and education to develop *new and effective classroom practices.*

In fact, the first paper to appear in the initial issue of *JABA* was by R. Vance Hall who studied the effects *contingent teacher attention* had on the academic engagement of students in general education classrooms (Hall et al., 1968). At the same time, Hill M. Walker demonstrated a very similar effect for students with behavioral disorders (Walker & Buckley, 1968). These were the first demonstrations that classroom teachers could be more effective if they provided their attention to students behaving appropriately, rather than waiting until they misbehaved.

At the same time, Thomas C. Lovitt began developing systematic instruction techniques for improving the performance of students with learning disabilities (Lovitt & Curtis, 1969). This research combined systematic prompting and feedback to improve the academic performances of students. Working on similar issues, but with people with severe intellectual disabilities, Joseph E. Spradlin was simultaneously conducting applied and basic research on learning processes (Spradlin et al., 1973). This work led to an improved understanding of the emergence of symbolic behavior and how to more effectively teach students who, at the time, were considered unteachable.

Ogden R. Lindsley continued to extend basic operant findings to ever more applied issues (Lindsley, 1991). Working separately, Lindsley and Owen R. White (Alper & White, 1971) developed techniques for teachers to base their instructional decision making on objective data (i.e., graphs) regarding student performance, rather than the teacher's intuition. Just like researchers in a laboratory, if teachers used objective information rather than their personal perceptions, it was demonstrated that they could be more effective at accomplishing their jobs. From this work, data-based decision making has become a hallmark of effective teaching practices throughout education (Kirschner et al., 2006).

Beth Sulzer-Azaroff and G. Roy Mayer produced a series of studies, together and separately, that demonstrated effective approaches for managing student behavior at a school-wide level (Sulzer & Mayer, 1972). Their work focused on the careful application of behavioral mechanisms derived from laboratory research. These researchers had a strong influence on how school psychologists and educational administrators approach school discipline issues, which served as a precursor to positive behavior interventions and supports.

During this early period of applying behavioral mechanisms to educational topics, Doug Guess, Wayne Sailor, Gorin Rutherford, and Donald M. Baer studied language development in people with severe intellectual disabilities (Guess et al., 1968). This work demonstrated that complex language forms could be taught to students who were typically characterized by the lack of language use. The success of this work was instrumental in focusing attention on providing meaningful educational opportunities for students with severe intellectual disabilities.

Phillip S. Strain and Richard E. Shores initiated the idea of teaching social skills to students with disabilities (Strain et al., 1976; Strain & Timm, 1974). These researchers used prompting and reinforcement techniques, much like those noted previously, to establish new socially competent behaviors. Their demonstrations were the first studies showing that appropriate social behaviors could be directly taught and used to gain entrée into a new set of social contexts that children might not otherwise contact.

All of the individuals mentioned in this chapter had highly productive careers as both behavior analysts and educators. Each person produced several generations of students too numerous to mention in such an abbreviated history. As a result, most colleges of education in the United States have several generations of behavior analysts among their faculty.

CONCLUSION

The foundations for single-case designs emerged in fields that many educators are not familiar with, such as biology, medicine, and psychology. These are the disciplines that took on the challenge of studying animate life in the 1800s. Researchers in these fields learned through a century of experience that the most productive means of studying their subject matter was to use techniques that focused on intensive analyses of individual cases, moving from there to establish their generality among larger populations. As noted previously, this is a conservative approach to knowledge production. However, if the alternative is false leads and misguided theorizing, research strategies such as single-case designs should not be viewed as conservative in the long term (Kennedy, 1995). Rather, these approaches have been repeatedly demonstrated to be productive strategies for learning about how human behavior works.

In translating these behavioral mechanisms to educational issues, researchers have made a great deal of progress in a relatively short period of time. Much has been learned about behavioral mechanisms, such as reinforcement, that underlie how we learn. Not only has this information yielded consistent and reliable results in the laboratory, but the application of these behavioral mechanisms has been repeatedly shown to change behaviors of relevance to educators. These techniques are effective enough that they have become standard practices in the training of most educators, even if some people might not be aware of their origins.

REFLECTION QUESTIONS

1. Describe differences between idiographic and nomothetic approaches to conducting experiments.

2. How do basic assumptions that underlie the research process shape the way investigators conduct and interpret research studies?

3. What were some of the very early research methods that led to the development of behavioral approaches to conducting experiments?

4. Using the idea of "translational research," provide some examples of behavioral mechanisms that are used in educational interventions.

5. Can you describe two or three researchers whose work was particularly influential in shaping the field of behavior analysis?

STRATEGIC ISSUES

3 FUNCTIONAL RELATIONS

LEARNING OBJECTIVES

After reading this chapter, you will be able to

3.1 Formulate independent and dependent variables according to their impact on functional relations.

3.2 Evaluate how extraneous variables might threaten the internal validity of an experiment.

3.3 Analyze baseline conditions and when to construct a controlled versus an uncontrolled baseline.

3.4 Introduce experimental manipulations that will establish functional relations in single-case designs.

When a person conducts a study, an important goal is to establish *experimental control*. You can think of experimental control as demonstrating that an intervention reliably produces a particular change in behavior. For example, if I am testing a new intervention to reduce talking out during mathematics instruction, I will need to accomplish several things to demonstrate experimental control. First, I will want to show that the student's behavior changes following intervention, when compared to preintervention. Second, I will want to show that if I remove the intervention, the student's behavior changes back to its preintervention pattern. Finally, if I reintroduce the intervention, I will expect to observe a change in the student's behavior similar to the first time I introduced the intervention. If these changes in student behavior only occur when I introduce or remove the intervention, then I am establishing experimental control.

Figure 3.1 shows an example of the process just described (Kuntz et al., 2020). The behavior of interest was the percentage of intervals of perseverative (closed squares) and appropriate speech (open circles) for a student with high-functioning autism.

The initial condition was a typical conversation occurring with a teacher. After observing the student's conversational speech for several sessions to identify a pattern of topics (BL), the experimenters introduced an intervention. The change introduced by the experimenters was an intervention that combined differential reinforcement, extinction, and prompting of appropriate conversational topics (D+E+P). The start of the intervention coincided with a decrease in

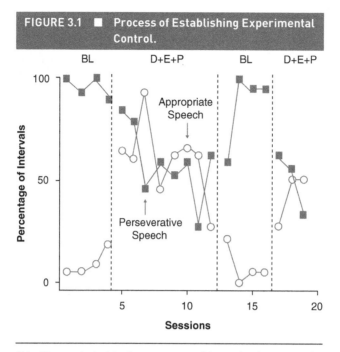

FIGURE 3.1 ■ Process of Establishing Experimental Control.

Note. The graph depicts the percentage of intervals of perseverative (closed squares) and appropriate speech (open circles) for a student with high-functioning autism. The student's conversational speech was observed for several sessions to identify a pattern of topics (BL), and then the intervention was introduced. The intervention combined differential reinforcement, extinction, and prompting of appropriate conversational topics (D+E+P). (Figure 2, p. 2426, from: Kuntz, E. M., Santos, A. V., & Kennedy, C. H. (2020). Functional analysis and intervention of perseverative speech in students with high-functioning autism and related neuro-developmental disabilities. *Journal of Applied Behavior Analysis, 53*(4), 2421–2428. Copyright 2019 by the Society for the Experimental Analysis of Behavior. Reproduced by permission.)

perseverative conversation to approximately 50% of intervals and an increase in appropriate conversational topics to 50% of intervals, with the change being sustained as long as the intervention was in place. The intervention was then removed, and both categories of conversational topics reverted to their baseline levels. After establishing an initial pattern of behaviors, introducing an intervention, removing the intervention, and observing the behaviors consistently vary in relation to the intervention, the experimenters had demonstrated experimental control.

INDEPENDENT AND DEPENDENT VARIABLES

When using single-case designs, establishing experimental control means demonstrating a *functional relation* (see Box 3.1). A functional relation can be defined as establishing a consistent effect on a *dependent variable* by systematically manipulating an *independent variable*. Dependent variables are typically estimates of the behaviors you are analyzing. For example, in Figure 3.1 the dependent variable was the mean percentage of perseverative and appropriate conversational topics. Often, the term *dependent variable* is synonymous with the measurement system being used to record behavior (see Part III). The reason it is referred to as a dependent variable is that if a functional relation is established, the level of the behavior being measured is dependent on the presence or absence of the independent variable. There is no limit, other than *tractability*, regarding the number of dependent variables you can use in a study.

BOX 3.1: USING PRECISE LANGUAGE WHEN ENGAGING IN RESEARCH

A common public stereotype is the researcher who is painfully precise in their use of language. Every word they use is carefully selected for its specific meaning, and only the minimum number of words needed to express an idea are used. Superfluous words and vagueness are avoided at all costs because they only lead to confusion, which is the opposite goal of conducting research. Unlike most stereotypes, this one is actually quite accurate. The reason is simple. Research is a very precise endeavor, but one in which the researcher is often studying a phenomenon that is not well understood. Therefore, as a researcher is breaking new ground, it is best to be as careful as possible in describing what is being done and what results from these activities. The researcher cannot be sure exactly what they are discovering or how it will be understood 10 or 15 years later.

In order to avoid as much confusion as possible, researchers use as few words as possible and carefully define what they mean. The only way to learn to do this is to monitor everything you say or write about your research and analyze it for *conciseness* and *clarity*. It also helps to solicit critical appraisals from others, although it is not always a pleasant experience. These are good practices to adopt, because researchers constantly monitor and discuss the meaning and appropriateness of terms. In other words, even if you do not critique your own technical language, other researchers *will critique your use of language*.

A good example of linguistic precision is use of the terms *functional relation* and *functional relationship* as if they are interchangeable. One of the first uses of the term *functional relation* was by Murray Sidman (1960) in his classic book on single-case designs, *Tactics of Scientific Research*. A functional relation, as previously noted, is the demonstration of control over the dependent variable by systematic manipulation of the independent variable. However, over time, language use has drifted, and some researchers now use the term *functional relationship* in a manner that is synonymous.

The issue is this. Merriam-Webster (2024) defines *relationship* as "(1) the state of being related or interrelated (studied the *relationship* between the variables); (2) the relation connecting or binding participants in a relationship: such as (a) kinship [or] (b) a specific instance or type of kinship; (3a) a state of affairs existing between those having relations or dealings (had a good *relationship* with his family); [and] (3b) a romantic or passionate attachment."

In essence, use of the term *functional relationship* assumes a social and interpersonal meaning that goes far beyond the demonstration of experimental control among independent and dependent variables. Use of the term *functional relation*, however, describes an abstract connection between two variables, with no additional connotations or inferences. In sum, a marriage can be a *functional relationship*, but the experimental control you demonstrate in your research is a *functional relation*.

The following are examples of dependent variables used in recent educational research: number of words read per minute, percentage of observations that a person was happy, duration of self-injurious behaviors, percentage of correctly executed football tackles, percentage of sight words accurately read, occurrence of precurrent behaviors for problem solving, percentage of questions correctly answered on a French language exam, latency to following requests, proportion of social interactions with appropriate social amenities, interresponse times between bites taken during snack time, and so on. These examples are far from exhaustive, being used only to highlight the concept of a dependent variable. Any variable that is of experimental interest and meets the requirements outlined in Part III of this book is an acceptable dependent variable.

An independent variable is the event that is of experimental interest in relation to the behavior(s) being studied. In Figure 3.1, the independent variable was a multicomponent intervention to promote conversational speech. Typically, your intervention is the independent variable. Use of the term *independent variable* is based on this part of the experiment being free to vary when the experimenter chooses to do so. That is, the experimenter decides when to apply it, when to remove it, or when to alter the intervention, and by this fact, the variable is independent of the experimental situation. Independent variables can be comprised of as many elements as are of experimental interest. Some independent variables are singular, as in the use of teacher praise to increase on-task work. Other independent variables contain multiple components, such as the inclusion of students with disabilities in general education settings. A critical issue, discussed at length in Chapter 8, is the need to operationalize all possibly relevant aspects of an independent variable. Obviously, the more complex the independent variable, the most difficult this task is.

Examples of independent variables include contingent teacher praise, behavior intervention plans, individualized literacy instruction, data-based teacher decision making, systematic prompting of correct responses, teaching problem-solving skills, time trials to increase mathematics fluency, classroom-based reward systems, errorless learning strategies, and so on. Independent variables are often used to improve an educational situation. At other times, independent variables are used as tools to understand why certain behaviors occur or do not occur (see Chapter 5).

So, to recapitulate, a functional relation is the demonstration of experimental control over the dependent variable by the independent variable. It is a convincing demonstration that your intervention is what changed someone's behavior. This observation raises an interesting issue. What about other events that might have changed the person's behavior that were not measured? For example, a child might have started, stopped, or changed a particular psychotropic medication; a student's family may have become indigent; an adolescent may experience turmoil in a romantic relationship; or a third grader's parents might enroll them in after-school reading instruction. Each of these events can have a profound effect on a student's behavior at school. However, as a researcher, you may not be aware of these events.

An example of how variables outside the experimenter's control can affect behavior is presented in Figure 3.2 (top panel). The data represent the problem behavior of an adolescent with severe disabilities, including self-injury and aggression (Kennedy & Meyer, 1996). The behavior was negatively reinforced by escape from instructional demands. In one condition, the demands

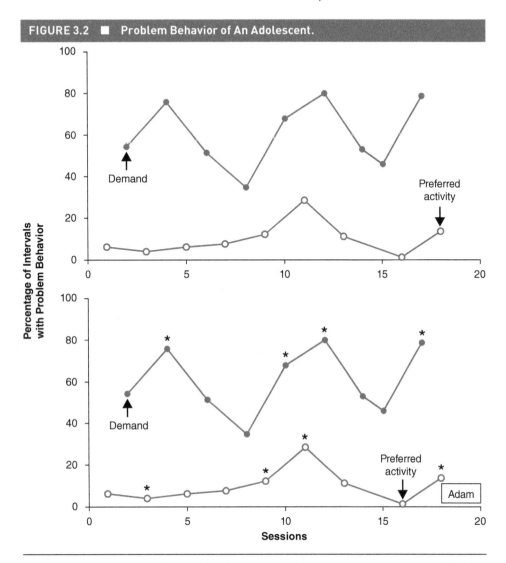

FIGURE 3.2 ■ Problem Behavior of An Adolescent.

Note. The *y*-axis shows the percentage of intervals with problem behavior, and the *x*-axis shows individual sessions. Open circles represent a condition in which preferred activities were available without demands, and closed circles represent an instructional demand condition. The data set displayed in the top panel shows information on problem behavior collected during an experimental session. The data set displayed on the bottom panel shows information on problem behavior collected during the experimental session and the student's sleep patterns at night. Asterisks indicate nights when he was sleep deprived. (Adapted from Table 1, p. 135, from: Kennedy, C. H., & Meyer, K. A. (1996). Sleep deprivation, allergy symptoms, and negatively reinforced problem behavior. *Journal of Applied Behavior Analysis, 29,* 133–135. Copyright 1996 by the Society for the Experimental Analysis of Behavior. Reproduced by permission.)

were terminated for a specific duration each time the student engaged in problem behavior (closed circles). In a second condition, the student engaged in a preferred task (open circles). Each condition was conducted once per day. Low levels of problem behavior were observed in the preferred task condition, but highly variable responding was observed in the demand condition. It appears as if the problem behavior is negatively reinforced by escape from task demands, but the effect changes from time to time. In this particular study, the authors were interested in the influence of sleep deprivation on behavior and, therefore, were documenting the amount of sleep the student received each night. When sleep deprivation is noted by asterisks in Figure 3.2 (bottom panel), it becomes clear that the variability in behavior is associated with nights of poor sleep. Such data illustrate how a variable outside of the experimental situation can influence a student's performance in the experimental context.

EXTRANEOUS VARIABLES

Events that can influence behavior, but that are not included as independent or dependent variables in a study, are referred to as *extraneous variables*. The sleep deprivation noted in Figure 3.2 is an example of an extraneous variable. To demonstrate a functional relation, researchers need to hold extraneous variables constant during an experiment. In laboratory settings, this is readily accomplished and is a primary reason why researchers find these settings so amenable to careful experimental analyses. However, educational research, by its nature, occurs primarily in real-world settings. Because of this, the control of extraneous variables becomes very important *and* very difficult. To the extent possible, a researcher should either hold constant extraneous variables or measure them to study their possible relation to behavior; otherwise these variables might *confound* the interpretation of the results.

The concern with extraneous variables is that they may be the source of behavior change, not the events that you, as the researcher, are referring to as your "independent variable." Take, for example, a 7-year-old child with attention deficit hyperactivity disorder (ADHD) who is disrupting their class by calling out to the teacher. Using an A-B-C chart (see Chapter 8), the classroom teacher conducts a functional behavioral assessment of the child's problem behavior. The results show a near-perfect correlation between the child's calling out and the delivery of a reprimand by the teacher. The teacher concludes from this process that the child's problem behavior is maintained by positive reinforcement in the form of adult attention. Following this conclusion, the teacher develops a functional communication training procedure (see Carr & Durand, 1985; Ghaemmaghami et al., 2021) designed to replace calling out with a more appropriate response that results in adult attention (e.g., raising their hand). The teacher implements the intervention, and on the first day the behavior drops to near-zero levels.

At this point, should the teacher conclude that their hypothesis-driven intervention has caused the dramatic change in behavior?

Let's say the teacher has heard the dictum that "every experimental finding should be checked and checked again." Following this advice, they continue collecting data for two more days. The result is a continued pattern of frequent hand raising followed by adult attention and almost no calling out. Then, on the fourth day the child's mother calls the teacher and asks how the child's behavior has been during the week. The teacher describes to the parent the functional behavioral assessment-derived intervention and the pattern of behavior that has occurred. After listening to the teacher, the parent informs them that the child's pediatrician had prescribed a test trial for methylphenidate (Ritalin®) for the child's ADHD. The child has been receiving the drug every day this week.

Such a series of events suggests that any conclusion drawn about the effectiveness of the behavioral intervention *or* medication would be premature. First, the behavioral and psychotropic drug interventions began at the same time, so both correlate with the change in behavior. It could be that one of the interventions is the source of the behavior change, their combination is needed for the effect to occur, or some other event produced the change. Second, although the drug and behavioral interventions were both introduced and their effects on behavior measured for several days, we have no idea if the withdrawal of one or both of the potential independent variables would coincide with a return to the baseline pattern of responding. Finally, we do not know if, following a return to baseline, whether the reintroduction of one or both interventions would change behavior.

In effect, the teacher needs to repeat these findings to better understand the source of change in the child's behavior. Again, it could be that the behavioral intervention changed behavior, the methylphenidate changed behavior, their combination was needed to change behavior, or some other event caused the behavior to change. Without repeating baseline and intervention, we will not know the source of the behavior change. Indeed, both interventions will need to be independently introduced and withdrawn if we want to learn about their separate and combined effects on behavior.

All of this involves *replication*. The teacher and parent could decide to hold medication constant and withdraw the behavioral intervention, or vice versa, and then reinstate both interventions. If this was done, it would be a test of the effects of the behavioral intervention. Let's say that when the communication-based strategy is withdrawn, behavior returns to preintervention levels. Can we conclude that the behavioral intervention is effective and the drug ineffective? "Maybe" would be the most prudent answer.

When *extraneous variables* influence behavior, they become *threats to internal validity*. Internal validity is a concept drawn from group-comparison designs and refers to the degree to which a researcher can be confident that an independent variable is what changed behavior and not an extraneous variable (Campbell & Stanley, 2015; Shadish et al., 2001). Using single-case designs, internal validity is demonstrated by establishing a functional relation between independent and dependent variables.

Following the nomenclature introduced by Campbell and Stanley (2015), threats to internal validity can be of eight types:

- *History effects* are events that occur outside of the experimental situation but can potentially influence the behavior under study. Examples include events such as sleep deprivation, health problems, or out-of-school mathematics tutoring. In addition, history effects in educational research encompass events such as substitute teachers, unanticipated fire alarms, and students being called out of class.

- *Maturation effects* are a second type of threat to internal validity. Children are notorious for maturing over time, and those developmental processes present a problem to researchers. Referred to as maturation effects, normal developmental processes can influence the behavior under study, particularly in experiments that occur over a long period of time. For example, when studying the effects of an intervention on language development, if the experimental effect from the independent variable is delayed, it may be unclear how much of the effect is from normal maturation versus the intervention.

- *Testing effects* are threats to experimental control resulting from changes in behavior that occur when exposed to a testing situation. The idea is that exposure to questions regarding the curriculum being taught to a student might, in fact, teach them something about the testing context (e.g., how to answer questions more accurately) or the testing situation may teach the student something about the material to be learned. In such instances, behavior can change simply as a result of testing, apart from any intervention being analyzed.

- *Instrumentation effects* take two general forms. First, malfunctions in software and/or hardware being used to record behavior might occur. For example, an app programming glitch or a stuck key on a keyboard during a computer-based assessment can alter the data that are obtained and produce unwanted changes in recorded behavior. Second, behavior being recorded by observers can result in inaccurate representations of responding. One example of this is poorly trained observers who inaccurately record the behaviors of interest. Another concern is that observers will gradually alter how they define and record behavior over the course of a study, a phenomenon known as *observer drift*. Each of these types of instrumentation effects will be discussed at length in Chapter 9.

- *Regression to the mean* is another threat to internal validity. This is a statistical sampling phenomenon in which highly unlikely outcomes ("outliers") occurring within a normal distribution tend not to reoccur when resampled (see Rucker et al., 2015). In behavior analysis, there is no such thing as an outlier behavior. All behavior occurs for a reason, and "outliers" are simply a manifestation of a behavioral process that has yet to be analyzed and understood. This makes the concept of statistical regression not very useful for a research approach based on repeated measures (see next section).

- *Participant selection bias* relates to the equivalence of people being assigned to different treatment groups. This threat, like regression to the mean, is derived from a group-comparison (i.e., nomothetic) approach to research taken from traditional psychological research (see Chapter 2) and does not easily map onto a single-case design logic focus on individuals (i.e., idiographic approach).

- *Selective attrition of participants* refers to individuals dropping out of, or being removed from, a study for some systematic reason that is unrecognized by the researcher. Although this is historically a concern of group-comparison designs, it also can affect single-case designs. For $N = 1$ designs, selective attrition is a concern because people with certain characteristics may not be able to complete an experiment. For example, the intervention may be too complex, it may not be socially acceptable, it may run counter to some cultural practices, or it may produce unwanted side effects. This is not so much a concern for the internal validity of a single-case design, but can be an important issue for systematic replication (i.e., establishing the generality or external validity of findings; see Chapter 4).

- *Interaction between selective attrition and other threats* is the final concern in regard to internal validity. In such cases, a threat such as history effects or testing effects systematically influences why participants do not complete a study. In single-case designs, because of their inductive nature, this type of threat is really an elaboration of the previously mentioned concern. This is because interactions between variables causing selective attrition are essentially a refinement in the potential experimental question: *"Why did some participants not complete the study, but others did?"*

Identifying when extraneous variables are threats to internal validity is a critical aspect of the research process. An experienced researcher will know when and where to look for extraneous variables and how to control for their influences on behavior. Perhaps the most effective guide to identifying extraneous variables comes from the data themselves. Anytime that there is variability in your data that you cannot account for by known events, that variability represents the influence of unknown (extraneous) variables on behavior. In this sense, *variability in data for single-case designs is not a nuisance to be ignored, but an indication of other sources of control over the behavior being analyzed.* For this reason, variability in the data often represents an opportunity to learn more about the types of events that can influence behavior.

There are obviously a large number of extraneous variables present in natural environments, including home, community, and educational settings, and many of them cannot be directly controlled like they can in the laboratory. However, there are systematic techniques for studying behavior that can allow for important questions to be answered via single-case design research in educational settings. And, as reviewed in Chapter 2, these designs have a long history of being used successfully. Because all the events just described are possible threats to the establishment of a functional relation, researchers use various types of *experimental designs* to try and control for their possible influences on behavior (see Part IV).

BASELINE

The starting point for most experimental analyses of behavior is the establishment of a *baseline*. "Baseline conditions serve as the background or context for viewing the effects of a second type of condition" (Johnston et al., 2020, p. 225). An experiment has to start somewhere, and a baseline, as we will see, is a logical starting point.

The notion of a baseline may seem simple, but it is actually a complex concept. How a researcher constitutes a baseline has important implications for what conclusions can be drawn from an experiment. A poorly designed baseline may render an experiment uninterpretable or severely constrain the interpretation of findings. To appreciate why this is, we will need to discuss what constitutes a baseline and how it is used in single-case designs.

There are several elements comprising a baseline. One aspect of a baseline centers on the *procedures* used. Procedures refer to specific aspects of the environment and how it is structured and functions. The physical setting, including the size of the room, arrangement of furniture, and general characteristics of the staff, are one component. For example, does the study take place in a small room with only a related-services staff person present, or does the study take place in a gymnasium with dozens of other students and several adults present? Another component relates to who interacts with the student of interest, including other students, educators, paraprofessionals, research staff, and so on. For example, are students working in teams of three or four people monitored by paraprofessionals, or are students working alone with an educator engaging in didactic instruction? In addition to who interacts with the focal student, another issue is what they do when interacting. What are adults doing in the classroom? How do they react to specific behaviors? How does a student's peers react to behaviors of interest? Are there explicit or implicit reinforcement contingencies in place for certain behaviors?

There are at least three additional aspects of educational baseline procedures that need to be explicitly described. First, what is the curriculum, if any, that students are contacting? Is there a structured curriculum with predefined units and tests? Second, what instructional procedures are in place? What type of instruction is provided to students? How is the instruction paced? How often does a teacher request information from students? How does the educator provide feedback regarding student performance? Third, what types of materials are provided in the context of interest? Are the students using tablets, paper-and-pencil worksheets, or manipulable objects?

The previous paragraphs have attempted to describe the basic elements of baselines in educational settings. However, each experiment is somewhat unique, and there are, undoubtedly, many other features that may be relevant to a particular study. In general, the more thorough the description of baseline procedures, the better able future readers will be to interpret any changes in behavior produced by the independent variable (as well as the pattern of behavior established in baseline).

An example of a good baseline description is provided by Dugan et al. (1995). These researchers were studying the effects of cooperative learning groups on the performance of two students with autism in a general education classroom. Their description of baseline procedures included the following:

> Participants were 2 students with autism and 16 fourth-grade regular classroom peers in an inner-city elementary school . . . The teacher rated the 16 peers for their knowledge and typical performance in social studies activities; 5 students were rated high, 8 average, and 3 low.

> All instruction took place in the regular classroom with the teacher monitoring the sessions and a special education paraprofessional assisting with monitoring and administering pretests and posttests. One or two experimenters were present and provided occasional directions but primarily served as monitors to ensure program fidelity and as data collectors.

> A 2-week initial baseline was conducted during 40-min teacher lecture on social studies material given four times per week. This traditional teacher-led format was one that the teacher was currently using for social studies as well as for other content areas. Sixteen students and the 2 students with autism were seated in assigned groups of 3 or 4 in the classroom. The presentation covered topics arranged as units in the text *States and Regions*, including the Northeast and the Southeast. The teacher's lecture and discussion format included introducing key words and facts, posing questions to individuals, and using maps. The students were expected to use texts and take notes. (Dugan et al.,

The previously mentioned research was all conducted with model systems in the laboratory to establish the existence of *basic behavioral mechanisms*, such as positive reinforcement, negative reinforcement, concurrent operants, behavioral contrast, and behavioral momentum, among others (see Catania, 2013). A new generation of research, initiated in the late 1950s and continuing through the 1960s, emerged from this work and translated basic behavioral mechanisms to the behavior of humans. Not surprisingly, these early studies on *human operant behavior* were conducted in laboratory settings, just like the previous research using model systems (see Box 2.3).

BOX 2.3: TRANSLATIONAL RESEARCH AND BEHAVIORAL MECHANISMS

"Translational research" emerged in the 1990s from policy initiatives put forward by the National Institutes of Health (Leschner et al., 2013; Nathan & Varmus, 2000). The initiatives focused on facilitating the translation of preclinical (basic) research into clinical (applied) interventions. Since then, translational research has become a common theme for many research teams working to exploit mechanisms of action discovered in the laboratory into effective treatments for people. Most of these efforts have emerged from the life sciences with an emphasis on basic biochemical findings (e.g., the identification and manipulation of targeted genes for disease processes). However, researchers using single-case designs in the experimental analysis of behavior have been translating model system findings into application since the late 1950s. These mechanisms of action are *behavioral*, rather than biological, and involve processes like positive reinforcement, negative punishment, and behavioral momentum, just as examples. Interventions such as the "good behavior game," "token economies," and "response cost" are directly translated from basic operant mechanisms. What is interesting is that basic behavioral mechanisms discovered using rodent and avian model systems have proven uniquely translatable into behavioral interventions for human beings. The translatability of behavioral mechanisms from laboratories to classrooms and clinics is an exemplar of translational research. It may also suggest that the emphasis on internal validity (experimental control) in single-case design research has aided in the identification of behavioral processes that are robust and readily translated across contexts (see also Chapters 1 and 4).

The first human operant study was conducted by Paul R. Fuller (1949) who studied reinforcement processes in a person with profound intellectual disabilities. His findings demonstrated that basic behavioral mechanisms could be translated to humans and showed that even people with the most profound disabilities could learn if taught in a systematic manner. Another early extension to human behavior was the dissertation research of Ogden R. Lindsley. Lindsley studied the effects of reinforcement schedules on the behavior of people with schizophrenia, finding similar effects to nonhuman research, and initiating the idea of "behavior therapy" (Lindsley, 1956).

1995, pp. 177–178. Copyright 1995 by the Society for the Experimental Analysis of Behavior; reproduced by permission.)

Baselines are used to *establish initial patterns of behavior*. That is, how often do behaviors occur, how long do they last, how much time passes between their occurrences, and do they co-occur with other behaviors that may be of interest? One characteristic of single-case designs is the use of *repeated measures* to document patterns of behavior. Repeated measures refer to a research method in which multiple samples of behavior are collected over time. Unlike group-comparison research, which often measures behavior at a single time point (e.g., a pretest), single-case designs repeatedly measure the behaviors of interest during baseline and intervention.

Depending on the situation, observations may occur throughout a school day, once per day, several times per week, once a week, or once a month. How frequently behaviors are sampled is related to the situation being studied. In general, the more frequently behavior is sampled, the more representative the resulting pattern of behavior. However, the amount of time and resources also increases as the frequency of behavioral sampling increases. As with most issues of experimental design, the researchers conducting the study need to use their best judgment about what is a *representative level of sampling*. If behavior is variable during the week, then multiple samples during the week will be necessary to capture that pattern. If behaviors are very consistent, then less sampling may be appropriate.

By using repeated measures, researchers can establish how often a behavior occurs and how much that behavior varies from observation to observation. Figure 3.3 shows two examples of baselines displaying different patterns of behavior. Cushing and Kennedy (1997) studied the effects of peer support programs on the task engagement of students without disabilities who served in these programs. The baseline was the student without disabilities individually work-ing at their desk while the general educator lectured. Students' task engagement was measured for the same class period each day of the week. For the purposes of this discussion, only the initial baselines will be discussed. Cindy showed a highly variable initial baseline with task engagement ranging from 0% to 76% (*M* = 38%). Kealoha, on the other hand, had a mean task engagement of 44%, with moderate variability (ranging from 25% to 53%).

In the baselines for Cindy and Kealoha, a *predictable pattern of behavior* was established prior to intervention. For Kealoha, the pattern of behavior was one of consistency, whereas for Cindy, the predictable pattern was one of high variability (see Chapter 16). A general rule of thumb in single-case research is that *the more variable the data pattern, the longer it takes to estab-lish a predictable baseline.* This observation raises two interrelated issues: (a) What are the mini-mal number of data points in a baseline? and (b) How stable should that pattern be? In keeping with the general theme of this book, the answer to these two questions is *"it depends."*

The question of how many baseline points constitute a minimum baseline is an interesting one. The default response among single-case researchers is "three data points." Whatever the original source of this dictum, it has been codified in many textbooks on single-case designs. However, I would argue that a baseline needs to be as long as necessary, but no longer. The goal of a baseline is to establish patterns of behavior to compare to intervention. Therefore, a base-line needs only to be long enough to adequately sample this pattern. This judgment depends on the variability of behavior and the pattern of responding relative to other conditions.

For example, in Figure 3.3, there were only two data points collected in the second baseline for Cindy, but there is a clear change in the pattern of behavior. Another exception is the use of brief experimental designs (see Chapter 14) in which only a single data point might be collected in a particular condition. Again, the number of data points needing to be collected depends on the pattern of behavior and the experimental situation.

FIGURE 3.3 ■ Effects of Peer Support Programs on Students Without Disabilities.

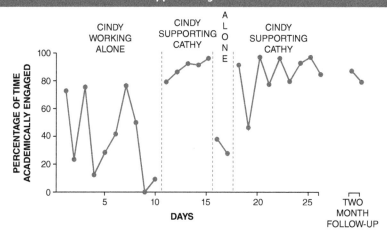

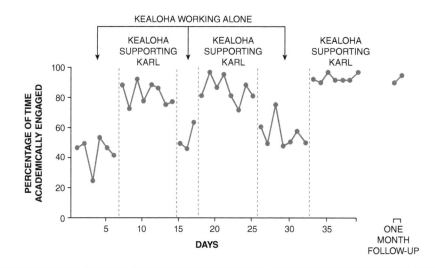

Note. The percentage of intervals in which students were academically engaged is shown along the *y*-axis. Data were collected once per day, five days per week (*x*-axis). The top panel shows the analysis of Cindy's behavior, and the bottom panel shows the data for Kealoha's behavior. Baseline consisted of the student working alone. Intervention was Cindy or Kealoha serving as a peer support for Cathy and Karl (students with severe disabilities), respectively. (Figures 1 and 2, p. 145, from: Cushing, L. S., & Kennedy, C. H. (1997). Academic effects of providing peer support in general education classrooms on students without disabilities. *Journal of Applied Behavior Analysis, 30,* 139–151. Copyright 1997 by the Society for the Experimental Analysis of Behavior. Reproduced by permission.)

A second issue has to do with baseline stability and the concept of a *steady state of behavior*. The idea of "steady states" was initially developed in laboratory research involving the experimental analysis of behavior (Sidman, 1960). Before introducing (or removing) an independent variable, it is desirable to have behavior occur in a highly predictable pattern, or steady state. Therefore, when the independent variable is altered, any changes in the pattern of responding can be indexed against the previously stable pattern of behavior. The logic of this approach is impeccable, but its requirements cannot always be met in applied contexts. An important limitation on the use of steady states in applied research is that some behaviors are so undesirable (e.g., biting another person) that exposing people to an extended baseline would be unethical. Because of this, applied researchers often rely on *changing the pattern of behavior* as an alternative method. In such instances, what the researcher looks for is whether the pattern of behavior is getting worse or better in baseline or intervention, respectively. In sum, when it is possible, steady states of behavior are analytically preferable, but because of constraints that are a part of applied research, they are not necessary if contraindicated for ethical reasons.

Uncontrolled Baselines

In general, there are two broad approaches to constructing baselines. The first approach is to adopt existing practices as the context for establishing baselines. Situations such as this can be referred to as *uncontrolled baselines*, and the term *business-as-usual* is often used. The defining characteristic of this baseline strategy is that nothing is changed from existing practices. For example, if studying the acting out of a student with behavior disorders in a self-contained classroom, researchers could simply enter the classroom and begin observing and recording behavior. Or, the social interactions of a student with extensive support needs might be recorded during a playground situation in which no systematic intervention is in place. Typically, once an uncontrolled baseline is established, an intervention package is then implemented, and improvements in the behaviors are noted.

Uncontrolled baselines are not optimal for at least two reasons. Often, behaviors are occurring at zero, or near-zero, levels, or they are occurring at very high levels. These *floor* and *ceiling effects*, respectively, are a concern because they limit the degree to which the occurrence of behavior can vary. That is, a highly restricted range of occurrence is all that is available as a baseline comparison. Optimally, behaviors vary around the midpoint of the measurement scale, allowing for both increases and decreases in behavior following introduction of an independent variable. In addition, uncontrolled baselines often establish highly artificial situations in the sense that there is no realistic expectation that behaviors might improve during baseline. For example, if a researcher exposes a child who cannot read to sight words without feedback as a baseline condition, the only surprise will be if the child actually begins to read. Uncontrolled baselines are reasonable for demonstrating the effectiveness of a new type of intervention, but they contribute little additional information to a systematic body of research (see Chapter 4).

This observation is related to another concern about uncontrolled baselines. Because the researcher is adopting currently existing, and often deficient, educational practices, there are often multiple changes that are introduced when the independent variable is applied to the baseline. Take, for example, the acting-out behavior of a student with behavior disorders, where an intervention might change social reinforcement contingencies (e.g., teacher praise), change tangible reinforcement contingencies (e.g., a token economy), alter the curriculum (e.g., use lesson plans and units), introduce a new teacher (e.g., a highly skilled graduate student), and alter classroom seating arrangements (e.g., all desks facing away from the windows). Although this multicomponent intervention may prove to be effective, it will be hard to know why it is effective, and, thus, little will be learned about effective teaching practices.

With these concerns noted, there are instances when use of an uncontrolled baseline is justifiable. As previously mentioned, if a line of research is at an early stage of development, the demonstration that a novel intervention can be effective is certainly warranted. This is a logical starting point for beginning the analysis of a new intervention. However, as soon as the new intervention has been demonstrated to be effective, these findings set the occasion for research on understanding *why* the intervention changes behavior under better-controlled conditions.

Controlled Baselines

A second approach to constructing baselines is to hold all conditions constant, except for the variable that is the focus of comparison between baseline and intervention. Such an arrangement can be called a *controlled baseline*, because specific conditions are created to constitute the baseline condition and are adopted in reference to the independent variable. For example, Kennedy et al. (2000) used a multiple baseline (see Chapter 12) across operant functions to study stereotypy. Each baseline was concurrently established to maintain stereotypy on a different reinforcer derived from a previous assessment: (a) positive reinforcement by adult attention, (b) negative reinforcement by escaping demands, and (c) nonsocial reinforcement when alone (see Figure 3.4). A functional communication training intervention (Ghaemmaghami et al., 2021) specific to each behavioral function in baseline was systematically introduced to analyze whether each reinforcer function would transfer to a novel behavior. Such controlled baselines held constant reinforcer functions throughout the study, allowing for an analysis of whether behavioral functions could transfer across topographies of responding (e.g., from stereotypy to sign language).

Controlled baselines provide a number of advantages over uncontrolled baselines. In particular, controlled baselines allow a researcher to move from demonstrating intervention effectiveness to asking more refined experimental questions. This issue is discussed at length in Chapter 5 but will be briefly reviewed here for purposes of explication. Controlled baselines can be used to *compare* one type of treatment with another treatment to contrast which aspect of the two interventions is responsible for producing specific outcomes. For example, use of constant time delay could be compared with constant time delay plus social praise. Controlled baselines can also be used to conduct *parametric* analyses, which contrast different amounts or degrees of an independent variable to establish their effects on behavior. Such a strategy could be used to study the effects of differing amounts of reading instruction on reading proficiency and fluency. A third type of analysis enabled by controlled baselines is *component* analyses. This approach to experimentation can establish a particular intervention as a baseline and then remove an individual component of the independent variable to analyze its effect on behavior.

Historically, controlled baselines have been the minority in educational research using single-case designs. A primary drawback to controlled designs is that the setting in which the

FIGURE 3.4   ■   Multiple Baselines to Study Stereotypy of Behavior.

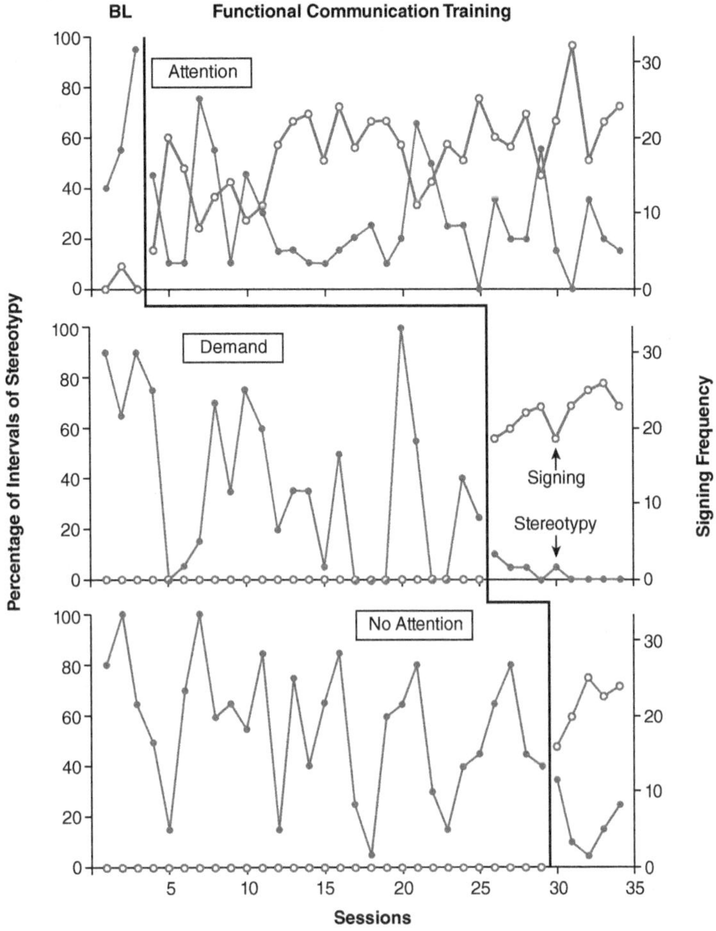

Note. The percentage of intervals of stereotypy is arrayed along the left-side *y*-axis, and the frequency of signing is displayed along the right-side *y*-axis. Consecutive 5-minute sessions conducted once per day are arrayed in the *x*-axis. Stereotypy was maintained on various reinforcers identified in a previous analog functional analysis. Functional communication training was used to transfer reinforcer functions to novel behaviors (i.e., signing). (Figure 2, p. 565, from Kennedy, C. H., Meyer, K. A., Knowles, T., & Shukla, S. (2000). Analyzing the multiple functions of stereotypical behavior for students with autism: Implications for assessment and treatment. *Journal of Applied Behavior Analysis, 33,* 559–571. Copyright 2000 by the Society for the Experimental Analysis of Behavior. Reproduced by permission.)

research is being conducted has to be reconfigured to establish a systematically designed baseline. Anyone familiar with educational environments knows the complexities involved in such an arrangement. However, the analytical benefits of establishing controlled baselines are worth the effort because they allow for more refined experimental analyses. Such analyses allow for the establishment of functional relations that tell us a great deal more about why behavior changed than simply demonstrating that the intervention can be effective.

DEMONSTRATING FUNCTIONAL RELATIONS

Establishing a clear pattern of behavior during baseline sets the occasion for introducing the independent variable and studying the effect on behavior. If the pattern of behavior changes following introduction of the independent variable, there is reason to suspect that the intervention may have influenced responding. However, at this point it would be premature to conclude that a functional relation has been demonstrated. At least one additional experimental manipulation is required to establish a functional relation.

As can be deduced from reading Box 3.2, the situation just described can be referred to as an A-B arrangement of conditions. This A-B arrangement is a necessary, but not sufficient, set of conditions for establishing a functional relation. Although there may be a correlated change in the level of the dependent variable from A to B conditions, a range of extraneous variables could have coincided with the onset of the independent variable. Because of this, researchers need to conduct at least one additional experimental manipulation, a return to the baseline condition (i.e., A-B-A).

BOX 3.2: THE ABCS OF SINGLE-CASE DESIGNS

At this juncture, it's time to introduce some technical nomenclature used in single-case research. In this type of research, baselines are often designated as the "A" condition. If a researcher in spoken or written communication refers to either the A condition or baseline, the terms are being used synonymously. Along the same line of thought, the initial intervention being analyzed is referred to as the "B" condition. Interventions, independent variables, and B conditions are typically synonymous. When we begin discussing different types of single-case design tactics, we will frequently refer to the arrangement of conditions using this alphabetic shorthand. For example, using an A-B-A design, the researcher would use baseline, intervention, and baseline as their sequence of conditions. Or, noting the use of an A-B-A-B design would imply that the following sequence of conditions occurred: baseline, intervention, baseline, and intervention. If additional interventions are introduced, those independent variables are designated using the next letter in the alphabet (e.g., C). An experimental design that tests two separate independent variables against a baseline condition might be designated as A-B-A-C-A-B-A-C. If two separate intervention conditions are combined, a plus (+) sign is typically added to note their combination (e.g., B+C condition). A hypothetical sequence might be this: A-B-A-C-A-B+C-A-B.

The planned return to baseline allows a second test of whether the independent variable actually influenced the dependent variable, rather than an extraneous variable influencing behavior. *This experimental manipulation is a form of replication.* If changes in the dependent variable are largely due to the independent variable and not extraneous variables, the presentation and subsequent withdrawal of the independent variable should strongly influence the pattern of behavior (see Box 3.3).

BOX 3.3: PLANNED EXPERIMENTAL MANIPULATIONS

It was previously noted that interventions are referred to as independent variables because the experimenter directly controls the implementation and withdrawal of these variables. Implicit in this observation is that *the implementation and withdrawal of independent variables is a planned event*. That is, the experimenter decides to start intervention because baseline stability has been achieved or data trends are in the opposite direction to anticipated intervention effects. This purposive process is also followed when removing or altering the independent variable. This can be contrasted with the unplanned, accidental, or serendipitous application or removal of an intervention. In such unplanned instances, the possibility that an extraneous variable may be associated with the changes cannot be ruled out, causing a potential confound in the study. If an extraneous event caused or was coincident with the change in the status of the independent variable, then it is possible that those extra-experimental events may also be responsible for some, or all, of the changes observed in behavior. For this reason, single-case researchers often specify the criteria for condition changes or present the rationale for a condition change prior to making a planned experimental manipulation. This aspect of single-case designs distinguishes it from case histories and other uncontrolled approaches.

Figure 3.5 shows four different patterns of data from A-B-A analyses. Some of the data in Figure 3.5 show functional relations, while others do not. Panel 1 of the figure shows the first baseline condition (A), where a low level of behavior was recorded, with little variability and no increasing or decreasing trend. When the intervention (B) was introduced, an immediate increase in the level of behavior was observed with little variability and no trend. At this point we have shown a clear change from A to B, but it is possible that an extraneous variable may have coincided with the introduction of the B condition. To test for this possibility, the researcher plans to withdraw the intervention (B) once a stable pattern of behavior is established. When the intervention is withdrawn and the experiment returns to baseline (A), behavior returns to a pattern consistent with the original baseline. At this point, we have met the minimal requirements for establishing a functional relation.

Would additional manipulations with correspondingly consistent changes in behavior be ever more convincing? Absolutely. However, how many experimental manipulations is necessary is a complex issue and is discussed in detail in Chapter 4. To presage that discussion, at least three issues enter into determining *how many replications are enough*. First, an A-B-A analysis that shows a clear pattern of behavior change in relation to the status of the independent variable is all that is needed to establish a function relation. However, if the researcher believes that there might be an extraneous variable covarying with the intervention, then additional manipulations are warranted. (In a case like this it is also desirable to directly measure the status of the potential confounding variable.) Finally, because we are discussing single-case designs within

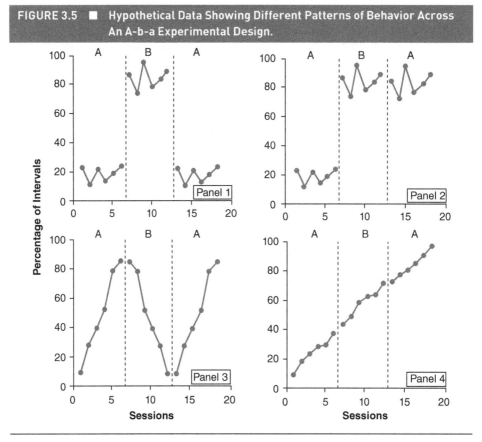

FIGURE 3.5   ■   **Hypothetical Data Showing Different Patterns of Behavior Across An A-b-a Experimental Design.**

Note. The dependent variables are arrayed across the ordinates, while the time course of the studies is arrayed across the abscissa. Each panel is labeled 1, 2, 3, or 4 to correspond with the discussion in the text.

an applied context, the issues of what can be tolerated by the environment and what is minimally intrusive for the participant are critical to consider.

Panel 2 in Figure 3.5 shows a baseline pattern of responding similar to the first panel. Introduction of the independent variable, a change from A to B conditions, produces a clear change in the pattern of behavior. However, when the B condition is withdrawn and a return to baseline occurs, there is no change in behavior. That is, the pattern of behavior in the second baseline is the same as during the intervention. In this instance, we have not replicated our initial A-B data pattern and thus failed to establish a functional relation. Such patterns are not uncommon and can be due to a range of possible interactions among variables. One common cause of such a result is that *the intervention changes behavior in a manner that cannot be easily reversed* (e.g., learning to read particular words). Another common reason for this pattern of data is that an extraneous variable, not your independent variable, was what made the dependent variable change.

Panel 3 of Figure 3.5 shows yet another data pattern. In this case, assume that increases in the dependent variable are a concern and decreases in this variable are desirable. In baseline, there is a consistently increasing trend in the data. The researcher, in this example, decided to introduce intervention even though a steady state of responding had not been achieved. However, an increasing number of undesirable behaviors were being emitted, and in applied contexts this can suffice if the intervention changes that pattern. In the case of Panel 3 of Figure 3.5, introduction of the B condition not only changed the pattern of behavior in baseline but completely reversed it. When the study was changed back to the A condition, the behavior immediately began to increase, session after session. Although there is complete overlap in the data across the A-B-A conditions, a functional relation was established because of the consistent changes in the pattern of the data.

Panel 4 of Figure 3.5 displays a final data set for consideration. Unlike the previous example, assume that increases in the dependent variable are highly desirable. In this hypothetical study, there was an increasing trend in behavior throughout baseline. When the intervention was applied, behavior continued to increase, and when the intervention was withdrawn, behavior continued to increase. The result of this study, for our hypothetical participant, is excellent. However, no functional relation was established, and no experimental control was demonstrated. Because of the continuously increasing trend in the data, there was never any change in the pattern of responding from one condition to the next. In more pedestrian terms, *we have no idea why things got better*.

A useful way of thinking about independent variable manipulations is in terms of additions and subtractions of discrete events to the baseline condition. When an intervention is introduced, something is added to the situation (e.g., error correction in sight word reading) or removed (e.g., noncontingent teacher attention). Often in educational research, several events are added and/or removed. Operationalizing your baseline condition and intervention will assist in explicitly identifying what aspects of your experimental situation are being altered. Such an understanding typically leads to an improved understanding of the nature of the experimental question and the effects on behavior that result from the analysis.

CONCLUSION

In educational settings (or laboratory settings, for that matter), you rarely see such clear findings as those in Figure 3.5. Instead, there is typically more variability, cyclical trends, and less dramatic change across conditions. How to interpret such results takes years of training and experience. We will be dealing with these issues throughout the remainder of the book, as we learn more about measuring behavior and using experimental designs, each of which, in and of itself, can influence your interpretation of the data. It is important to understand that the initial goal of an experimental analysis is to establish a functional relation. However, pursuing that goal is complex, and it is best to be skeptical of findings that are consistent with your anticipated results. Human nature as it is, we often critically scrutinize negative findings but quickly accept positive findings (Simmons et al., 2011). Part of learning to be an effective researcher is to remember that *you are seeking to understand how nature works, not telling nature how it works*.

That means that errors can occur at any time in a research study and being objective and vigilant is required. It's a humbling experience to be a researcher, but well worth the effort in many respects.

The broad goal of research is to explain the world we live in. Part of the process necessary for arriving at explanations is identifying the causes of the phenomenon being studied. The establishment of functional relations is an important step toward such an outcome. When a study is conducted and believably demonstrates that the independent variable influenced the dependent variable, something has been learned. As more and more functional relations are established, a body of evidence accumulates that begins to provide researchers with clues about how some behavioral processes influence behavior. These multiple findings are then interpreted by researchers and used to assemble an explanation for why humans act the way they do (Kennedy, 2004). In the next chapter, we will begin discussing how research proceeds from specific functional relations to the assemblage of larger bodies of evidence using two distinct but related experimental strategies, *direct replication* and *systematic replication*.

REFLECTION QUESTIONS

1. Why would creating a clear experimental question be beneficial when creating the ideas for a study?

2. Explain different approaches to creating a "baseline" condition and how those different approaches may influence what conclusions can be drawn from the investigation.

3. What does it require for an experimenter to claim that they have established a "functional relation" as a result of conducting a study?

4. Can you explain why it is important to identify and control for threats to internal validity?

5. When you use single-case designs, why is it desirable to plan an intentional change in experimental conditions rather than allowing for extraneous events to change conditions?

4 DIRECT AND SYSTEMATIC REPLICATION

LEARNING OBJECTIVES

After reading this chapter, you will be able to

4.1 Define the various ways in which direct replication of an experiment may be conducted.

4.2 Discuss the two primary forms of systematic replication, the design implications for generality, and other factors that influence design choice.

4.3 Identify patterns of negative findings in a failure to replicate an experiment.

For researchers, the term *replication* means "performance of an experiment or procedure more than once" (Merriam-Webster, 2024). Explicit in this definition is that some type of experimental manipulation is conducted *once* and then repeated *once again*. As we will see in this chapter, replication has many facets and derivations, but all these aspects of replication are based on this seemingly simple concept. In fact, replication pervades the research enterprise. Almost every facet of research activity involves repeating an experimental activity. This has led some people to observe that replication is the foundation of science. Without replication, experimentation could not exist.

If I arrange to introduce an independent variable on a steady-state dependent variable performance and the level of the dependent variable changes, I might conclude that my experimental manipulation was the cause of the change in behavior. However, although I would like to conclude that my prowess as an experimenter was the source of behavior change, I would be very naïve to assume so. I would be much wiser to replicate the independent variable manipulation with the same person to see if I get a similar effect a second time, and maybe even a third or fourth time. Even if I get the same effect again, it would be advisable to conduct this experiment again with another person to see if I get a similar effect, perhaps even with a third or fourth person.

The reason for being so careful before rushing to judgment about an experimental finding is that a multitude of events could have co-occurred with the independent variable and any one of those events could be the cause of the behavior change. Such issues beg the question, "How many replications are sufficient to establish a functional relation?"

The answer is that there is no fixed amount (see Box 4.1). The degree to which a finding needs to be replicated depends on the experimental context, nature of the independent variable, characteristics of the population being studied, status of the literature on the particular topic, and experience of the researcher, among many other factors. In essence, a researcher has to rely on their own judgment regarding what degree of replication is acceptable. In addition, the findings need to be sufficiently replicated to convince others that a functional relation has been established.

BOX 4.1: HOW MANY REPLICATIONS ARE ENOUGH?

When asked how many times a finding needs to be replicated, whether within an individual analysis or across participants, most applied behavior analysts would answer, "Two"—that is, the initial demonstration and two more (for a total of three demonstrations). Ask the same question of behavior analysts trained in laboratory settings, and you are likely to get a different answer—that is, the initial demonstration and one more (for a total of two demonstrations). The basic researcher's response is based on economy, logic, and efficiency. A replication, by definition, is an initial demonstration that is repeated once. In some cases, it might be wise to attempt more replications, but it is not necessary. Why have applied behavior analysts arrived at a different and somewhat idiosyncratic answer to the question of replication? Are two replications that much better than one? What about three replications, or four?

There are probably as many answers (and rationales) to this question as there are single-case researchers. Conventions such as these develop over time and often become reified and not critically questioned. The critical issue under discussion is not which number is best, but how to think about the issue of replication. As repeated several times in the text of this chapter, there is no easy answer to how many replications are enough. In some cases, one replication will be the only justifiable amount. In other cases, attempting two, three, four, or more replications may be the only justifiable experimental approach. Which of these is the case for any particular experiment is dictated by the experience and knowledge of the researcher and the nature of the experimental data. What needs to be remembered, though, is that research is a public endeavor and all aspects of an experiment need to be justified to a critical audience. How much is enough, but not too much, is a complex decision.

Although there is no simple answer to how many times to replicate an experimental result to establish it as a believable finding, there is a clear minimum number of times a finding needs to be repeated to qualify as a replication. Numerous research journals (e.g., *Journal of the Experimental Analysis of Behavior* and *Science*) have explicitly stated what qualifies as a minimally acceptable unit for replication. A finding needs to be demonstrated once and then once again. From a logical perspective this is the essence of replication and provides the basis for being able to claim the existence of a functional relation. Whether this amount convinces the researcher that their finding is accurate is left to that individual's experience with the subject matter.

Ideally, researchers would have the luxury of repeating an experimental finding over and over again to their heart's content. However, several factors argue against an almost limitless approach to replication. First, repeatedly exposing a student to experimental manipulations may not be in the best interest of the individual. It is possible that repeatedly presenting and withdrawing an independent variable may have deleterious effects on behavior (although it is possible that positive benefits may also result). Second, the environment(s) that an individual behaves in may not tolerate repeated manipulations. Third, repeating the same experiment numerous times with other individuals may keep the researcher from discovering new functional relations that would further benefit others. Finally, research resources (research participants, materials, classroom time, etc.) are typically limited and mitigate against excessive repetition of an experimental finding.

It is probably best when wrestling with the issue of replication to apply *Occam's razor* or the *rule of parsimony* as a decision-making guide. That is, a researcher needs to decide when enough is enough and more is not necessary. Obviously, this is a moving target depending on a range of experimental factors. One does not want to rush to judgment that an important new finding has been made and then not be able to replicate the phenomenon or have others fail to replicate it. On the other hand, excessive replication is wasteful and potentially harmful. Each replication that is undertaken needs to be evaluated using the criteria mentioned earlier so that a believable finding is arrived at but excessive replication is avoided.

The previous discussion illustrates why replication is so important. By using replication as a focal point for experimental activities, researchers establish a self-correcting system. If someone is conducting an experiment with one participant, observes a positive finding, and then seeks to show the effect again with the same individual, the researcher is checking their results. If a replication is obtained, they can have more confidence in the robustness of their findings. If they fail to find an effect the second time, their initial finding may have been due to some behavioral process other than their independent variable. Similarly, if a researcher is able to replicate their findings with a particular student but cannot obtain a similar effect with other students, concerns are raised. This process allows those involved in the research enterprise to check their own results before publicly presenting them. In addition, the findings of one research team can be checked by other researchers. If the original findings are confirmed, the field has greater confidence in the integrity of the functional relation. If the original findings are not confirmed, a red flag is raised that will require further explanation of the discrepant findings.

As the astute reader will have surmised at this point, there is no single type of replication, but multiple types of replication. In the sections that follow we will distinguish between *direct replication* and *systematic replication*, as well as various subtypes and issues specific to each approach to replication.

DIRECT REPLICATION

A fundamental requirement for conducting an experiment is direct replication. Without this type of replication there can be no experiment. Direct replication refers to the repetition of an experimental manipulation either *within* or *between* participants. For example, changing from baseline to the introduction of an independent variable allows a researcher to evaluate the effects of the intervention on the dependent variables of interest. If the experimenter then returns to baseline and reintroduces the independent variable, that would be an attempt at direct replication. We say "attempt" because we are testing to see if the same effect can be produced again. If we again see a similar effect on the dependent measures as a result of reintroducing the independent variable, then we have replicated our original finding. This example illustrates the use of *direct replication within a participant*, also referred to as *intraparticipant replication*.

Figure 4.1 shows an example of this approach to estimating the effect of an experimental manipulation on behaviors of interest in an effort to establish a functional relation. The figure shows the amount of time that a student—given the pseudonym Allie—emitted behaviors that were deemed indicators of happiness (Logan et al., 1998). Arrayed along the horizontal axis are the specific days on which data were collected. Along the vertical axis is the percentage of intervals of smiles. In this experiment, two types of independent variables were studied: (a) social interactions with students without disabilities (closed circles) and (b) social interactions with students with disabilities (closed squares). On April 14, the dependent measure was studied in relation to social interactions among students with disabilities, with smiles occurring in approximately 55% of the intervals. On April 16, Logan and colleagues (1998) arranged for social interactions with peers without disabilities, resulting in smiling occurring in approximately 90% of the intervals.

If the researchers had stopped the study at this point, they would have shown a large difference between the two experimental conditions. However, at this point, that experimental effect would be unreplicated. As was discussed in Chapter 4, to establish a functional relation

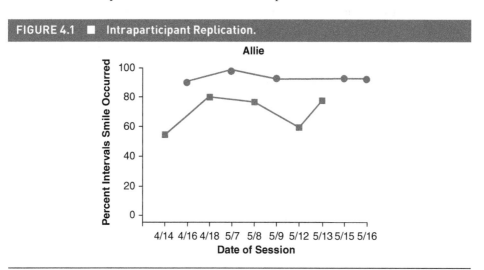

FIGURE 4.1 ■ Intraparticipant Replication.

Note. Comparison was made of the percentage of intervals with smiling by a student with multiple disabilities (Allie). Arrayed along the horizontal axis are the specific days on which data were collected. Along the vertical axis is the percentage of intervals of smiles. Closed circles represent interactions with students without disabilities. Closed squares represent interactions among classmates with multiple disabilities. (Figure 1, p. 315, from: Logan, K. R., Jacobs, H. A., Gast, D. L., Murray, A. S., Daino, K., & Skala, C. (1998). The impact of typical peers on the perceived happiness of students with profound multiple disabilities. *Journal of the Association for Persons With Severe Handicaps, 23*, 309–318. Copyright 1998 by TASH. Reproduced by permission.)

between independent and dependent variables, a consistent and believable pattern needs to be established. Because of this, Logan and colleagues (1998) repeated their experimental comparison. On April 18, peers with disabilities were interacted with, and during the next observation, peers without disabilities were interacted with. The result was a direct replication of the effects shown earlier, although the levels of behavior varied somewhat. At this point the original finding was directly replicated within the participant (i.e., Allie). However, in this instance the researchers opted to repeat several more times the comparison between independent variables. It is possible that they were concerned about the upward trend in the data on April 18 and were not convinced that this was a pattern that would continue if repeated. In addition, they were working with interventions that could easily be replicated with little concern for harm occurring to anyone.

Overall, the original findings from April 14 and 16 were replicated four times. In each of these replications, Allie smiled more when she was interacting with peers without disabilities. This would appear, then, to be a convincing demonstration that Allie was happier among peers without disabilities than among other students receiving a special education. By using direct replication within the participant, this research group was able to make a very believable case about the existence of a functional relation.

However, to further convince themselves that they had a robust finding, Logan et al. (1998) opted to engage in a second form of experimental confirmation, *direct replication across participants*, also referred to as *interparticipant replication*. This type of replication involves the repetition of an experimental finding with a second, and perhaps additional, participant. It helps establish whether an experimental finding extends across one individual to others. Or, put another way, does the functional relation demonstrated through direct replication within a participant generalize to other participants?

An example of direct replication across participants is shown in Figure 4.2. After showing an initial experimental effect with Allie, Logan and colleagues (1998) sought to extend their finding to a second student. This person, given the pseudonym Kay, attended the same school as Allie and had similar characteristics. The same independent and dependent variables used with Allie were used with Kay. These included the same physical settings, peers, activities, time of day, and adults supervising the interactions. In essence, every aspect of the experimental preparation that could be reasonably controlled for was held constant across research participants. Such an arrangement allows for a relatively straightforward test of whether what was found for Allie would also occur for Kay.

A similar experimental design was used to test the two independent variables for the two participants (see Chapter 11, "Multielement Designs"). The results for Kay show a pattern very similar to what was found for Allie. Kay consistently smiled more when she interacted with peers without disabilities than with her peers with disabilities. This finding suggests that the phenomenon originally found for Allie's behavior was not entirely idiosyncratic. Instead, it was also found to extend to a second student, Kay. At this point the finding has been replicated within a participant and across participants. All the basic requirements of experimental replication have been met.

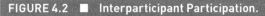

FIGURE 4.2   ■   Interparticipant Participation.

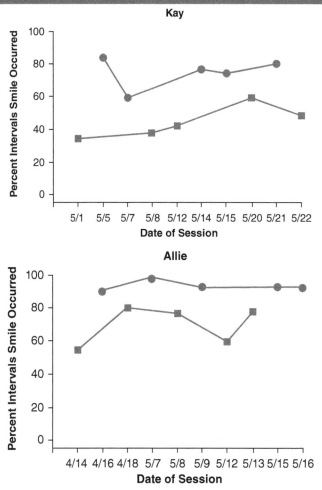

Note. Comparison was made of the percentage of intervals with smiling by two students with multiple disabilities (Kay and Allie). Arrayed along the horizontal axis are the specific days on which data were collected. Along the vertical axis is the percentage of intervals of smiles. Closed circles represent interactions with students without disabilities. Closed squares represent interactions among classmates with multiple disabilities. (Figure 1, p. 315, from: Logan, K. R., Jacobs, H. A., Gast, D. L., Murray, A. S., Daino, K., & Skala, C. (1998). The impact of typical peers on the perceived happiness of students with profound multiple disabilities. *Journal of the Association for Persons With Severe Handicaps, 23*, 309–318. Copyright 1998 by TASH. Reproduced by permission.)

These findings, therefore, beg the question, "Is this degree of replication enough?" There is not a yes or no answer to this question. It depends on a range of issues discussed in this chapter. Two quotes from Sidman (1960) might be particularly apropos at this point in relation to the foregoing discussion: "The value placed on specific replicative techniques results not from a priori logical consideration but from a background of scientific accomplishment. The experience and judgment of the individual scientist are always involved in the evaluation of data"

(p. 71). "Eventually, the experimenter will reach a point at which he decides that further replication would be less profitable than a new experiment" (p. 87).

SYSTEMATIC REPLICATION

In this section, we will discuss what considerations go into extending initial research findings through a process referred to as *systematic replication.* This approach to replication differs substantially from direct replication. As we have seen in direct replication, the exact same experimental preparation (independent variable, dependent variables, experimental procedures, participant population, etc.) is repeated within or between research participants. In systematic replication some aspect of the experimental preparation is changed and its effect on behavior analyzed. For example, in the Logan et al. (1998) study, the findings could be tested for a student population with a different type of disability than the one that Allie and Kay had (e.g., attention deficit hyperactivity disorder, or ADHD). Or, the Logan et al. study could be systematically replicated with a different age range of students. Or, a different set of dependent measures could be developed that more adequately reflect the behavior of interest (i.e., positive affect). The potential number of permutations on the original experiment is only limited by the experimenter's imagination and the complexity of the phenomenon being studied.

Systematic replication takes two general forms. First, variations in experimental preparations can be introduced *within a particular experiment.* The researchers might make a slight variation in the task required of the participants or the behaviors that are measured. A second type of systematic replication occurs *across experiments.* That is, some aspect of the experimental procedure is varied from one analysis to the next, and the similarities and differences in behavioral patterns are studied.

Replication Within an Experiment

Figure 4.3 shows an example of systematic replication within an experiment. The figure reports data from a study of adults with disabilities who had a job performing office duties (e.g., stuffing envelopes or folding letters). Because the workers had very substantial disabilities, they required a high level of support from a job coach. Typically, job coaches were assigned individually to a particular person. A basketball analogy would be playing "man-to-man" defense. The researchers—Parsons et al. (1999)—thought there might be an alternative approach that would be more effective and efficient (i.e., *efficacious*). The experimental question was whether a more dispersed supervisory approach, analogous to a "zone" defense, would work as well (i.e., one job coach switches back and forth between coworkers in an office area). Two dependent variables were of interest: work productivity and work assistance. (We will arbitrarily focus on the latter, since both variables reflect the same systematic replication issues.)

Parsons et al. (1999) established baselines for specific tasks and workers using a traditional one-to-one support arrangement (see Chapter 12, "Multiple-Baseline Designs"). From a systematic replication perspective what is particularly interesting about this experiment is that Parsons and colleagues varied both tasks and workers to assess the robustness of their new intervention.

FIGURE 4.3 ■ Systemic Replication within an Experiment.

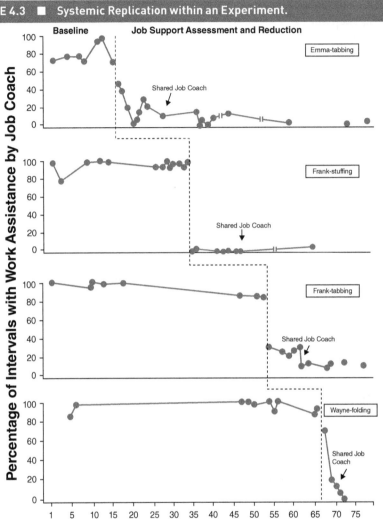

Note. Percentage of observation intervals with work assistance provided by job coaches to adults with disabilities in an office work setting (y-axis) across sessions (x-axis). Three different adults (Emma, Frank, and Wayne) were working on three different tasks (tabbing files, stuffing envelopes, and folding brochures). (Figure 1, p. 296, from: Parsons, M. B., Reid, D. H., Green, C. W., & Browning, L. B. (1999). Reducing individualized job coach assistance provided to persons with multiple severe disabilities in work settings. *Journal of the Association for Persons With Severe Handicaps, 24,* 292–297. Copyright 1999 by TASH. Reproduced by permission.)

They could have studied one worker across multiple tasks. This would have allowed them to draw conclusions about the generality of their findings across specific types of jobs (but not workers). Or, they could have focused on multiple workers and a single task type. This would have allowed them to draw conclusions about the generality of their findings across workers (but not work tasks).

Instead of varying one aspect of the experimental procedure, Parsons et al. (1999) varied two so that they could draw conclusions about the generality of the intervention across workers and job tasks. They did this by having three employees (Emma, Frank, and Wayne) work on three different jobs ("tabbing," "stuffing," and "folding"). Emma worked on tabbing, Frank on stuffing and tabbing, and Wayne on folding. The results of the experiment showed that the job coach intervention was effective across these various permutations. The authors' design allows readers to judge the robustness of the independent variable across two parameters of the experimental preparation (i.e., job types and workers), thus extending their findings across variables within a single experiment. (It should be noted, however, that conclusions regarding job types are limited because two of the tasks were not directly replicated within the experiment.)

Replication Across Experiments

The study by Parsons and colleagues (1999) provides an example of how systematic replication can be used within an experiment to allow researchers to claim a more robust set of functional relations from a single study. An alternative approach is to extend functional relations by systematically replicating across experiments. Because there are logistical constraints on how many systematic replications can be designed into a single experiment, systematic replication across experiments is the primary means by which single-case researchers establish the *generality* of their findings.

Generality refers to the degree to which the findings of one experiment can be extrapolated to other circumstances (Birnbrauer, 1981; Walker & Carr, 2021). Put another way, it is the extent to which a functional relation extends to other behavior–environment relations that vary along some dimension. Those dimensions can include variables such as the grade level of a student, curriculum type, time of day, or degree of teacher training, among many others. Or, those dimensions can be expressly behavior analytic and include variations in magnitude of reinforcement, changes in stimulus dimensions, rate of reinforcement, or alterations in motivating operations, among many others.

The generality of a functional relation is an important focus for researchers. After conducting an experiment, one should rightfully wonder if what has been discovered can be replicated by other researchers. Because the replication of one experiment by another research group necessarily entails some small variation(s) in the experimental preparation (e.g., different school, teachers, or curriculum level), it is typically considered systematic replication. This type of replication helps develop confidence that the original findings are veridical.

However, there is another reason that researchers concern themselves with the generality of their findings (see Box 4.2). In the natural sciences, the extent to which a research finding extends to other instances is not simply something to be confirmed to show that the original finding is generalizable to other samples of participants. Instead, additional studies (i.e., systematic replications) vary some aspect of the experimental preparation to determine the boundary conditions of the functional relation. This aspect of establishing the generality of functional relations via systematic replication uses experimental analyses to determine under what conditions a particular functional relation exists and when it begins to change or no longer exists. So, the more important aspect of a research finding is not if the results can be reproduced (that is only a starting point), but how functional relations change as you alter some aspect of the independent variable.

BOX 4.2: SYSTEMATIC REPLICATION AND EXTERNAL VALIDITY

Because the historical antecedents of single-case designs are based in the biological sciences, there are certain ways in which this approach differs from mainstream educational research, which has its foundations in sociology and psychology. An excellent example of this difference involves the interrelated issues of systematic replication and external validity. Most research methods textbooks in psychology define external validity as the extent to which a finding from one experiment can be extrapolated to other participants, places, and conditions. Implicit in this definition is the logic of *samples* and *populations* derived from group-comparison designs and related statistical analyses (Campbell & Stanley, 2015; Cook et al., 2002). In group-comparison designs a researcher draws a sample (e.g., undergraduates in a research methods course) with the goal that they represent a larger population (e.g., adults in the general population).

A study has high external validity if the findings of the experiment are highly representative of the larger population of interest. Obviously, this is an important issue. If a researcher conducts an experiment with 11-year-olds in a suburban midwestern middle school, the extent to which those findings are representative of other instances is an important question. However, for single-case design researchers, there is a more important question: What makes those 11-year-old suburban midwestern middle schoolers act the way they do? To answer such a question requires an intense focus on internal validity and the behavioral processes that cause people to behave the way they do. Once those behavioral processes have been experimentally analyzed (using direct replication), then the question becomes in what instances do those functional relations exist, and to what degree, under other conditions? For behavior-analytic researchers the generality of a functional relation requires experimental demonstration in the context of altering certain variables. This allows a researcher to establish the robustness of a functional relation. Given that all functional relations have parameters at which they no longer hold, there does not appear to be any other process that can be used to find out how nature actually works. This process is referred to in single-case research as *systematic replication*.

External validity has its origins in hypothetico-deductive reasoning, and statistical inference and systematic replication have their origins in inductive reasoning and natural science. These are terms that refer to related processes but are rooted in distinct epistemologies. It is not surprising that the terms are often used as if they are synonymous, nor is it surprising that people are often confused about what they refer to and how to use the concepts. It is probably fair to say that if a researcher wants to know how something works, systematic replication is the appropriate strategy. However, if a researcher wants to know the extent to which a finding is representative of what would be found in a larger population, then external validity is the appropriate focus. For researchers using single-case methodologies, the latter question makes little sense until the former question has been answered.

For example, take an experiment showing that 6-year-olds who are poor readers can improve their reading performances by receiving 15 minutes per day of peer-mediated instruction (i.e., adult-supervised instruction by a classmate). An obvious question for additional research that could be asked is, "How would parametric variations in the amount of peer-mediated instruction influence reading performance?" A systematic replication of the original finding might compare 30 minutes of peer-mediated instruction with 15 minutes and 7.5 minutes of the same intervention. Hypothetical outcomes from such a parametric analysis are arrayed in Figure 4.4. The data from this hypothetical analysis show reading performances improved by 20% with 7.5 minutes of exposure to the independent variable, 50% after exposure to 15 minutes of instruction, and 55% following 30 minutes of instruction. These data not only confirm that peer-mediated instruction improves reading performance over baseline but establish an interaction between the amount of instruction and gains in student performance. Such a finding better characterizes the relation between independent and dependent variables in a manner that an initial study focusing on demonstrating the effects of one level of the independent variable could not.

This type of inductive approach to replication builds the research literature on a particular topic by replicating the effects of previous experiments and extending them in new directions. In addition to broadening the range of effects a particular behavioral process may encompass, systematic replication allows for establishing the limits of a procedure. For example, in Chapter 1 we discussed applied and basic research on the effects of sleep deprivation. Initial findings replicated the effects of sleep deprivation on negatively reinforced responding for humans and nonhumans. Such a finding established the interspecies generality of the phenomenon through systematic replication. However, when tests of sleep deprivation were conducted with positively reinforced behavior, very different results emerged: Little, if any, effect was observed on behavior when exposed to sleep deprivation. This inductive approach to replication was able to identify where the effects of sleep deprivation did and did not occur. Demonstrating this type of generality is the purpose of systematic replication.

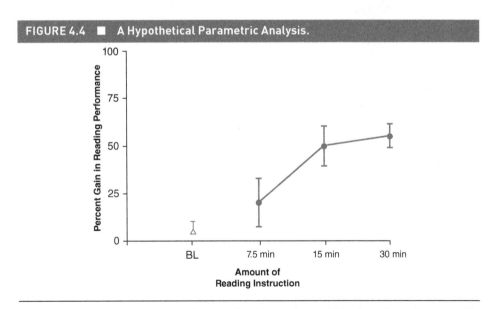

FIGURE 4.4 ■ A Hypothetical Parametric Analysis.

Note. The object of study was the effect of peer-mediated instruction on children's reading performances. The amount of instruction is arrayed along the *x*-axis along with the baseline (BL) procedure. The *y*-axis displays the percentage of improvement in reading from testing the previous week. Data points are the mean performance for the children (bars represent 1 standard deviation).

Another example comes from the field of kinesiology, of which we will selectively review only three studies to highlight the process of systematic replication. In 1974, McKenzie and Rushall provided an initial demonstration of how competitive swimming performances could be improved by publicly posting the number of laps adults swam each day. Critchfield and Vargas (1991) replicated the earlier finding with collegiate swimmers (extending the earlier findings to a new participant population). In addition, they made an important comparison to separate the effects of swim instructor feedback and public posting of swimming performance. The earlier experiment had combined these two procedures as part of the independent variable. When Critchfield and Vargas disembedded these two procedures, they found that instructor feedback did not influence swimming, but public posting improved swimming performances. These results replicated the previous results of McKenzie and Rushall and refined those findings by showing that only a single element of their original component intervention was necessary to improve swimming.

The findings of McKenzie and Rushall (1974) and Critchfield and Vargas (1991) were replicated and extended by Ward and Carnes (2002). The Ward and Carnes study differed in several aspects from the previous studies, but for clarity we will highlight only two dimensions: (a) a new athletic population and (b) the type of performance feedback athletes received. Ward and Carnes studied the role of performance feedback on the athletic performances of collegiate football players. In addition, they studied a variant of earlier procedures: Athletes selected their own goals (formerly, coaches had selected the goals), and the only aspect of their performance that was publicly posted was whether their goal had been met (previously, the absolute level of performance had been posted). The findings of Ward and Carnes showed this approach was effective with another participant population and that only the overall outcome of a personally selected goal needed to be publicly posted.

As a collection, these findings replicated each other in key aspects. For example, each experiment operationalized athletic performance, used similar recording procedures, and publicly posted athletic performances. In each instance this combination of procedures was demonstrated to be effective in changing behavior. However, these experiments also varied in at least two key dimensions. First, each study extended the findings of the previous experiment to a new group of participants. Across the three studies there is evidence that these procedures improved the performances of football players and different types of competitive swimmers (i.e., adult versus collegiate). Each new study also refined previous experiments by further isolating what were the effective components of the original independent variable. Critchfield and Vargas (1991) showed that public posting was critical for improving behavior, but incidental feedback by coaches was ineffective. Ward and Carnes (2002) further refined the intervention by showing that athletes could set their own goals and the only information that needed to be posted was whether the goal was met.

In this sport psychology example, systematic replication was used both to extend the generality of findings across participant populations and to clarify the functional dimensions of the independent variable. In each experiment, the research groups built on previous findings that incorporated replication of previous results and extensions of the existing literature. This example highlights the dual function of systematic replication: (a) replicating on previous experimental results and (b) elaborating and/or refining previous findings. No single experiment in such a process can answer all the relevant questions regarding an educational or psychological phenomenon. However, through the process of systematic replication a research literature emerges that can adequately characterize the phenomenon of interest.

Factors In Designing Systematic Replication

So, how does a researcher know when and how to systematically replicate previous experimental findings? As with direct replication there are no absolute rules. There are a number of factors that enter into decisions regarding what form a systematic replication can take (see also Johnston et al., 2020; Sidman, 1960). Factors that can influence the decision of when to replicate another experiment include the *novelty of the finding*. If a finding is new and unreplicated, having another research group repeat the experiment provides an important check on the integrity of the original findings. For example, if an investigator reports a new technique for teaching phonemic awareness to 4- and 5-year-olds, other researchers may want to see if it works for students in other schools.

The *context of experimental findings* also influences judgments about when to replicate. An extremely well-developed literature may require fewer additional replications than a relatively new area of research. For example, the use of curriculum-based measurement (Deno et al., 2001; Kame'enui et al., 2006) has received considerable research attention over several decades. Because of the large body of literature on this procedure, the need for additional replication is less compelling than an area of research in which the first experimental report has recently appeared.

Another factor is the research group's *familiarity with the experimental preparation*. This can entail either incorporating new techniques into a researcher's activities (e.g., a new computerized measurement system) or the need to repeat previous findings when working in new settings (e.g., in a new school system or with a different student population). In the former example, the replication might be undertaken so that the new system can be checked against the previously established system to compare the consistency or efficacy of the two data collection strategies. In the latter example, repeating a previously established functional relation allows the researcher to verify that a new experimental preparation can yield similar results.

Yet another factor influencing the decision of when to replicate is the *existence of alternative explanations* for a finding. If a new, or even well-established, experimental finding exists and a research group suspects that there are alternative explanations, replication may be warranted. In this instance, the new experiment may use a new dependent variable, use a more sensitive or reliable measurement system, or include an additional control condition that helps clarify the effect of the independent variable.

Systematic replication can also be used to establish the generality of research findings *across participant populations*. Not surprisingly, educational researchers tend to focus their experimental efforts on specific student populations, such as individuals with gifts and talents and/or from low socioeconomic backgrounds. Establishing a functional relation among experimental variables with one population of students often raises questions about how robust the finding is. Part of answering this question is to test the generality of the finding across a range of learner characteristics.

Typically, when researchers engage in systematic replication they are seeking to *extend or refine an independent variable* that has previously been shown to enter into a functional relation with some behavior(s) of interest. Chapter 5 goes into detail regarding specific types of experimental questions, but we will note some general issues here. By its nature, systematic replication varies some aspect of the experimental preparation and can include variations in an intervention(s). In some instances, it may be of interest to remove some component of the independent variable and see how behavior changes or does not change. In other cases, some aspect of the intervention may be increased or decreased, as in our previous example using peer-mediated instruction (see Figure 4.4). Another possible approach to systematic replication is to compare one technique with another. Finding answers to each of these questions provides potentially important information about the functional properties of an independent variable and helps establish a better understanding of the behavioral processes involved.

Sometimes researchers seek to better understand a phenomenon by *improving the way in which it is measured*. In some instances, a researcher may develop a more efficient measurement system and want to establish its usability and accuracy. In other instances, additional measures of behavior may be incorporated to extend the scope of the analysis. In other cases, researchers may develop new measurement techniques that are more sensitive to the events of interest. In each of these examples systematic replication can be used to better capture the behavioral events of interest by analyzing how various behaviors are measured.

A final area where systematic replication can occur is in the *repeating of research findings using different approaches to establishing experimental control*. This is a growing area of replication because of the increase during the past decade in educational researchers using a wide variety of approaches to conducting research. Given that each approach to research has strengths and limitations, checking experimental findings that used group comparisons, surveys, or ethnographic techniques helps researchers better understand the nature of the original findings. In particular, the use of single-case designs to replicate findings that used different methodologies allows for a more careful check on the behavioral processes that might be influencing behavior.

FAILURES TO REPLICATE

What happens if an experimental effect is not replicated via direct or systematic replication? For example, what could be concluded if in the Logan et al. (1998) experiment an effect was achieved with Allie, but no difference or an opposite effect was achieved with Kay? Or, in the Parsons et al. (1999) experiment, what conclusion could be drawn if experimental effects had not been replicated with Frank's working on envelope stuffing? Such findings are not unusual and require a great deal of attention from a researcher when they occur in order to accurately understand their reason for occurring (Branch, 2019; Maxwell et al., 2015).

In general, negative findings resulting from attempts to replicate take on three patterns: (a) finding no effect, (b) finding an opposite effect, or (c) finding a partial or mixed effect (Simmons et al., 2011). Any of these outcomes can occur as a result of attempts at direct or systematic replication. Failure to replicate an experimental effect is relatively self-explanatory: No change in behavior occurs when the experiment is replicated. Finding an opposite effect entails the independent variable inducing an effect that is the inverse of the original experimental outcome. Partial or mixed results occur when there is variability in the effect of the intervention.

Outright failures to replicate seem to be relatively rare, or at least they are rarely reported in peer-reviewed journals (Stroebe & Strack, 2014). This is probably because failures to replicate usually raise more questions about the replicative attempt than the original experiment itself. Typically, failures to replicate are interpreted as suggesting that some aspect of the new experimental preparation was not appropriately followed when attempting the replication. It is not uncommon when attempting to replicate another investigator's work that some small but crucial aspect of the previous experiment is omitted or altered in the replication attempt. For this reason, when experienced researchers encounter a failed replication, their initial bias is to check to see if some procedural detail was omitted or inaccurately conducted in the replication. However, if the researchers can make a compelling case that they have faithfully followed the original experimental protocol yet repeatedly fail to obtain an experimental result, significant concerns are raised about the integrity of the original finding.

Similar issues are raised when a researcher replicates another person's experimental preparation and obtains results opposite to the original investigation. The first round of questions raised by such an outcome focuses on how carefully the original experimental protocol was followed in the attempt to replicate. If the original experimental methods are being faithfully replicated, then opposite findings suggest that there is some type of interaction effect occurring that was previously unidentified (see Hains & Baer, 1989). That is, the experimental replication has identified some type of interaction between behavioral processes that the original experiment did not. Such results can occur because one or more of the behavioral processes was not present in the original research, the measures used were not sensitive to the phenomenon, or some aspect of the procedures did not permit the effect to occur. Unlike outright failures, replications that find different experimental outcomes are usually viewed as possible discoveries of new behavioral processes or novel interactions between behavioral processes.

The interpretation of mixed outcomes from a replication largely follows the same logic as the finding of opposite results. That is, if the experimental methods were accurately followed (and the burden of proof of this is always on the researcher conducting the replication), then a new process or a more complex interaction between or among variables may have been identified. Again, such an experimental result is usually greeted by the research community—if not always the original investigator—as an exciting source of new discoveries.

Failures to replicate or incomplete replications are some of the most complex and difficult issues a researcher can face (Camerer et al., 2018; Freese & Peterson, 2017). A large part of this complexity stems from the interpretation of negative findings. What exactly can be concluded when somebody fails to find an experimental effect? The number of possible sources of influence on such an experimental outcome and the resulting speculations are only limited by a person's ingenuity in concocting possible explanations. Because there are often many plausible alternative explanations in these cases, such experimental outcomes are best interpreted with a great deal of caution and the results considered tentative until further replications are conducted. I would suggest that when failures to replicate occur or alternative results are obtained, the best course of action is to conduct further experimental analyses of behavior to identify the sources of behavioral variability. By following such a course of action, the researchers place themselves in a position of potentially demonstrating new functional relations, rather than simply reporting contradictory findings that might have multiple interpretations.

CONCLUSION

Replication is a complex topic that is at the core of the endeavor we call research. Its complexity arises from the nature of the research act itself. Every facet of an experiment can potentially be directly and/or systematically replicated. These facets include variables that are currently poorly understood or have yet to be discovered. In addition, because there are no absolute rules regarding when to replicate, what form a replication should take, or when to move on to a new analysis, researchers are forced to use their own judgment. Replication requires researchers to make informed judgments that have no guarantee of being successful, but those decisions are guaranteed to be critically analyzed by the investigator's peers.

Although replication is a difficult issue to grapple with, it is also the process through which research literatures emerge and thematic lines of research develop. By carefully crafting experimental questions, finding answers to those questions, and then moving on to the next set of experimental questions, empirical findings accumulate. Through this process, we gain a better understanding of what comprises a particular educational issue, how it is structured and functions, and ways to improve it. Both direct and systematic replication play a fundamental role in this process.

REFLECTION QUESTIONS

1. Can you describe different approaches to replication and explain why they are important?

2. How does replication relate to the notion of experimental control or internal validity?

3. Why do researchers' studies using single-case designs place such a high value on internal validity?

4. What steps should investigators take if they fail to replicate a previously established functional relation?

5. What is the relation between an investigator using systematic replication and the external validity of their findings?

5 EXPERIMENTAL QUESTIONS

When a researcher decides to conduct an experiment, they usually start with some type of experimental question—that is, some general statement about what type of question will be asked when conducting the experiment. For example, the researcher may be interested in a new method for teaching young children with autism to produce more complex language. A general experimental question might ask whether a naturalistic language instruction technique, such as milieu therapy (Garfinkle & Kaiser, 2003), increases the length and complexity of a child's utterances. The basic question in this instance takes the form of "Is the teaching technique effective?"

Formulating an experimental question is important for a number of reasons. First, it requires the researcher to clarify what they are attempting to accomplish by conducting an experiment. Research often starts with an innovative idea and a great deal of enthusiasm. However, in the rush to analyze the new idea, the researcher may not adequately define what the study is about. This is important because a range of issues need to be dealt with when moving from an exciting idea to a successful experiment: (a) Has another research team conducted a similar investigation? (b) What were the procedural details of related experiments that might provide important information about what to include or avoid in conducting a related study? and (c) Is the new idea tractable, meaning could the experiment actually be conducted in a reasonable amount of time? Asking questions like this before an experiment is begun substantively increases the probability of conducting a successful, interpretable, and important study.

Prematurely starting an experiment can also result in problems implementing the study and developing procedures that will allow for the demonstration of a functional relation. Most experienced researchers have learned the hard way that rushing to conduct a new experiment often leads to a flawed investigation and uninterpretable findings. Following up on an innovative idea with a carefully crafted experimental question can help avoid such errors. The reason for this is that explicitly stating an experimental question forces the researcher to think through various procedural issues that might have not initially been considered.

Developing an experimental question also forces a researcher to be able to clearly communicate their idea to other people. This, again, requires the researcher to think clearly about the nature of the experiment. What precisely is the experiment about? What will be measured? Exactly what is it about the independent variable that will result in behavior change? Will the measures adequately capture the effects of the intervention on behavior? Will the experimental design adequately control for plausible confounds? Not only does developing an experimental question require further evaluation of an idea by the researcher, but it allows others to critique the proposed experiment, which often results in an improved experimental plan.

Experimental questions can vary in their specificity but should contain a certain set of elements that are necessary to properly characterize what will be tested. These elements include (a) the student population, (b) the nature of the independent variable, and (c) the dependent variable(s) to be measured. The student population refers to the relevant characteristics of the people who are the focus of the experiment. For instance, in the earlier example, the student population could be characterized as children with autism. Depending on the nature of the experimental question, additional details might be necessary, such as standardized estimates of expressive and receptive language or the extent of each student's autistic characteristics. The specification of independent and dependent variables should be self-explanatory. As with the population under investigation, the degree of specificity used to characterize the intervention and behaviors being studied follows from the nature of the experimental question. For example, an initial experiment to investigate the behavioral effects of a new instructional procedure might be much more general than an experiment in a well-characterized area of research that is exploring the behavioral processes that cause a particular intervention to be effective.

Putting all of this information together with the example mentioned in the first paragraph, the experimental question might be "What effect will milieu language therapy have on the requesting of children with autism?" Such a statement makes clear to an informed reader what will be done in the experiment, what types of behavior will be measured, and who the focal participants are. Formulating such explicit experimental statements also allows the researcher to clarify what they intend to do and take their experimental interests from an exciting idea to a precisely defined experimental question.

In addition to the elements just discussed, a researcher may specify the effect the independent variable will have on behavior. However, such a statement is not necessary to formulate a clear experimental question. It does, on the other hand, add a predictive element to the formulation of the question. For example, the researchers could change their experimental question to include a prediction about the effect of the intervention on behavior: "Will milieu language therapy increase the requesting of children with autism?" When a researcher adds the predicted outcome to an experimental question, they are specifying a hypothesized outcome for the experiment.

As was discussed at length in Chapter 1, hypotheses take various forms, with some being more useful than others. Many researchers believe that specifying a precise effect on behavior is necessary for an adequately formulated experimental question, while others would say that such predictions are unnecessary and might even be counterproductive. The basis for the former opinion is the belief that a researcher should know what effect their intervention will have on a person's behavior before conducting the experiment. Supporting arguments for the latter opinion often note that by specifying a predicted outcome a researcher may be unnecessarily committing to one particular experimental outcome and, thus, might not be as aware of other possible outcomes. Again, different research groups adopt different practices regarding experimental questions. There is probably no right or wrong answer on this issue. As always, the final arbiter is the effectiveness of one experimental practice over another in leading to meaningful findings.

Another aspect of experimental questions is the nature of the question itself. That is, at a more abstract level, *what type of question is being asked?* Researchers do not always think about their questions in this way because they are focused on the day-to-day issues of effectively conducting successful experiments. However, if you reflect on this issue, you will find that there are a fairly small number of categories that experimental questions can be characterized as, with each having its own merits and uses. In the remainder of this chapter, we will discuss the four basic types of experimental questions: (a) *demonstration*, (b) *comparison*, (c) *parametric*, and (d) *component*. These four types of experimental questions provide a complete characterization of the types of experiments that people conduct in single-case design research (see Table 5.1).

TABLE 5.1 ■ Types of Experimental Questions and Examples	
Question Type	**Question Examples**
Demonstration	• Will the independent variable alter the dependent variable?
	• Will an error correction procedure that repeats math problems that a student answers wrongly improve the student's math skills?
	• Will modeling fluent speech decrease a child's disfluencies?
	• Will written cues, videotaped feedback, and the use of children's stories improve a child's social interaction skills?
Comparison	• Will Independent Variable 1 or Independent Variable 2 alter the dependent variable to a greater degree?
	• Will sign language alone or sign language plus spoken language differentially affect a child's expressive and/or receptive communication?
	• Will an intervention derived from functional behavioral assessment improve the problem behaviors of a student more than an arbitrarily selected intervention?
	• Will error correction improve a student's spelling when compared to a traditional spelling strategy?

(Continued)

TABLE 5.1 ■ Types of Experimental Questions and Examples *(Continued)*	
Question Type	**Question Examples**
Parametric	• What effect will incremental increases in the level of the independent variable have on the dependent variable?
	• What changes in reading fluency will result from 7.5 minutes, 15 minutes, or 30 minutes of peer-mediated instruction?
	• What effect will variable-interval (VI) 6-second, VI 12-second, VI 30-second, and VI 60-second schedules of reinforcement have on the math performances of students with attention deficit hyperactivity disorder (ADHD)?
	• What effect will 5 seconds, 15 seconds, and 45 seconds of escape from instruction have on the rate of negatively reinforced problem behavior?
Component	Will removal of one element from a multicomponent intervention change the level of the dependent variable? Will removal of the "rule statements" component from the good-behavior game change the frequency of students' problem behaviors? Will adding a response-extinction component to functional communication training reduce the self-injury of a child? Will the removal of public posting from a goal setting plus public posting intervention alter the tackling accuracy of collegiate football players?

DEMONSTRATION QUESTIONS

The first type of experimental question focuses on *demonstrating* the existence of a particular functional relation. In its most basic form this type of question asks, "Will the independent variable alter the dependent variable?" For example, does an error correction procedure that repeats the mathematics problems a student gets wrong improve their mathematics skills? Or, will modeling of fluent speech decrease the disfluencies of a child who stutters? In general, demonstration questions seek to answer how a particular intervention affects various behaviors of interest. Hence, as noted in Box 5.1, they are the type of experimental question most frequently addressed in educational research.

BOX 5.1: THE PROBLEM WITH BEING EFFECTIVE

One of the hallmarks of behavior analysis is its effectiveness (see Baer et al., 1968; Fisher et al., 2021). Multiple examples exist of the substantive progress that has been made by researchers working in this tradition over the many decades. However, there is an important concern with being so effective. That is, because so much progress is being made in demonstrating the effectiveness of new techniques, less experimental attention is focused on *why* the techniques are effective. Hayes et al. (1980) referred to this as the "technical drift" of applied behavior analysis. The concern is that new techniques are being described and their effects on behavior documented, but researchers do not understand what causes them to be effective (i.e., why they work). The concern is that researchers may be developing a "bag of tricks" that cannot be related back to basic learning processes. Discovering why interventions are effective, and why they are not effective, may allow researchers to develop a science of learning that will be more effective than a simple catalog of techniques. This is particularly the case for instances where complex interactions among experimental variables will need to be identified and analyzed. It is likely that many of our current failures to change interventions may be due to these unknown complex interactions. It may seem paradoxical, but in the short term being very successful in changing behavior may result in limited effectiveness in the long term.

Figure 5.1 presents an illustrative example. Thiemann and Goldstein (2001) studied the effect of a multicomponent intervention on the social behavior of children with autism. The independent variable used by the authors included written cues of when and how to socially interact, videotaped feedback of the child's social interaction, and the use of children's stories to teach appropriate social skills. The behavioral measures included social skills such as securing the attention of another child, initiating a comment about the play activity, requesting the other child to play with them, and responding to the other child's requests. The former three dependent variables each increased only when the multicomponent intervention was introduced by the research team, indicating a functional relation between intervention and social behavior. The only response that increased without intervention was responding to the other child's requests. As a result of this analysis, Thiemann and Goldstein concluded that "following implementation of the visually mediated treatment, the children with social impairments demonstrated improved and more consistent rates of targeted social behaviors compared to baseline performance" (p. 442).

Such experimental questions are used to demonstrate whether an intervention changes behavior in some way. Such questions are the foundation of an evidence-based educational literature (see Chapter 7). These types of questions allow researchers to study how a particular independent variable will change a learner's performance. The cumulative effect of asking such questions is the ability of researchers to respond to practitioners', families', and administrators' requests for information about various educational practices by showing them what interventions work and which do not. This type of experimental question also allows researchers to describe the type of effect that an intervention can be expected to have on responding. In addition, this type of experimental question sets the stage for more complex analyses of how and why interventions change behavior (see the following section).

COMPARISON QUESTIONS

Another approach to experimental questions is *comparing* independent variables. Typically, two, or more, independent variables are studied in relation to a fixed set of dependent variables. That is, two, or more, distinct environmental arrangements are studied in relation to the same set of

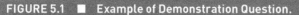

FIGURE 5.1 ■ Example of Demonstration Question.

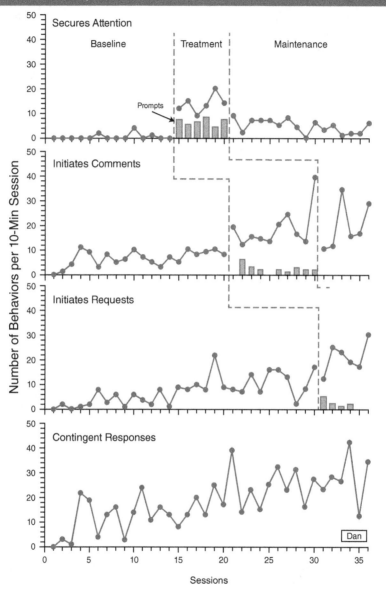

Note. Researchers measured the number of times a child with autism used appropriate social skills to interact with a playmate without disabilities. The behaviors included "secures attention," "initiates comments," "initiates requests," and "contingent responses." Closed circles represent the number of times each behavior occurred during a 10-minute session. The shaded bars represent the number of prompts provided by a teacher. (Figure 2, p. 436, from: Thiemann, K. S., & Goldstein, H. (2001). Social stories, written text cues, and video feedback: Effects on social communication of children with autism. *Journal of Applied Behavior Analysis, 34*, 425–446. Copyright 2001 by the Society for the Experimental Analysis of Behavior. Reproduced by permission.)

behaviors. For example, researchers might study the effects of two different interventions on the communicative development of children who are deaf. One intervention might be comprised of learning to communicate using American Sign Language (ASL). A second intervention might be comprised of ASL and spoken English (i.e., "total communication"). The experimental question might be "Do the two different interventions produce differential effects on receptive and/or expressive communication?"

Figure 5.2 shows another example of a comparative analysis. In a study of reading performance, Kim et al. (2023) compared three conditions for teaching sight word reading to second-grade students. The first strategy presented students with reading words and provided praise and/or corrective feedback based on the individual's performance (Set Analysis [SA]). The second strategy, Operant Analysis (OA), used similar procedures to the SA condition, but re-presented words until a mastery criterion was met. The OA condition was subdivided into two different trial presentation formats: five presentations of each sight word (OA5) and three presentations of each sight word (OA3). This comparison strategy was replicated across multiple word lists. As can be seen in the figure, the OA3 procedure was more effective for all four students. Such a finding led Kim et al. to recommend that teachers use a presentation format for sight word reading that used fewer trials of the re-presentation format (OA) along with a standard error correction format.

Researchers use comparative analyses for a number of reasons. One reason is to study the *effectiveness* of different educational interventions. A very practical reason for comparing independent variables is to find out which intervention is more effective in changing behavior. How effective an intervention is refers to the absolute change in behavior that resulted from being exposed to the independent variable. That is, after repeated exposures to the intervention, how much behavior change has occurred? For example, Baer et al. (1968) noted that an intervention that raised a child's grades from Ds to As is more desirable than a strategy that changed the same child's grades from Ds to Cs.

Researchers are also interested in the *efficiency* of interventions. An important concern in educational contexts is the amount of time or effort required to teach students specific elements of the curriculum. Because educational resources, including time, are limited, the faster a student can be taught something, the more time they have for learning additional material. Or, in instances such as self-injurious behavior, the faster an intervention has an effect, the less harm the individual can cause to themself. When researchers are interested in analyzing both the effectiveness and efficiency of interventions, the term *efficacy* is used. In these cases, the comparative analyses are conducted in terms of both overall level of behavior change and how rapidly that change occurs.

Another reason why researchers ask comparative questions is to explore the behavioral processes that are responsible for behavior change. As was noted in Box 5.1, being effective (or efficacious) is important, but such efforts are ultimately limited if researchers do not know the behavioral processes that bring about changes in responding. Comparative analyses provide researchers with a tool for exploring *why* behavior is changing. For example, if a research team believes that task difficulty is the reason a child avoids doing mathematics problems, they could compare conditions in which task difficulty is varied. If the child attempts to escape instruction when hard mathematics problems are presented, but not when easy mathematics problems are

FIGURE 5.2 ■ Example of Comparative Analysis.

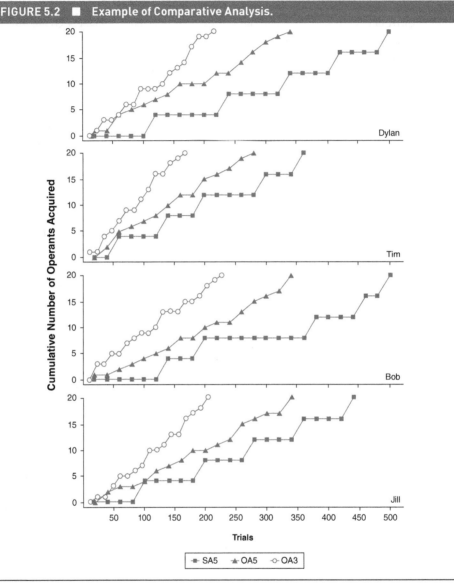

Note. The graph shows the cumulative number of sight words acquired during three different experimental conditions that varied presentation conditions (i.e., Set Analysis [SA] and Operant Analysis [OA]) and trial presentation formats (i.e., 3 versus 5). Students acquired sight words most quickly under the OA3 condition compared to the SA5 and OA5 conditions. (Figure 1, p. 393, from: Kim, J. Y., Fienup, D. M., Draus, C. J., & Wong, K. K. (2023). Differential mastery criteria impact sight word acquisition and maintenance: Application to individual operants and teaching trial doses. *Journal of Applied Behavior Analysis, 56*(2), 388–399. Copyright 2023 by the Society for the Experimental Analysis of Behavior. Reproduced by permission.)

provided, then task difficulty may be the noxious stimulus dimension negatively reinforcing the child's avoidance behavior (Common et al., 2019; Spooner et al., 2019). *By carefully arranging conditions that compare possible variables responsible for behavior change, a researcher can discover the causes of behavior.*

PARAMETRIC QUESTIONS

One of the most important analyses that a researcher can conduct is to identify how behavior changes in relation to *parametric variations* in some dimension of the independent variable. Such an analysis establishes a far more thorough understanding of the relation between an intervention and behavior than can be accomplished through asking whether an intervention is effective or not. For instance, consider the classic example of peer-mediated instruction provided in Medland and Stachnik's (1972) replication of the good-behavior game. The investigators originally focused on demonstrating that 15 minutes of peer-mediated instruction could improve reading performance by 50% above the baseline practices used in the classroom. This finding is important but does not provide any information about the interrelation between the intervention and behavior change. It is an all-or-nothing finding. However, when the researchers parametrically varied the amount of time spent in peer-mediated instruction, a much more complete picture emerged. The functional relation that was established showed that 7.5 minutes of instruction produced a 20% gain in performance (but with increased variability in those gains) and 30 minutes produced only a 5% gain over 15 minutes of exposure to the independent variable. Such a finding demonstrates that there is not a linear relation between the intervention and behavior change. This finding is significant because it means that "more" is not necessarily "better." In addition, the parametric analysis suggests, from a practical standpoint, that 15 minutes seems to provide the best outcome for the effort involved.

The hallmark of parametric analyses is the systematic increase or decrease in the value of some dimension of the independent variable. Figure 5.3 shows such a manipulation in relation to the use of methylphenidate (Ritalin®) for a child with attention deficit hyperactivity disorder (ADHD) named Willis. The dependent variable was the number of mathematics problems solved by Willis per minute. In addition, the researchers (Murray & Kollins, 2001) alternated across school days between the child receiving a placebo and methylphenidate (MPH). What Murray and Kollins (2001) were particularly interested in was how the schedule of positive reinforcement that maintained Willis's math work would interact with the placebo and MPH conditions. To accomplish this analysis the authors parametrically varied the variable-interval (VI) schedule of reinforcement (i.e., 6 seconds, 12 seconds, 30 seconds, or 60 seconds). The researchers found that MPH interacted with the VI schedule of reinforcement so that the denser the schedule of reinforcement, the more problems solved per minute. However, the different VI values of the reinforcement schedule had no differential effect on problem solving during placebo conditions.

Any aspect of the independent variable that can be quantified can be subjected to a parametric analysis. Possible dimensions for a parametric analysis might include the amount of exposure, the magnitude of exposure, or the density of exposures, among other permutations. In addition, two (or more) different dimensions of an independent variable can be parametrically manipulated in relation to each other to establish how the dimensions interact. For example, researchers could vary the temporal dimension of VI reinforcement schedules and reinforcer magnitude.

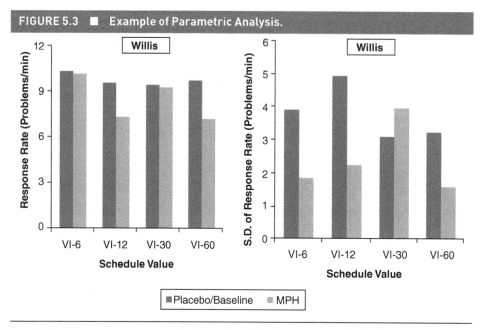

FIGURE 5.3 ■ Example of Parametric Analysis.

Note. Problem responses per minute emitted by a child with ADHD were recorded. Black bars in the histogram represent instructional sessions in which Willis received a placebo pill. Shaded bars represent instructional sessions in which Willis received methylphenidate (MPH). The effects of the psychoactive drug were studied across parametric variations in the schedule of reinforcement for appropriate behavior (VI-6 seconds, VI-12 seconds, VI-30 seconds, or VI-60 seconds). *S.D.* on the right-hand vertical axis refers to standard deviation. (Figure 2, p. 581, from: Murray, L. K., & Kollins, S. H. (2000). Effects of methylphenidate on sensitivity to reinforcement in children diagnosed with attention deficit hyperactivity disorder: An application of the matching law. *Journal of Applied Behavior Analysis, 33*, 573–592. Copyright 2000 by the Society for the Experimental Analysis of Behavior. Reproduced by permission.)

How a specific dimension of an independent variable is parametrically altered is another matter. Typically, researchers opt for a systematic approach to parametric variation in interventions. Options for how to vary the metric being analyzed include the following manipulations: (a) additive progression (e.g., 10 seconds, 20 seconds, and 30 seconds), (b) multiplicative progression (e.g., 10 seconds, 20 seconds, and 40 seconds), or (c) logarithmic progression (e.g., 1 second, 10 seconds, and 100 seconds). In general, which sequence is used depends primarily on logistical constraints on levels of the independent variable, sensitivity of the dependent variable metric, and the nature of the experimental question.

Often parametric analyses follow from initial demonstrations of the effectiveness of a particular intervention. In this sense they constitute a form of systematic replication. The reasons for conducting a parametric analysis are multiple. In some cases a researcher may want to simply establish the form of a functional relation between responding and the environment. In other cases a researcher may want to find out if a complex functional relation discovered in the laboratory also holds in applied settings (e.g., the effects of deprivation induced shifts in dose-effect functions). In yet other cases a researcher may want to know the cost-benefit ratio between the amount of an intervention and how much educational progress results. Each of these is a valid experimental question that makes use of parametric variations in the independent variable.

COMPONENT QUESTIONS

Researchers also find it useful to "pull apart" independent variables. This approach is referred to as *component analysis*. The reason this type of question is asked is typically to discover *what* makes an independent variable work and/or *why* it works. When trying to identify what aspect of an intervention is necessary, researchers often remove one, or more, components of the independent variable. This is particularly important in educational research because most interventions have multiple components. By removing a select number of elements researchers can determine how that particular component(s) affects behavior.

Component analyses can be used to conduct efficiency experiments in the sense that they can identify the necessary components of an intervention. An example of a component analysis is provided in Figure 5.4. Medland and Stachnik (1972) studied an intervention

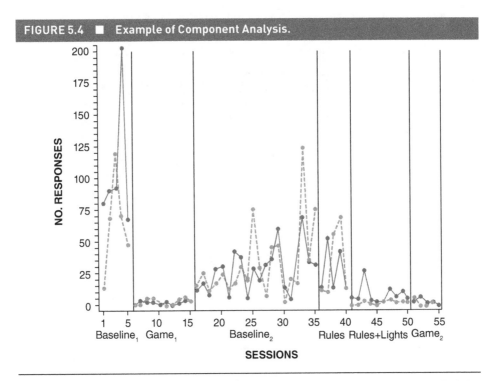

FIGURE 5.4 ■ Example of Component Analysis.

Note. The experimenter measured the number of problem behaviors occurring during a class period. Each data symbol represents a different class "team." The component analysis occurred between Sessions 36 and 55. The treatment package (Games 1 and 2) consisted of "rules," "lights," and access to a reward. (Figure 1, p. 49, from: Medland, M. B., & Stachnik, T. J. (1972). Good-behavior game: A replication and systematic analysis. *Journal of Applied Behavior Analysis, 5,* 45–51. Copyright 1972 by the Society for the Experimental Analysis of Behavior. Reproduced by permission.)

called the good-behavior game (Barrish et al., 1969). This game was developed in the 1960s but is still used today because it is effective. In the Medland and Stachnik experiment the independent variable was comprised of (a) rule statements, (b) a light box that signaled when the class was being "good" or "bad," and (c) a group contingency that provided differential reinforcement for meeting goals. The experiment was conducted in a fifth-grade general education classroom that had 28 students. As shown in Figure 5.4, a baseline was established with problem behaviors frequently occurring (e.g., talking out in class or not being in your assigned seat). The good-behavior game was then introduced, with problem behaviors virtually eliminated. On Session 36, one component of the intervention was introduced alone (i.e., rule statements), with little effect on classroom behavior. However, when two components of the original intervention were used (i.e., rule statements plus performance feedback), problem behaviors occurred at near-zero levels and were the same as when the entire treatment package was used. These findings suggested that only two of the three intervention components were necessary for the independent variable to be effective. Although this analysis does not show why the intervention was effective in terms of specific behavioral processes influencing behavior, it does show which components are necessary for the intervention to be useful.

An example of a component analysis that did identify why an intervention was effective is provided in Figure 5.5. In this experiment, Wacker and colleagues (1990) initially conducted an assessment that identified a child's problem behavior as occurring as a function

---

FIGURE 5.5   ■   Example of Component Analysis that Identified why Intervention was Effective.

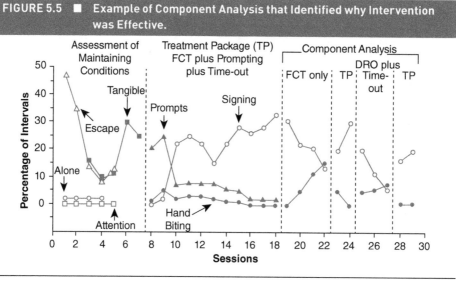

Note. The figure indicates the percentage of intervals in which various responses occurred. The responses included hand biting, signing, and prompting by an adult. The component analysis occurred between Sessions 19 and 29. The treatment package (TP) included functional communication training (FCT) and differential reinforcement of other behavior (DRO) plus time out. (Figure 1, p. 424, from: Wacker, D. P., Steege, M. W., Northup, J., Sasso, G., Berg, W., Reimers, T., Cooper, L., Cigrand, K., & Donn, L. (1990). A component analysis of functional communication training across three topographies of severe behavior problems. *Journal of Applied Behavior Analysis, 23,* 417–430. Copyright 1990 by the Society for the Experimental Analysis of Behavior. Reproduced by permission.)

of positive reinforcement in the form of access to a tangible object (i.e., a favored toy). Following this assessment, a treatment was developed called functional communication training (FCT) that prompted and reinforced the child to sign for the toy and placed hand biting on a schedule of negative punishment (i.e., removal of access to the toy). The results show that by Session 18, the child was independently signing to gain access to the toy and not biting his hand. During Sessions 19 through 29 a component analysis was conducted. The first component removed was the differential reinforcement and negative punishment contingencies, resulting in the child once again resorting to hand biting. This effect was reversed when the reinforcement and punishment components were reinstated. Then, when the prompting and signing components were removed, similar increases in problem behavior were observed. This analysis showed that each component of the intervention was necessary for it to have a beneficial effect on communication and problem behavior. Removing any one of these components rendered the intervention ineffective, suggesting that each of the behavioral processes that comprised the intervention were necessary. That is, the reason the FCT intervention worked was because it placed problem behavior on extinction and differentially reinforced the occurrence of signing.

The general process is the same whether a research team uses component analyses to identify (a) necessary versus superfluous components of an intervention or (b) the behavioral processes that make an intervention effective. The independent variable needs to be operationalized and the individual elements identified. Then the researchers need to decide on an experimental plan for which component(s) will be removed and when (see Part IV: Design Tactics). This decision can be complex because some elements of an independent variable are dependent on the presence of other elements. In cases such as this, the removal of one component may necessitate the removal of another component. Such situations will necessarily constrain what can ultimately be said about the intervention, but at the same time they clearly identify for the researchers and future readers what interdependencies exist within the intervention package. This is important because as with parametric analyses, component analyses typically follow demonstrative and comparative analyses. In the latter type of experiments, the focus is more on being effective than on systematically analyzing each aspect of an intervention.

CONCLUSION

When conducting research, a range of experimental questions can be posed. In this chapter we have reviewed four general types of experimental questions: demonstration, comparative, parametric, and component. Explicitly stating experimental questions assists an investigator to improve what they are proposing to study. Such a process typically results in refinements in the initial experimental question and an increased likelihood of experimental success. In addition, different types of experimental questions can be combined to pursue even more complex experimental analyses. The posing of experimental questions is an often overlooked aspect of the experimental process, but one that is integral to the activity.

1. Can you describe each of the four types of experimental questions that are studied using single-case designs?

2. Thinking of your own teaching or clinical experiences, can you formulate a hypothesis to answer a "demonstration" question?

3. How would you change the answer to the previous question so that you are posing a "comparative" experimental question?

4. From your knowledge of the research literature, how common is it for investigators to ask "parametric" research questions?

5. Thinking of an evidence-based practice you have recently used, how would you conduct a "component" analysis to test which variables are key to the success of the method?

6 EVIDENCE-BASED PRACTICES

LEARNING OBJECTIVES

After reading this chapter, you will be able to

6.1 Apply evidence-based practices in research.

6.2 Compare the roles by which single-case designs determine the effectiveness of an intervention.

6.3 Explain the best available current standards for establishing the quality of an experimental design.

6.4 Articulate the significance of thresholds for cumulative evidence in evidence-based practice as defined by independent professional organizations.

As research findings demonstrating whether interventions are effective or ineffective have accumulated in recent decades, the opportunity to assess which treatments can be considered recommended interventions has emerged. Researchers, practitioners, and policymakers realized that educational research had matured to the point that recommendations regarding what were, and were not, effective interventions could be based on extant data, rather than less objective bases. This opportunity has come to be referred to as *evidence-based practices* (EBPs).

EBPs emerged as an emphasis in clinical medicine in the early 1990s (Guyatt et al. 1992; Woolf, 1992). As Sackett et al. (1996) noted, EBP was "about integrating individual clinical expertise and the best external evidence" (p. 71). The overall goal was to integrate existing scientific evidence regarding the efficacy of treatments with clinicians' knowledge and experience regarding how certain patient populations and characteristics would intersect with specific interventions. EBP in clinical medicine quickly become a growing area of inquiry focused on guiding improved intervention practices and outcomes (Greenhalgh et al., 2014).

Applied psychology quickly adopted EBPs within the context of mental and public health. In 2005, the American Psychological Association (APA) created the Presidential Task Force on Evidence-Based Practice. The task force report (2006) noted parallels with previous efforts in clinical medicine and provided a rationale and expanded criteria that could integrate EBP efforts into psychological interventions. As with clinical medicine, EBP efforts for psychological interventions have emphasized a careful analysis of the existing research literature, areas where interactions occur between treatment types, and individual characteristics with the goal of guiding informed clinical intervention (Gambrill, 2005).

Parallel with these efforts in psychology, educational researchers and policymakers began emphasizing EBPs in school, community, and clinical contexts. Policymakers specified that "scientifically proven practices" be the basis for selecting interventions when the national legislation for elementary and secondary education was reauthorized in the early 2000s (No Child Left Behind Act, 2001). Contemporaneously, the National Research Council issued a report on scientific research in education (Shavelson & Towne, 2002) that noted a range of acceptable methodologies and that different research questions required different methodological approaches—similar to the recommendations of the APA task force in 2006. At the same time, with the founding of the Institute of Education Sciences in the U.S. Department of Education, there was a clear emphasis on scientific rigor and outcomes in federally funded education research (Whitehurst, 2003).

All of these efforts have transpired to create a contemporary context in which educational interventions must meet various requirements to be considered EBPs. What specifically those criteria are and how various methodologies contribute to the designation of an intervention as an EBP are still evolving (Bauer & Kirchner, 2020; Byiers et al., 2012; Toste et al., 2023). However, what is clear is that for researchers and practitioners the focus on what to recommend and use as educational interventions is firmly established within the framework of EBPs.

DEFINING EVIDENCE-BASED PRACTICE

While there is a high degree of concordance that EBPs are essential for defining best practices in educational research, *defining what qualifies as an EBP is more challenging.* In many respects, when defining EBPs, you know it when you see it. The intervention has been shown through repeated research studies to be effective and produced outcomes for various student populations that can be defined and measured. The accumulation of research evidence for an intervention and its range of effective applications *becomes compelling at a certain level of evidence.* However, what that level is remains to be definitively operationalized in educational research (Cook & Odom, 2013; Odom et al., 2005).

Perhaps the best working definition to adopt is that offered by Dunst and colleagues (2002) who defined EBPs as "informed by research, in which the characteristics and consequences of environmental variables are empirically established and the relationship directly informs what a practitioner can do to produce a desired outcome" (p. 3). Defining what "informed research" is has produced three parallel efforts relating to EBPs. One area of development has been to focus on *which types of experimental designs qualify as contributing to evidence for intervention effectiveness* (APA Presidential Task Force on Evidence-Based Practice, 2006; Odom et al., 2005).

Table 6.1 shows a broad constellation of research methodologies that are viewed as contributing to research evidence in the social sciences. The methods range from systematic clinical observations to randomized controlled trials (RCTs). If the reader notices a hierarchical characteristic to the list, you would be correct. Two key variables interact in establishing the degree to which research methods contribute findings to establish an intervention as effective—*internal*

TABLE 6.1 ■ Types of Research Evidence	
Experimental Design	**Rigor/Generality**
Systematic Clinical Observation	(weaker internal/external validity)
Qualitative Research	
Systematic Case Studies	
Single-Case Research Designs	
Epidemiological Studies	
Process-Outcome Studies	
Clinical Intervention Studies	
Randomized Controlled Trials	(stronger internal/external validity)
Meta-Analyses	

Note. Based on the APA Presidential Task Force on Evidence-Based Practice (2006, p. 274).

and external validity (see Chapter 3). The table lists, in a qualitative sense, how at least one set of scholars (APA Presidential Task Force on Evidence-Based Practice, 2006) viewed the cumulative gravitas of each research method in terms of its rigor in experimental control and population generality. Overall, systematic clinical observations are viewed as weaker in internal and external validity but useful in generating observations that can lead to testable hypotheses, and RCTs are viewed as the highest in combined internal and external validity characteristics.

Because this is a book on $N = 1$ methodology, we will focus on the role that single-case designs can serve in EBPs. As noted previously in Chapter 3, single-case research designs are generally the strongest type of experimental design when it comes to establishing internal validity. The precise definition of independent and dependent variables and the emphasis on direct replication makes $N = 1$ designs the raison d'être of methods for establishing rigorous experimental control. However, as noted in Chapter 4, that strong focus on internal validity limits the external validity of findings from single-case designs. While focusing on the establishment of experimental control with a single participant, the design approach eschews much of what is needed to establish representativeness in a larger participant population (see also Byiers et al., 2012; Johnston et al., 2020; Riley-Tillman et al., 2020).

CONTRIBUTIONS OF SINGLE-CASE DESIGNS

Given the characteristics of single-case designs just noted, and the caveat that no single research method defines an EBP, what roles can $N = 1$ designs serve in developing the evidence that an intervention is effective? One role is to take advantage of the experimental rigor inherent in single-case designs to demonstrate that an intervention is effective in the individual case and the degree to which that effect can be quantified (e.g., through effect-size estimates; see

Chapter 17). Ruling out potential threats to internal validity (e.g., history or instrumentation effects) plays to the strength of $N = 1$ designs. This aspect can contribute to the early development of data supporting an approach as effective. A second role can be to inductively test the boundaries of how different participant populations are impacted by the intervention and test the boundaries of its effectiveness (e.g., people living in city versus rural locations). Both of these contributions presage larger-scale efficacy studies that are the hallmark of RCTs. A third role is to identify why participants in large-scale investigations do not respond to the intervention in a way that is characteristic of the larger sample. When some people do not respond to what has been shown to be an effective intervention, it is likely that investigators are identifying interactions between "individual differences" and some dimension of the independent variable (see Box 6.1). By using single-case designs to identify a "mechanism" that causes the intervention to be less effective with some individuals and/or contexts, $N = 1$ designs can contribute to the refinement of interventions in specific situations and enable them to be more effective in a larger set of cases.

BOX 6.1: INDIVIDUAL DIFFERENCES AND RESPONSE TO INTERVENTION

In the development of any EBP there are participants who respond positively to the intervention and those who respond partially or not at all. Sometimes the initial reaction of investigators has been to treat varied outcomes as outliers and focus on the positive results. However, it is becoming increasingly clear that participants who do not respond optimally to an emerging intervention can be viewed as "guides" for how to refine the instructional approach and ultimately increase the treatment's external validity. For example, most students who are struggling to read respond to more intensive reading interventions (Fuchs & Fuchs, 2007; Griffiths & Stuart, 2013). However, some participants do not successfully respond. Why this latter group of students are not successful provides the opportunity to study what mechanism(s) might be responsible for the nonoptimal effects—an ideal opportunity to use single-case designs to test hypotheses. In regard to reading, reasons might include a lack of instructional fidelity in a school with limited resources or the mismatch between reading content and students' out-of-school experiences. Discovering information like this helps identify why some students do not respond to intervention and often provides a clear cause that needs to be remedied by refining the intervention to better fit specific learning contexts.

RESEARCH DESIGN QUALITY INDICATORS

A second area of development in establishing EBPs is the specification of *research design quality indicators* (e.g., Lloyd & Therrien, 2023). The concept of quality indicators for experimental designs is one that has high face validity (i.e., it seems an intuitive idea). Such an effort seems very reasonable: Simply outline the core components of a rigorous experimental design and assess the degree to which a particular experiment has met the quality indicators. For single-case designs, several efforts have been made to specify criteria to differentiate a study with "high rigor" in its methodology from studies with "less rigor" and to set a clear threshold of acceptability. For example, the What Works Clearinghouse (WWC) *procedures and standards handbooks* (Version 4.1, 2020a, 2020b) identified a set of characteristics of what constitutes a rigorous single-case design (see also Horner et al., 2005; Kratochwill et al., 2013). Some examples of the WWC (2020a, 2020b) standards include an objective set of behavioral definitions and a measurement system that meets accepted standards for interobserver agreement. Other examples of the WWC standards include the requirement that three specific replications occur within an $N = 1$ design to establish internal validity and three or more data points must be collected in each phase of the experiment (see Chapter 3).

These types of a priori design requirements may make sense for experimental and quasi-experimental group designs that are based on procedures established before an experiment starts (e.g., RCTs; Gersten et al., 2005), but the history of single-case designs has been one of design flexibility without preset standards for design practices (e.g., Johnston et al., 2020; Sidman, 1960). Remember the quote at the beginning of this book about single-case designs: "There are no rules of experimental design" (Sidman, 1960, p. 214). This ethos has guided generations of researchers using $N = 1$ experimental design through discovery after discovery (see Chapters 10 through 15 for examples using various design types). In many instances the initial discoveries may have used a new single-case design created for the requirements of the particular experiment. This ethos of design plasticity has met the pragmatic criterion of successful utility having been shown to be effective across many thousands of experiments.

Therefore, it is not surprising that a priori standards for single-case designs have been received with a wide range of reactions from general acceptance (e.g., Ledford et al., 2023) to substantive concerns (e.g., Maggin et al., 2022; Wolery, 2012). A case for accepting such standards is that individuals without expertise in $N = 1$ designs can apply objective quality criteria to assess experimental rigor and that such standards provide uniformity in design expectations. Such a view is highly consistent with the intent and purpose of EBPs. In contrast, researchers voicing concerns about existing standards note the arbitrariness of many design requirements (e.g., the number of replications and number of data points) that conflict with well-established design practices and replicable experimental outcomes.

Researchers who frequently use single-case designs have put the proposition that a priori standards inappropriately constrain experimental designs to an empirical test. One approach, used by Moeller et al. (2015), was to compare published $N = 1$ design studies that have been successfully vetted through peer-reviewed journals and assess them using standards and procedures such as the WWC (2020a, 2020b) criteria. Moeller et al. found that only 33% of published single-case design experiments met the WWC a priori design standards. Similar efforts have been offered by other researchers questioning the viability of a priori design requirements (e.g., Natesan Batley et al., 2023; Tankersley et al., 2008; Tincani & Travers, 2017). The general conclusion from such critiques has been that many published experiments are judged by experts as having successfully demonstrated experimental control, but do not meet preset standards such as the WWC. *This raises the question of whether the experiments do not have acceptable internal validity or whether they may be too restrictive or not relevant.*

Whichever view the reader adopts on the topic of preset experimental design standards for single-case designs, it is safe to conclude that no definitive answer to what constitutes acceptable $N = 1$ design criteria has been established. This observation may change given future events and findings, but for now a priori design standards for these types of designs remain in question. Thus, the second element in the development of EBPs—clear and objective design standards— is not clearly established at this juncture in time for single-case designs. *Perhaps the best available current standard is whether an experiment is successfully vetted by experts prior to publication (i.e., peer review) and the degree to which published single-case designs are replicated by the same investigators and by other researchers.*

THRESHOLDS FOR CUMULATIVE EVIDENCE

The final area of development for identifying EBPs has focused on the *threshold of cumulative evidence* for identifying when an intervention qualifies as an EBP or, conversely, when a practice should be designated as *not* being an effective intervention. Across disciplines like medicine, psychology, and special education, the primary vehicle for identifying whether a particular intervention meets EBP standards is through *professional associations* and *research synthesis organizations* (Cook & Odom, 2013; Lonigan et al., 1998; Smith et al., 2002). Professional associations, such as the APA and Division for Early Childhood of the Council for Exceptional Children, have formed structures within the organizations to vet evidence that may make an intervention an EBP. A second approach has been to establish independent organizations whose goal is to review and evaluate research evidence that may, or may not, support a particular intervention as an EBP. For example, organizations such as the National Clearinghouse on Autism Evidence and Practice (NCAEP), the Oxford Centre for Evidence-Based Medicine (OCEBM), and the U.S. Department of Education's WWC provide explicit standards for classifying EBPs.

The evidence typically used in evaluating interventions as EBPs includes criteria for *internal validity, external validity*, and *systematic replication* (see Chapters 3 and 4). An example of a dichotomous approach to EBP designation (i.e., it is an EBP, or it is not) is used by the NCAEP (Steinbrenner et al., 2020), which looks at particular types of evidence (e.g., the type of experimental methodology and number of replication studies) and uses expert review committees to evaluate existing evidence. Such an approach allows the designation of an intervention as an EBP. Although many approaches specify a dichotomous approach to EBP designation, the general trend over the last two decades has been to *view EBP status along a continuum of evidence*. One reason for using a continuum of evidence is that just because an intervention has not met an organization's threshold for being an EBP does not mean the treatment is ineffective—it only means that it has not yet accumulated enough research evidence to qualify as an EBP. Conversely, in some instances there is a conspicuous lack of evidence that an intervention could be an EBP and, in some cases, there may be multiple studies showing a null or negative outcome for the intervention. A frequently cited example of a continuum is the OCEBM (Howick et al., 2009) use of a five-level classification system in which Level 1 interventions have the highest level of evidence (i.e., meta-analyses with multiple RCTs) and Level 5 interventions have very limited evidence of effectiveness (i.e., expert opinion without additional evidence). Whatever approach is used, these efforts rely on independent organizations not affiliated with specific interventions using objective and verifiable criteria to classify treatments in relation to the existing research evidence. Such a process and set of outcomes is at the core of EBP designation.

An Example of EBP Status: Time Delay

Time delay is "a practice used to systematically fade the use of prompts during instructional activities by using a brief delay between the initial instruction and any additional instructions or prompts" (Hume et al., 2021, p. 4025). Time delay was first demonstrated in the experimental analysis of behavior in an effort to measure the moment in time when stimulus control transferred from a previously effective stimulus to a novel stimulus. Touchette (1971) demonstrated that individuals with intellectual disabilities could be taught to respond to novel stimuli by delaying a prompt "linking" the new and established stimuli (see Terrace [1963a, 1963b] for a model system precursor).

The Touchette experiments were then extended to applied behavior analysis by Halle et al. (1979) to facilitate language use by adults with intellectual disabilities during a mealtime routine (see also Halle et al., 1981 for a systematic replication). Following these initial experiments, time delay has been systematically manualized, replicated, and extended to many instructional contexts for students with and without disabilities (see Wolery et al., 1992). In fact, the laboratory development and subsequent extension to clinical situations of time-delay procedures stands as a hallmark of translational research in applied psychology (see Chapter 2).

The current status of time delay is that multiple organizations have conducted literature reviews relating to its empirical status and determined it to be an EBP. For example, the NCAEP published a report assessing frequently used behavioral interventions for people with autism spectrum disorder (ASD) (Steinbrenner et al., 2020). In their review of time delay, the report identified 15 research studies conducted between 2012 and 2017 that met criteria for empirically supporting the effectiveness of time delay and 31 experiments from 1990 to 2017 demonstrating positive outcomes (see also Hume et al., 2021). The NCAEP conclusion was that time delay met the criteria for designation as an EBP.

The designation of time delay as an EBP is a straightforward example of an instructional intervention that has been demonstrated to be effective. Across five decades of applied research, based on basic research identifying the mechanism of action, the effects of time delay have been replicated across hundreds of experiments, conducted by a broad range of investigators globally, and with many different participant populations. This brief review of the time-delay literature provides an exemplar of an EBP. However, for some interventions the status of their effectiveness is less clear, and the empirical evidence may lead researchers to question whether the practice has any utility as an intervention. The following example illustrates this complex process of accumulating evidence to demonstrate that an intervention has not been demonstrated to be effective (i.e., attempting to prove a negative).

An Example of EBP Status: Weighted Vests

In 1972 Ayers published a theoretical outline for what was termed sensory integration (SI) that focused on how children process sensory information and how disruptions in SI can lead to changes in behaviors from increased stereotypy to reading deficits such as dyslexia. The term *SI* has changed over time to also include reference to sensory processing (SP) and is often referred to as SI/SP therapy and uses multiple sensory modalities (e.g., olfactory, vestibular, and touch senses) to treat a wide variety of behaviors that include social, communication, and daily living difficulties (Miller et al., 2007). As an example of its widespread use, Green et al. (2006) noted that 38% of children with ASD were currently receiving SI/SP therapy and that another 33% had previously received the therapy.

One treatment that emerged early in the development of SI/SP therapy was a technique using *weighted vests*. The use of weighted vests was based on the theoretical perspective that some children were over- or understimulated by their environments and use of the vests (typically 5%–10% of the child's body weight) provided sensory input that alleviated the sensory dysfunction within the central nervous system (Deris et al., 2006; Olson & Moulton, 2004). As estimated by Green et al. (2006), 15% of children with ASD were actively receiving weighted vest interventions, and 26% had previously received the intervention (see also Case-Smith et al., 2015).

However, despite the very broad adoption of weighted vests as an intervention, for decades researchers have noted the lack of empirical evidence supporting the use of this intervention (e.g., Camarata et al., 2020; Taylor et al., 2017). *Of particular interest in the weighted vest literature is the presence of several experimental studies conducted by a variety of investigators using a range of methodologies that have produced mixed results.* For example, a research review by Bodison and Parham (2018) critiqued eight research reports on weighted vest outcomes published between 2007 and 2015. The experiments documented largely negative outcomes relating to possible weighted vest effects and, interestingly, noted that the studies that did report positive results contained clear methodological flaws (e.g., nonrandomized assignment in a RCT or lack of interobserver agreement in observational measures). Bodison and Parham concluded "insufficient evidence is available at the present time regarding whether weighted vests are helpful for children with ASD" (p. 190040p6). A similar set of outcomes were reported for seven studies by Stephenson and Carter (2009)—published a decade before the papers reviewed by Bodison and Parham—who found a similar pattern of mixed results with positive outcomes associated with flaws in the researchers' methodologies. Similarly, the authors concluded "weighted vests cannot be recommended for clinical application at this point" (p. 105).

The cumulative evidence in regard to weighted vests as an intervention has been demonstrated through experiments and independent reviews to *not meet the requirements of an EBP*. Most findings have indicated no effect for the intervention, but the findings noting positive outcomes have contained methodological limitations. Although researchers cannot recommend the use of weighted vests, the process that has been undertaken is a good illustration of how the EBP literature can over time accumulate evidence that a particular intervention should not be used by practitioners because of a lack of research support.

CONCLUSION

The past four decades have seen a surge of interest in EBPs. Researchers, practitioners, and policymakers from medicine, psychology, and education have worked in their respective disciplines to develop standards with which to vet interventions regarding their effectiveness. In educational research, often following the efforts in other disciplines, a consensus continues to develop regarding what methods should be used to assess the effectiveness of various practices. Three key areas in this effort include (a) designating certain *design methods* as acceptable and delineating the type of evidence they provide, (b) defining *quality criteria* for specific experimental approaches, and (c) *strategies for assessing evidence* to designate interventions as EBPs.

In terms of research methodology, significant advances have been made in establishing a broad range of acceptable methods, but work continues on how each research methodology contributes evidence regarding internal and external validity (see Box 6.2). In education, there has not yet been an integration of research methods and how they cumulatively contribute to the designation of an EBP. Instead, the methods have been treated as distinct and independent (e.g., Lloyd & Therrien, 2023; WWC, 2020a, 2020b). For single-case designs this evolution has been a significant step forward in recognizing the strengths of this design type (APA Presidential Task Force on Evidence-Based Practice, 2006; Shavelson & Towne, 2002).

BOX 6.2: DIFFERENT EXPERIMENTAL METHODS, DIFFERENT EXPERIMENTAL EVIDENCE

An often stated dictum is "for the experimental design to fit the experimental question and not vice versa" (see Chapter 5). This truism fits very well with the emerging notions of EBPs and the range of research methods that can contribute meaningful information for identifying effective educational practices (e.g., Shavelson & Towne, 2002). However, in reviewing Table 6.1 the reader undoubtedly noted the wide variety of design types from systematic clinical observations to meta-analyses. How does someone make sense of all these various methods? The best approach is likely to use the method that will provide you, as the researcher, with the information you need at that point in the development of an intervention. For example, in refining an intervention, investigators might want to understand why some students do not respond to the current iteration of a treatment. They could choose an inductive research method such as qualitative or $N = 1$ methodologies to explore possible hypotheses. In the use of qualitative methods, the researchers may be developing and exploring hypotheses regarding response to intervention. For the use of single-case designs, researchers may directly test those hypotheses with a focus on internal validity and experimental control. These studies could then be followed up with an RCT focusing on the newly identified mechanism and refined intervention to more clearly establish the external validity of the intervention. In efforts like this, there is not a correct or incorrect research method. Rather, as interventions are developed there are different types of experimental needs that become apparent, and investigators should use the research method that meets the need of the question at that moment. Over time, a body of findings emerge regarding intervention effectiveness that can lead researchers, practitioners, and policymakers to designate such cumulative findings as meeting the threshold of an EBP.

The second area of standards has been successful in establishing quality criteria for research designs, particularly in the area of group-comparison methods. However, for $N = 1$ designs there is still a broad range of perspectives on what constitutes quality criteria and the role of a priori assumptions in an experimental design approach that was developed from inductive experimental methods (see Chapter 2). Perhaps continued efforts to reconcile single-case design assumptions and explicit quality standards will emerge in the future.

Finally, great strides have been made in establishing systems to review interventions and weigh evidence regarding specific interventions being designed as EBPs. Professional associations and research synthesis organizations to assess specific interventions in the context of EBP status have emerged and are being actively pursued. One question that will remain for the foreseeable future is whether to use a continuum to designate EBP status or a binomial designation system. In medicine and psychology, the emphasis has shifted toward using a continuum to note EBP status, while in education the focus has been on a dichotomous designation approach. Again, time will tell which approach best fits the needs of educational research.

Overall, educational research has made significant progress in establishing a foundation for EBPs. The gains include designating some interventions as clearly effective, some interventions as practices with emerging evidence, and some interventions as lacking evidence despite repeated experimental efforts to establish their effectiveness. While it has been noted that progress on EBP designation is still needed, one might look at the efforts thus far in educational research as a successful *first-generation effort* that will continue to be improved over time. Education has benefited substantially from developing a system for establishing EBPs, and single-case design methods have an important role to serve in this process.

REFLECTION QUESTIONS

1. What field(s) began the process of developing the concepts we now call "evidence-based practices"?

2. When you consider the various elements that go into creating an evidence-based practice, are there any elements you consider particularly important? Why?

3. Since there are a range of research methods that can contribute important information to the establishment of evidence-based practices, how does an investigator go about selecting an experimental approach?

4. Can you make an argument in favor of and against using a priori criteria in evaluating the adequacy of single-case research design?

5. In evaluating whether a particular intervention qualifies as an evidence-based practice, why might experts want to set a fixed threshold versus a continuum of evidence when considering an intervention as evidence based?

MEASUREMENT

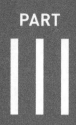

7 QUANTIFYING BEHAVIOR

LEARNING OBJECTIVES

After reading this chapter, you will be able to

7.1   Describe the benefits of precise measurement of behaviors in single-case research design.

7.2   Compare and contrast the dimensional quantities of individual behaviors and how these dimensions are quantified.

7.3   Articulate the "rules of thumb" when selecting dimensional quantities for a research study.

Quantifying behavior is a fundamental aspect of the single-case research process. However, before we discuss the quantification of behavioral events, we need to examine what behavior is. This may seem like an obvious question, but there is actually a great deal of confusion in the behavioral sciences about what constitutes behavior. Mistakenly, many people believe that behavior is only comprised of the motoric acts a person engages in. Examples might include running across a playground, picking up a pencil, foot tapping, arm wrestling, or opening your laptop while sitting down in a chair. These are behaviors, but they are only a subsample of what constitutes behavior.

As noted in Chapter 2, John B. Watson (1924) developed what has become known as *classical behaviorism* (Todd & Morris, 1994). In that approach to behavior analysis, Watson focused on overt behaviors that people engaged in, as opposed to subjective inferences about what a person was thinking or feeling. This analytical strategy was an attempt to make the fledgling field of experimental psychology more objective by focusing on events that people could directly measure. Unfortunately, it had the unintended consequence of directing researchers' attention away from other interesting behaviors, like solving mathematics problems, learning complex concepts, expressing emotions, and developing language. Hence, this approach came to be called black box psychology.

By the time that B. F. Skinner had become an active researcher, it was becoming clear that confining behavior analysis to only overt motoric behaviors was too limiting (see Todd & Morris, 1995). Therefore, Skinner (1945, 1950) proposed what he referred to as *radical behaviorism*. In this new conceptualization, Skinner proposed that anything a person did should be an allowable datum for experimental analysis. That is, behavior was anything that a person did, whether it occurred overtly or covertly. This rethinking of behavior analysis included thoughts, problem solving, talking, emotions, bodily sensations, and brain activity. Indeed, Skinner (1985) foresaw the integration of behavior analysis and neuroscience as mutually compatible, scientific approaches to understanding human and animal psychology. The only caveat Skinner proposed for radical behaviorism was that the event being analyzed had to be directly measurable and amenable to being operationalized.

Following the logic of radical behaviorism, in this book we will define behavior as "anything an organism does" (Catania, 2013, p. 380). However, in order for a behavior to be able to be counted—which is the whole point of measurement—it has to be amenable to certain conventions. First, the behavior has to be defined so that it can be physically characterized. That is, an operational definition of the behavior needs to specify its key physical qualities. Second, the behavior needs to be rendered as a physically measurable event. In some way, the behavioral event needs to be measured by observational, electromagnetic, or biochemical methods. Finally, the measure of the behavioral event needs to be physically recorded in some manner. Such events could include marks on a piece of paper, storage in a cloud server, an auditory recording, or written transcription, to name only a few types of media. If these characteristics of behavior can be met, then anything that a person does can be considered behavior and subjected to an experimental analysis (see Box 7.1).

BOX 7.1: WHY COGNITIONS AND MENTALISMS DO NOT COUNT IN SINGLE-CASE DESIGNS

Behavior analysts avoid cognitive and mentalistic references, not because they want to avoid what goes on inside a person, but because such references do not have physical existence and, hence, are of little use in understanding what goes on inside someone's head, for example. Or, to put it another way, *cognitions and mentalisms are only metaphors*, not events. A metaphor, according to Merriam-Webster (2024), is "a figure of speech in which a word or phrase literally denoting one kind of object or idea is used in place of another to suggest a likeness or analogy between them (as in *drowning in money*); *broadly*: figurative language." In general, cognitions and mentalisms are metaphors for events that occur in a person's nervous system or other tissues but do not need to be physically demonstrated to exist. For example, a child does not remember their multiplication tables because they have a faulty short-term memory or are unmotivated because they have poor self-esteem. The figurative language of cognitive and mentalistic explanations is intuitive and satisfactory at a superficial level. However, explaining human behavior by references to things that do not exist as physical events is a risky approach to arriving at an understanding of why people do what they do (see Chapter 2). Because of this, behavior analysts have opted for the more conservative approach of focusing on material events that can be directly measured. Continuing developments in functional neuroimaging, often used in cognitive neuroscience, are rendering brain activity as physical entities that meet the requirements of directly measurable events. The neuroimaging of events can include electrical potentials from changes in cellular firing rates, visualization of changes in blood flow resulting from cellular activity in certain brain nuclei, and radiological imaging of the activation of certain neurotransmitter receptors in various brain regions. Only time will tell whether physical events or metaphors have more explanatory power when trying to explain human behavior.

BENEFITS OF COUNTING BEHAVIOR

Assigning numbers to behavior has several benefits. Often referred to as *direct measures* of behavior, the quantifying properties of responding for analysis are a benchmark characteristic of behavior analysis. There are multiple reasons that researchers using single-case designs insist on counting the behavior of people they are studying. One reason is the fallibility of human memory. It has been demonstrated across multiple disciplines that what people observe, and later report, often differs dramatically from what actually occurs. For example, eyewitness accounts of events at a crime scene often differ substantially from one another, even though all individuals observed essentially the same events. Compounding this problem, the recall of events continues to become more variable over time (Ross et al., 2003).

If researchers had to rely on the memory of participants and/or observers, systematic progress would be extremely difficult because of the variability such an approach would introduce into the data. By directly measuring the behaviors of interest in a research study, investigators have a permanent product of what occurred that was produced as the events unfolded. This provides an accurate recording of behavior and related events that does not change over time. It also has the additional benefit of being available for reanalysis.

A second reason to directly measure behavior is that it provides an unambiguous way of communicating your experimental results to others. Because the behaviors were recorded as they occurred and are stored in a medium that does not change over time, the information can be shared with others. This information sharing may come in the form of a graph, a table, an appendix, or some other medium, such as a website, that allows access to the original data. This approach allows multiple individuals to look at the same data and arrive at their own conclusions about what happened to behavior during the experiment.

This very process also increases the accuracy of reporting what occurred in a study. Because the data are directly measured and publicly reported, other individuals are allowed to scrutinize the research activities and the resulting data. This also introduces a level of transparency into the research process that forces researchers to not overinterpret their findings. In general, this means that a researcher will offer a relatively conservative interpretation of their findings, given that more adventuresome interpretations may be critically questioned by others.

Without a doubt the most exciting reason for directly measuring behavior is the opportunity it provides for exploring patterns of events. Although educational researchers sometimes study the effects of an independent variable in relation to a single dependent variable, often a more complex set of dependent measures is used. Given the richness and complexity of human behavior, this should not be surprising. By having permanent records of the actual activity that occurred during a study, researchers can study which behaviors regularly occurred before or after other behaviors in an attempt to better understand interdependencies among variables.

An early pioneer in behavior analysis, William N. Schoenfeld, once referred to the complexity of human behavior and its interrelatedness with the environment, including other people's behaviors, as "the stream of behavior" (Schoenfeld, 1995). As a person behaves, there is a continual sequence of antecedent and consequent events surrounding their behavior. Some of those events enter into functional relations with their behavior, resulting in some behaviors becoming more likely and others less likely. Discovering the nature of those events and their effects on behavior is the primary goal of behavior analysis.

An example of this stream of behavior is provided in Figure 7.1 (from Baer, 1986). This graphic shows the behavior of two people: a child and an adult. Each capital letter (e.g., *A* or *L*) is an individual *topography* of aggressive behavior (e.g., hitting others or screaming). Each

FIGURE 7.1   ■   Graphing Streams of Behavior: Child and Adult.

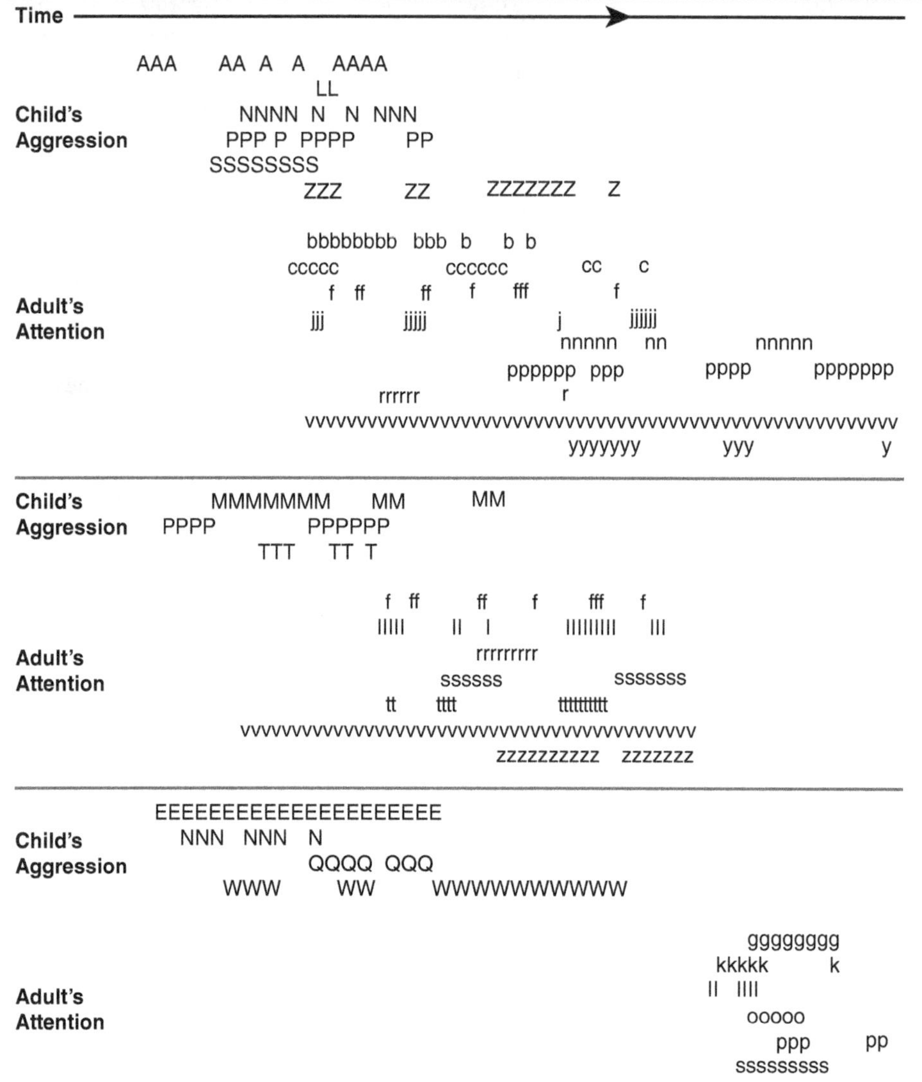

Note. The figure displays three graphic examples of the kinds of contingencies that can operate between the clusters of topography, subsets, sequences, interresponse times, and concurrencies that make up both a child's "aggression" and an adult's "attention." Time flows steadily from left to right. Each topography of the child's "aggressive" class is represented by uppercase letters, and of the adult's "attention" class by lowercase letters. Each topography's duration is indicated by the unspaced repetition of its symbol letter (e.g., AAAA represents twice as long a duration as AA). Spaces between symbol letters indicate interresponse times. (Figure 1, p. 125, from: Baer, D. M. (1986). In application, frequency is not the only estimate of the probability of behavioral units. In T. Thompson & M. D. Zeiler (Eds.), *Analysis and integration of behavioral units* (pp. 117–136). Lawrence Erlbaum Associates. Copyright 1986 by Lawrence Erlbaum Associates. Reproduced by permission of Routledge, an imprint of Taylor & Francis Ltd. https://doi.org/10.4324/9781315620060)

lowercase letter (e.g., *b* or *c*) is a single topography of adult attention (e.g., saying "stop" or turning away from the child). Some of the child's behaviors co-occur among themselves (e.g., *N* and *P*), while other behaviors tend to occur less dependably with others (e.g., *E* and *Z*). Such patterns suggest some behaviors share certain functional properties, despite having different response topographies, suggesting the existence of *response classes* (see Box 7.2). Similar patterns exist among the behaviors emitted by the adult. In addition to patterns of individual behavior, there are sequential dependencies between the child and adult behaviors that might suggest functional relations between their behavior (e.g., *Z* and *b*, respectively). Whether there are response classes for each individual's behavior and functional relations between their responses is a matter for experimental analysis. However, directly measuring behavior enables this experimental process to occur.

BOX 7.2: RESPONSE CLASSES AND THE ORGANIZATION OF BEHAVIOR

Response classes are of particular interest in behavior analysis because they reveal properties of behavior that are not readily visible to the casual observer. Like most concepts in behavior analysis, the notion of a response class is defined by its functional properties. Response classes are individual topographies of behavior that are maintained by a similar set of reinforcers. The response topographies (i.e., the form of the response) can be nearly identical or completely different, or both. What links them together is that the behaviors have similar effects on the person's environment. For example, an adolescent may learn to correctly answer difficult questions in mathematics class or talk with a friend to gain the attention of another student they are romantically interested in. They might also directly pass notes in class to the student they have amorous intentions for. If all three of these response topographies occasioned the young person's favorable attention, then they might all be members of the same response class. And, just to make things more interesting, the concept of response class can also be extended to antecedents (e.g., discriminative stimuli) and consequences (e.g., negative reinforcers).

DIMENSIONAL QUANTITIES OF BEHAVIOR

Most people think of the occurrence of a response as a singular event. Every response, however, has multiple dimensions that can be quantified for measurement. Each of these dimensions represents a different aspect of how behavior occurs in space and time. Referred to as *dimensional quantities* (see Johnston et al., 2020), we will discuss five fundamental types. Dimensional quantities are important because they allow you to count different physical characteristics of a response. For example, in some instances you might be interested in how many times a behavior occurs in a period of time. In other instances, you might be interested in how much time is taken up by the occurrence of a response. In yet other situations, you might be interested in the time between behaviors. Identifying the dimensional quantities used to describe patterns of behavior is a first step in developing measurement systems when using single-case designs.

Figure 7.2 shows the hypothetical occurrence of a response as an event log. Along the horizontal aspect of the figure is time expressed in seconds. The vertical aspect of Figure 7.2 denotes the occurrence of individual responses. When a response occurs, the level of the line increases and remains increased for as long as the response occurs. When the response ends, the line decreases and remains at that level until the behavior occurs again. We will use this specific pattern of behavior in Figure 7.2 to exemplify each of the dimensional quantities described in the following section.

Frequency (Rate)

Frequency counts of behavior are the most common dimensional quantity and the most intuitive. The frequency of a behavior can be defined as the number of occurrences of a response in a period of time. For example, a researcher could count the number of times a student talks to a peer during English class. If the class is always of a fixed duration, this datum could simply be reported as the number of times the student talks to a peer each day in class. Or, the researcher could report the rate of behavior as indexed against some *unit of time* (e.g., number per minute). Either approach to summarizing this dimensional quantity is an index of its frequency.

Figure 7.3 shows how frequency is used as a dimension of responding to identify individual occurrences of a behavior. The figure shows that the onset of each response is counted as an occurrence of the behavior, regardless of other aspects of responding. In this instance, seven responses were counted in Figure 7.3. Again, this could be counted as 7 occurrences during the fixed time of observation or 14 times per minute.

Another example of using frequency counts comes from a study by Christle and Schuster (2003) who analyzed a response card intervention for prompting active participation of elementary school students during whole-class instruction. Figure 7.4 shows sessions (class periods) along the abscissa and the number of student-initiated opportunities to respond (filled squares) and student responses (open squares) along the ordinate. Baseline

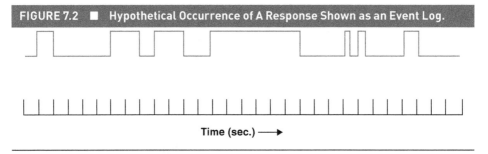

FIGURE 7.2 ■ Hypothetical Occurrence of A Response Shown as an Event Log.

Time (sec.) ⟶

Note. Along the horizontal aspect of the figure is time expressed in seconds. The vertical aspect of the graph denotes the occurrence of individual responses. When a response occurs, the level of the line increases and remains increased for as long as the response occurs. When the response ends, the line decreases and remains at that level until the behavior occurs again.

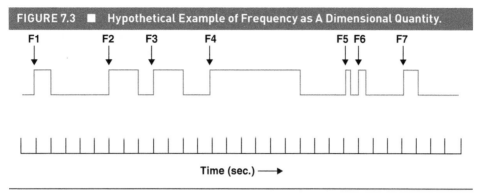

FIGURE 7.3 ■ Hypothetical Example of Frequency as A Dimensional Quantity.

Note. Each *F* indicates the onset of a response that will be counted as an occurrence of the behavioral event. See Figure 7.2 for additional details.

consisted of the typical whole-class instruction approach that relied on students' raising their hand (HR) to answer questions. The intervention was the use of response cards (RC) for students to write down their answers before initiating a response. As can be seen in Figure 7.4, the number of initiations and responses increased in frequency when the RC intervention was used.

It has become common practice to distinguish between frequency and rate of behavior, but this practice is more linguistic than substantive. Both terms refer to the number of occurrences of a response, with one noting occurrences in reference to a fixed amount of time (*frequency*) and the other expressing the frequency as occurrences per unit time (*rate*). Either way, the frequency of behavior is the dimensional quantity of interest since occurrences per unit time are a fixed, rather than dynamic, quantity. Rather than engage in a tortured verbal argument about how to differentiate these two ways of counting responses, I have opted in this book to consider them as isomorphic.

Counting the frequency of a behavior is an excellent and straightforward index of how many times a behavior occurs. In cases where this is the primary datum of interest, then frequency is an appropriate dimensional quantity. However, in instances where the primary characteristic of behavior that is of experimental interest is the pacing of responding, how long responding occurs, or the physical force of responding, then other dimensional quantities would better characterize those behaviors. As we will discuss later in this chapter, it is often wise to use multiple dimensional quantities to more completely characterize responding.

Duration

Duration as a dimensional quantity allows for the estimation of the temporal extent of a response. Duration can be defined as the amount of time that elapses from the onset of a response to the offset of the same response. For example, a preschooler might begin to work at a particular activity center and continue working for 540 seconds. In this instance, their working at the activity center has a duration of 9 minutes. A researcher can summarize individual response durations (e.g., how

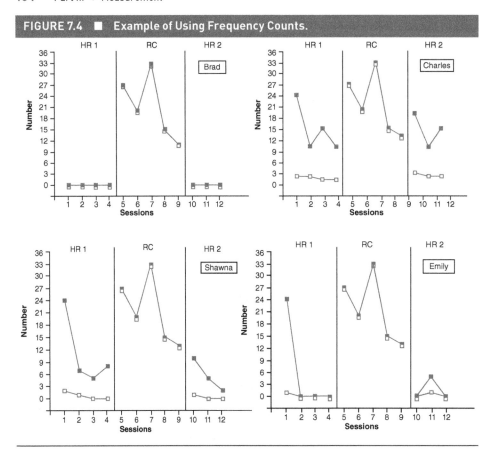

FIGURE 7.4   ■   Example of Using Frequency Counts.

Note. Sessions (class periods) are shown along the abscissa, and the number of student-initiated opportunities to respond (filled squares) and student responses (open squares) along the ordinate. Baseline consisted of the typical whole-class instruction approach that relied on students raising their hand (HR) to answer questions. The intervention was the use of response cards (RC) for students to write down their answers before initiating a response. (Figure 1, p. 158 from: Christle, C. A., & Schuster, J. W. (2003). The effects of using response cards on student participation, academic achievement, and on-task behavior during whole-class, math instruction. *Journal of Behavioral Education, 12*, 147–165. Copyright 2003 by Human Sciences Press, Inc. Reproduced with permission from Springer Nature Customer Service Center.)

long each response lasted), compute an average duration (e.g., mean duration of response), or note the percentage of time units occupied by responding (e.g., percentage of time).

Figure 7.5 presents a hypothetical example of duration as a dimensional quantity. In Figure 7.5, the duration of each response is indicated by the dashed line noting the number of seconds from the onset of each response to its offset. In this example, response durations were 1, 2, 2, 6, 0.5, 0.5, and 1 seconds, a total duration of 13 seconds, or 43% of the time.

Hagopian et al. (2001) present an example of duration as an index of behavior, as shown in Figure 7.6. Hagopian et al. studied the duration of staying seated during an academic work task for a young woman with autism (Natalie). Over brief work sessions (*x*-axis), the percent duration in chair was measured (*y*-axis). The independent variables consisted of rewards for working that were high preference (closed circle), moderate preference (open square), low preference (open circle), and control (open triangle). Each phase of the study assessed different combinations of

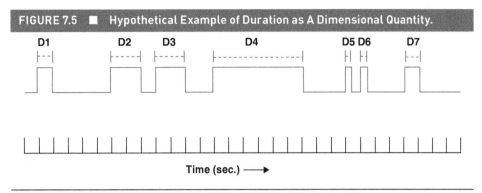

FIGURE 7.5 ■ Hypothetical Example of Duration as A Dimensional Quantity.

Note. Each dashed line indicates the duration from the onset of a response until the offset of the response. See Figure 7.2 for additional details.

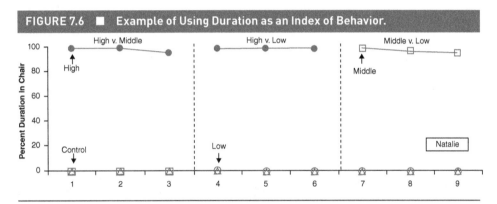

FIGURE 7.6 ■ Example of Using Duration as an Index of Behavior.

Note. Sessions are shown on the *x*-axis, and the percent duration in chair is shown on the *y*-axis. The independent variables consisted of rewards for working that were high preference (closed circle), moderate preference (open square), low preference (open circle), and control (open triangle). (Figure 2, p. 478, from: Hagopian, L. P., Rush, K. S., Lewin, A. B., & Long, E. S. (2001). Evaluating the predictive validity of a single stimulus engagement preference assessment. *Journal of Applied Behavior Analysis, 34,* 475–485. Copyright 2001 by the Society for the Experimental Analysis of Behavior. Reproduced by permission.)

rewards on Natalie's in-seat working. The duration of Natalie staying in her seat was highest when she was reinforced with high or moderate preference rewards, relative to the low preference or control conditions.

Duration is an appropriate dimensional quantity when a researcher is interested in how long a particular behavior is occurring or the amount of observation time that the response occupies. For example, if a behavior such as screaming only occurs a few times per day but continues for an extended period of time on each occurrence, then duration may be a more relevant dimension of behavior than frequency. In general, researchers use duration to estimate how long each behavior occurs.

Latency

This dimensional quantity can be defined as the amount of time between the onset of a stimulus and the occurrence of a response. Latency is a characteristic of behavior that allows for the estimation of how long it takes for a behavior to occur in relation to some salient event in the environment. For example, a researcher may be interested in the amount of time that elapses between the ringing of the classroom bell signaling the start of class and the student being seated. Reporting latencies can include each response latency or the average response latency.

Figure 7.7 shows a hypothetical example of response latency. The figure shows the occurrence of two events of experimental interest (E1 and E2) in relation to the occurrence of behavior. In the first instance 2 seconds elapsed between E1 and the response, and in the second instance the response did not occur until 1 second after E2. The average response latency was 1.5 seconds.

Figure 7.8 shows a study by Wehby and Hollahan (2000). In this study, Wehby and Hollahan analyzed the effects of different sequences of requests on the latency to engage in

---

FIGURE 7.7 ■ Hypothetical Example of Latency as a Dimensional Quantity.

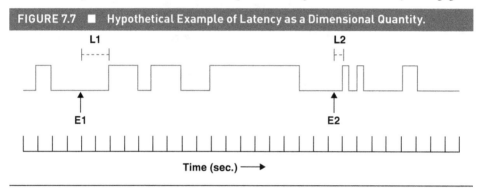

Note. Each latency (L1 and L2) from an event of experimental interest (E1 and E2) to the first response. The dashed line indicates the number of seconds from the stimulus to the onset of a response. See Figure 7.2 for additional details.

FIGURE 7.8 ■ Example of Response Latency.

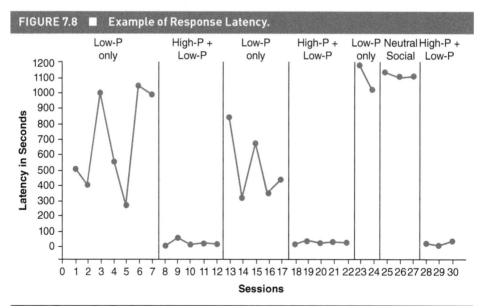

Note. Daily sessions (horizontal axis) and the latency of responding (vertical axis). Interventions included a sequence of low-probability requests (Low-P) and high-probability requests preceding a low-probability request (High-P+Low-P). (Figure 1, p. 261, from: Wehby, J. H., & Hollahan, M. S. (2000). Effects of high-probability requests on the latency to initiate academic tasks. *Journal of Applied Behavior Analysis, 33,* 259–262. Copyright 2000 by the Society for the Experimental Analysis of Behavior. Reproduced by permission.)

academic work for a girl with a learning disability (Meg). Across daily sessions (horizontal axis), the latency of responding was analyzed (vertical axis). When a series of requests that she was unlikely to comply with were made before asking her to start work (Low-P only), Meg had an average latency of 677 seconds before she began work. When a series of high-probability requests were made prior to asking her to do work (High-P+Low-P), there was an average latency of 21 seconds before Meg began working. As shown in Figure 7.8, the high-probability response sequence reduced Meg's latency to begin work.

Latency is of interest as a dimensional quantity when the temporal relation between two different events is a focus of the experiment. In particular, researchers use latency to study how much time elapses before the occurrence of one event (e.g., a teacher's request) and the onset of some other behavioral event (e.g., compliance). Although such relations do not, in and of themselves, show a functional relation between events being measured, this characteristic of responding allows for the quantification of the temporal relation between events.

Interresponse Time

Douglas Anger (1956) was the first behavior analyst to use interresponse times (IRTs) as a dimensional quantity when he was a doctoral student studying with B. F. Skinner. Unlike latency, IRTs are estimates of the time that elapses between occurrences of a response. IRTs can be defined as the time that elapses between the occurrence of two instances of a single response. The number of seconds that elapse between bites taken during lunch would be an example of an IRT. Let's say the first bite occurred at time zero and the second bite occurred after 25 seconds. In this instance, there was an IRT of 25 seconds. IRTs can be summarized as individual occurrences or the average time between responses.

A hypothetical example of IRTs as a dimensional quantity is displayed in Figure 7.9. In this example there are a total of six IRTs (number of responses minus one) as indicated by the dashed lines between each response. Each IRT is denoted by a number. The IRTs, in succession, were 4, 1, 2, 3, 1, and 3 seconds in length. Overall, there was an average IRT of 2.3 seconds.

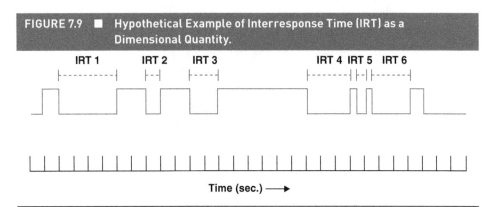

FIGURE 7.9 ■ Hypothetical Example of Interresponse Time (IRT) as a Dimensional Quantity.

Note. Each IRT is measured as the time that elapses from the onset of the behavior at one point in time and the onset of the next behavior. The dashed lines indicate the number of seconds from one response to the next response. See Figure 7.2 for additional details.

An example from the basic research literature of how IRTs can be used is provided by Lippman and Tragesser (2003). These authors studied the effect of magnitude of reinforcement on the choice making of college students. The arbitrary response selected for analysis was button pressing on a computer. The independent variables consisted of a positive reinforcement contingency that provided the largest magnitude of reinforcement either for brief IRTs or longer IRTs. Figure 7.10 shows how the reinforcement contingencies influenced response patterns. The percentage of responses (*y*-axis) that fell within certain IRT time bins (*x*-axis) is arrayed in the figure for each reinforcement contingency. The results of the Lippman and Tragesser study show that behavior was sensitive to reinforcer magnitude, with briefer IRTs or longer IRTs being emitted in accordance with the reinforcement schedules.

Quantifying behavior in terms of IRTs is particularly valuable when a researcher wants to establish how a response is distributed in time in relation to other occurrences of the same behavior. The value of such an analysis is that IRTs show whether behaviors occur in clusters

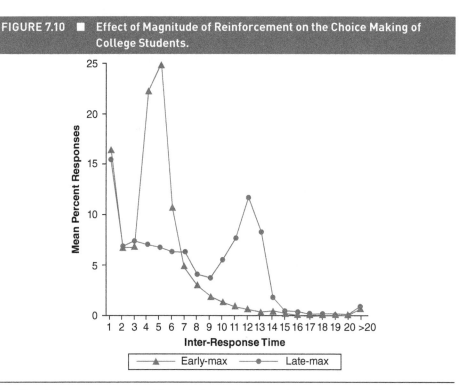

FIGURE 7.10 ■ Effect of Magnitude of Reinforcement on the Choice Making of College Students.

Note. The arbitrary response selected for analysis was button pressing on a computer. The mean percentage of responses is indexed against particular IRT lengths. The independent variables consisted of a positive reinforcement contingency that provided the largest magnitude of reinforcement for either brief IRTs or longer IRTs. (Figure 4, p. 440, from: Lippman, L. G., & Tragesser, S. L. (2003). Contingent magnitude of reward in modified human-operant DRL-LH and CRF schedules. *The Psychological Record, 53*, 429–442. Copyright 2003 by Association of Behavior Analysis International. Reproduced with permission of Springer Nature Customer Service Center.)

(i.e., brief IRTs), are evenly distributed around some time parameter (e.g., paced responding), or occur in a bimodal or more complex distribution (e.g., two different temporal peaks). Although not often used as the only dimensional quantity for characterizing behavior, IRTs provide a means of describing the temporal organization of responding that other dimensional quantities cannot provide.

Celeration

Celeration is a dimension that allows for the quantification of the change in response rate over some unit of time. This index of responding is directly analogous to the concepts of acceleration and deceleration used in physics and engineering. Celeration is defined as the frequency of responding for a particular time unit divided by unit time. That is, it is the change in average IRTs for a period of time (e.g., seconds) as indexed against another time period (e.g., minutes). For example, correctly solving mathematics problems could be characterized as the number per second per minute. This would allow for the analysis of changes in the rate of problem solving across one minute intervals during mathematics instruction.

Figure 7.11 presents a hypothetical example of celeration as a dimensional quantity. The figure shows the number of responses per 5-second unit indexed against 15-second intervals. This arrangement allows for a description of the number of responses per second interval and how that rate changes every 15 seconds. In this example, responding changed from 0.1 to 0.07 responses from one time unit to the next.

Kostewicz et al. (2000) present an example of using celeration to index behavior change over time. Kostewicz et al. examined the occurrence of aggressive thoughts and feelings of a newly arrived university graduate student. Counts of these behaviors (*xs*), as well as pleasant thoughts (dark circles), are displayed across days on a *logarithmic scale* (see Lindsley, 1991). The baseline rates of occurrence

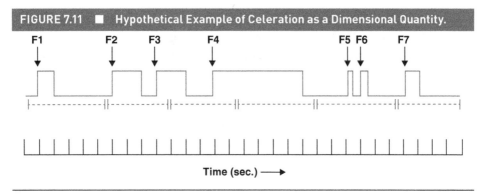

FIGURE 7.11 ■ Hypothetical Example of Celeration as a Dimensional Quantity.

Time (sec.) ⟶

Note. Celeration is measured as the number of times that a particular response occurs in a unit of time indexed against a unit of time. The dashed lines indicate the number of seconds from one response to the next response. In this example, the first unit of time is 15 seconds indexed against 30 seconds. See Figure 7.2 for additional details.

FIGURE 7.12 ■ Example of Using Celeration to Index Behavior Change Over Time.

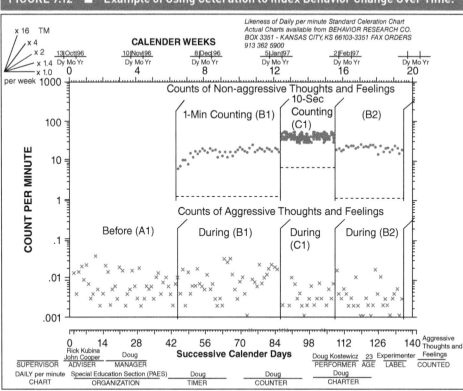

Note. The occurrence of aggressive thoughts and feelings of a new university graduate student. Counts of these behaviors (xs), as well as pleasant thoughts (dark circles), are displayed across days on a *logarithmic scale*. (Figure 1, p. 182, from: Kostewicz, D. E., Kubina, R. M., & Cooper, J. O. (2000). Managing aggressive thoughts and feelings with daily counts of non-aggressive thoughts and feelings: A self-experiment. *Journal of Behavior Therapy and Experimental Psychiatry, 31,* 177–187. Copyright 2001 by Elsevier Science Limited. Reproduced by permission.)

for these behaviors are shown in Figure 7.12. On average, the student counted 40 to 50 pleasant thoughts or feelings during baseline and fewer angry or aggressive thoughts.

The analysis of celeration is particularly useful in educational contexts because it captures what we often talk about as *fluency*. Fluency is the well-practiced, fluid, accurate performance we try to establish in students (Evans et al., 2021). Celeration accurately captures this pattern of responding by showing changes in behavior in relation to time. Celeration is also similar to what we have uncritically adopted in everyday usage as "rate." That is, changes in the frequency of behavior in a period of time as it changes over time.

CHOOSING DIMENSIONAL QUANTITIES

As this chapter has shown, behavior is not a monolithic entity that is unidimensional. Instead, even in the analysis of a single topography of behavior, there are multiple facets to each response that provide important information regarding various dimensions of its occurrence. Because of this multidimensionality of behavior, when designing a research study, you need to make some important decisions about how to best characterize the responding you are interested in analyzing. This is not an easy decision, and there is no rulebook to refer to for a definitive answer. Instead, a researcher needs to use their cumulative experience with the phenomenon being studied and their knowledge of other researchers' experiences with similar phenomena.

Adding to the difficulty in arriving at a decision about how to appropriately quantify behavior is that individual behaviors typically do not occur alone, and in most research the primary experimental question is the interrelation of different behaviors. That interrelation may be between how two different topographies of behavior from the same individual enter into the same, or independent, response classes or how behaviors from different people enter into various reinforcement contingencies. As illustrated in Figure 7.1, the behavioral stream of a single individual is complex, and that complexity is only multiplied by the interactions that person may have with others. Given this complexity, choosing the dimensional quantity(ies) that will adequately characterize the functional relations your experimental question is seeking to establish is imperative.

The first rule of thumb in selecting dimensional quantities is to directly observe the behaviors you are interested in and look at different aspects of those responses. This need not be a highly technical task. My experience would suggest simply spending time in the situation you are interested in studying, watching people carefully, and jotting down notes as appropriate are all that is required. When you do this, what are you looking for? What is it about a particular response that seems relevant to your experimental question? Is it the pacing of the behavior, the rapidity with which it is emitted following a stimulus, how frequently it occurs, how it changes in frequency over time, or the persistence of the behavior when it does occur?

Once you have an idea about which dimensional quantities may be of most interest to your research question, discuss your observations with others whom you will be working with and/ or researchers who are familiar with the area of research. Start by reviewing your experimental question and what it is you are hoping to learn by conducting your study. Are they relevant to your experimental question? Are the behaviors you are identifying good candidates for experimental analysis? Have you selected dimensional quantities that reflect meaningful characteristics of the behaviors of interest? By enlisting the feedback of others, you gain different perspectives on how to quantify behavior that may help you refine your ideas and improve how you are going about characterizing behavior in your study.

A third rule of thumb is to choose multiple dimensions of responding. In laboratory research, it is common for a researcher to characterize behavior in terms of multiple dimensional quantities. This allows as complete a picture of behavior in relation to the experimental environment as is possible. However, a hallmark of laboratory research is the automated recording of behavior, and that recording usually occurs in highly simplified environments. The settings in which educational research is conducted are more complex and may not permit the ubiquitous recording of all possible dimensional quantities. However, with that said, selecting more than one dimension of behavior to study is a wise experimental tactic. For example, it might be that the frequency and duration of a particular response interact and one, the other, or both might be particularly sensitive to the intervention you are going to analyze (see also Box 7.3).

BOX 7.3: ARE THERE OTHER DIMENSIONAL QUANTITIES?

Given the excitement engendered by discussions of dimensional quantities among most researchers, the reader is undoubtedly thinking, "Are there other dimensional quantities that have not been discussed in this chapter?" *The answer is yes.* A dimensional quantity is a way of characterizing some physical aspect of a behavior in space and time. The dimensional quantities discussed in this chapter are those most commonly used in educational research and most relevant to educational contexts. However, there are other dimensional quantities and means of quantitatively analyzing them that are beyond the scope of this discussion. An example of another dimensional quantity is *force*. A response clearly generates properties that could be physically measured relating to the force of the behavior. For instance, responses might generate a certain number of newtons of force or obtain a certain number of decibels as a quantifiable unit. In addition, there is the largely untapped issue of characterizing behavior using ratios of dimensional quantities (see Johnston & Hodge, 1989). An example of ratios would be quantifying behavior as a ratio of frequency and duration. Overall, there is a great deal of research that remains to be done regarding new dimensional quantities, and the utility of using different ratios of these quantities can be used to discover new aspects of responding.

The final arbiter in all research regarding the adequacy of the decisions you make, whether about hypotheses, measurement, or experimental design, is the data that are obtained. Do they show orderliness? Are they interpretable? Do they reveal something about the phenomenon you are studying that has not previously been revealed? Unfortunately, these questions cannot be answered a priori, but, instead, like all operant behavior (and research, itself, is a form of operant behavior), you have to learn from the consequences of your behavior. The phenomenon you are studying and the data that result from your choice of experimental arrangements will be the ultimate guide about the adequacy of your choices and how you should proceed in future studies attempting to systematically replicate your results.

REFLECTION QUESTIONS

1. What would happen if researchers used their memory of what events occurred and did not occur, rather than using direct observation and recording of events?

2. Investigators have developed clear criteria for operational definitions. Why do experts emphasize defining both positive and negative examples of behavior for operational definitions?

3. When would you consider using two or more dimensional quantities to describe behavior rather than using a single dimension?

4. What types of information are provided by interresponse times that differ from the dimensional quantities of frequency or duration?

5. When noting what a dimensional quantity is, why would "force" be considered a dimension, but not response "topography"?

8   RECORDING SYSTEMS

LEARNING OBJECTIVES

After reading this chapter, you will be able to

8.1   Illustrate the significance of recording systems in an experimental process.

8.2   Determine appropriate observational codes and measurement techniques for a recording system.

8.3   Utilize seven types of data collection procedures.

8.4   Explain additional research considerations for recording systems, including the recording medium, sampling settings, and training observers.

A foundation of behavioral approaches to educational issues is rigorous measurement. Measurement is a critical component of any effort to empirically study a phenomenon and involves (a) choosing dimensional quantities, (b) using recording systems to document behavior and stimuli, and (c) conducting integrity checks on data collection. The reason such care is taken with measurement is that accurately documenting the level of a dependent variable is required to reveal the potential effects of an independent variable. For example, if I were to measure events with $\pm35\%$ accuracy of the veridical level, then any effect produced by the experimental variable would have to have an effect much larger than $\pm35\%$ to be revealed. If the independent variable did not produce such an effect, its influence on behavior would be masked by the variability induced by poor measurement. However, if I measure events that are within $\pm5\%$ of the actual value, then more subtle effects produced by an intervention can be detected.

RECORDING SYSTEMS

A key component in developing a rigorous approach to measurement is the *recording system* to be used (Thompson et al., 1999). A recording system includes several different components. First, a recording system needs to adequately code the behaviors and other events of interest. That is, what is being recorded needs to accurately reflect what the experimenter is trying to study. This may seem obvious, but in practice it is extraordinarily challenging. Second, a recording system needs to accurately document the events of interest. Some type of measurement technique needs to be used to record what events occurred or did not occur. Third, some physical medium needs to permanently capture the recording of events. Fourth, events need to be sampled that reflect the scope of the experimental question. Finally, the recording system needs to be implemented and maintained. This includes recording behaviors and stimuli as accurately as possible and continually updating the recording system to preserve this level of precision. If all of this can be accomplished, then data will be gathered that can be analyzed in a meaningful way (see Parts IV and V of the book).

The process of recording events involves incorporating each of these aspects into the daily activities of a research study. Recording systems are a means to an end in the sense that without an adequate system, no study can yield interpretable results. Therefore, recording responses and stimuli occupies a somewhat unique role in all fields of research. Because of its importance, some scholars choose to specialize in the study of recording systems in and of themselves (e.g., Schall, 2007; Trout, 1998; Whaley, 1973), while others use the products of this work as tools to pursue other research interests.

In this chapter, we will discuss how behavior and stimuli are recorded. This information will be presented in a linear manner that reflects the process from start to finish. We will discuss developing observational codes, selecting measurement techniques, choosing a medium for recording, sampling behavior, and, then, training observers. This process will focus on the dependent variables used in an experiment. Once this is completed, we will turn to a separate but related issue—recording the independent variable(s) used in a study in Chapter 9.

STEPS IN DEVELOPING A RECORDING SYSTEM

Observational Codes

The first step in developing a recording system is to develop an *observational code*. This refers to the types of behaviors and other events that will be the focus of observations. Carefully developing an observational code is important because it provides the framework for what events can be documented during the experiment. If something is left out of the observational code or is poorly conceptualized, the result may require the experiment to be reconducted with an improved recording system. Therefore, this initial step in developing a recording system should be given considerable attention (Bijou et al., 1968).

What will be recorded? Generally, two categories of events need to be identified. First, the *behaviors* of interest need to be selected. This can include not only the behavior of the focal student, but the responses of other individuals in that person's environment. Behaviors could include completing mathematics problems, the occurrence of stereotypical behavior, steps used to solve a puzzle, types of social greetings used, and so on. As was noted in Chapter 8, the limitation on what can be considered a behavior is the ability to operationalize and directly measure the response. The second general type of event included in observational codes is *stimuli*. Like behavior, stimuli can take on a potentially infinite number of topographies. Anything that is not a behavior, but occurs, can be considered a stimulus. Examples include the presentation of materials, the presence of certain objects, sounds that might occur, and so on. Like behaviors, stimuli need to be operationalized and directly measured (cf. Cooper et al., 2020).

The particular behaviors and stimuli that will be included in a recording system are derived from the experimental question. If you are studying how students solve mathematics problems, then the focus of the observational code will be on various behaviors and stimuli associated with solving mathematics problems. Similarly, if you are studying aggression, the focus of the observations will be on types of aggressive behaviors and associated stimuli. One important way of identifying what behaviors and stimuli might be of interest is to repeatedly observe the situations you want to study and take notes about what occurs. Another source for identifying relevant events comes from previous experiments on similar topics. The observational codes that other researchers have developed may be adequate for your purposes or may need to be adapted to fit your experimental interests. If appropriate, a researcher should not hesitate to use previously developed observational codes because their use allows for the findings from various studies to be readily integrated at the level of the data collected.

Whatever behaviors and/or stimuli are used, they will need to be defined into discrete categories (Mayer et al., 2012). It does not make sense to simultaneously record social interactions and positive verbal statements, because the latter is a subset of the former. Instead, researchers developing observational codes need to make sure their operational definitions of behaviors and stimuli are nonoverlapping. For example, social interactions could be subdivided into positive, negative, or neutral verbal statements. An additional issue is whether the observation code will contain elements that are *exhaustive* or *open-ended* (Bakeman & Gottman, 1997; Bakeman & Quera, 2012). An exhaustive code defines events so that all events have a category for being recorded. The previous example of positive, negative, or neutral verbal statements is an example of an exhaustive set of categories. An open-ended category system focuses on particular events and does not attempt to inclusively define a logically exhaustive set. For example, if a researcher were only interested in greetings to other peers and that was sufficient to address the experimental question, there would not be a need to use a more complex observational code.

The simplest observational code that could be developed would focus on a single response. More complex codes can include dozens of behaviors and stimuli. Tang et al. (2003) provide an example of a very simple system. These researchers studied students with extensive support needs who engaged in a single topography of stereotypical behavior (e.g., hand waving). Because the experimental question was to identify the environmental causes of the behavior, a more complex observational code was not necessary. On the other end of the continuum is an observational code developed by Walker and colleagues (Walker & Severson, 1992) to study antisocial behavior in school settings. This observational code includes multiple categories for student behaviors, types of environmental contexts, various stimulus events, and how others react to the behaviors of a focal student. As in many aspects of research, the application of Occam's razor is an important consideration. The observational code needs to identify relevant behaviors and stimuli in order to adequately address the experimental question. However, the more complex the code, the harder it is to train observers and obtain acceptable levels of interobserver agreement (see Chapter 9). *Basically, you want the observational code to be as simple as possible, but no simpler.*

Measurement Techniques

Once an observational code has been established, researchers need to determine which dimensional quantity or quantities they will need to document the occurrence of each response and stimulus represented in the code (see Chapter 7). For example, if screaming is the response of interest, would frequency or duration or both dimensions be the most appropriate way of representing the response? If the behavior is brief, then frequency might be an appropriate index. If each time the behavior occurs it lasts an extended period of time, then duration may be a more relevant dimension. Or, it might be concluded that both indexes of screaming need to be used to adequately characterize the nature of the behavior. Deciding what dimension(s) of responses and stimuli to measure requires that the researchers be familiar with the behavior they will be recording prior to developing a recording system. Such a process needs to occur for each response and stimulus included in the observational code. It is possible that different dimensional quantities need to be selected for different responses and stimuli.

After dimensional quantities have been selected for the observational code, researchers will need to decide what measurement technique(s) they will use. Two general categories of measurement techniques can be used to sample behavior and stimuli. The first requires *direct measures*, and the second requires *indirect measures*. Direct measures sample events through observation of the behaviors and/or stimuli themselves. That is, the events are directly observed. This can be contrasted with indirect measures, which sample events via products of events and/or stimuli. For example, in a vocational work setting, the number of dishes washed could be used as an indirect measure of dishwashing. It should be noted that direct versus indirect measurement is a different topic than automated versus manual recording (see Box 8.1).

BOX 8.1: AUTOMATED RECORDING IN EDUCATIONAL SETTINGS

A hallmark of the experimental analysis of behavior is the use of an automated apparatus to record the occurrence of responses and stimuli. For example, each time a lever is pressed or a food pellet delivered in an operant conditioning chamber, the event is separately recorded by a computer (see Catania, 2013). Such an arrangement allows the events that occur during an experiment to be recorded without human intervention (e.g., recording discrete events using paper and pencil). This arrangement removes the possibility of human error from the recording of events of experimental interest, although it does not remove the possibility of hardware or software errors.

In educational settings there is a long history of using human observation to record the behaviors and stimuli of interest (see Bijou et al., 1968). This is because educational environments do not easily lend themselves to automated recording. For example, it would be extremely difficult to find a mechanical means of recording the occurrence of social initiations or obscene gestures in school hallways. Such behaviors, however, can be easily recorded by human observers. This aspect of educational settings has required researchers since the 1960s to develop sophisticated recording procedures that rely on humans to record behaviors and stimuli. Because of this feature of educational settings and the history of using human observers, this chapter focuses on this approach to recording events. However, with the increasing use of computer software and web-based applications, it is likely that there will be an increase in the use of automated recording in educational settings in the future.

TYPES OF DATA COLLECTION PROCEDURES

Once dimensional quantities and a general measurement technique are selected, the type of data collection procedure needs to be selected. We will discuss seven different procedures that are well established in the research literature. Each type of data collection procedure will be described, its use illustrated, and its advantages and disadvantages discussed (see also Springer et al., 1981).

Event Recording

Event recording documents individual occurrences of a response or stimulus during an observation period. Each time an event of interest occurs, that instance is recorded. At the end of an observation, the number of events for a particular category can be counted and the total number of occurrences reported as a measure of the behavior of interest. Figure 8.1 shows an example of an event recording system. The observation period was 20 minutes, and the numbers of questions asked and questions correctly answered during a classroom lecture were recorded. The figure shows that 12 questions were asked during the lecture and 9 correct answers were observed. In this instance the event recording system documents two separate events.

The observation period used with event recording can be of either a *fixed* (e.g., 50 minutes) or *variable length* (e.g., 45 to 60 minutes). In some instances, particularly in classroom settings, a fixed observation length is not possible because the length of instruction may vary from one day to the next. In such cases, researchers typically choose to use a variable length of observation that matches the duration of the educational activity being studied. For instances in which a fixed amount of time is used, the dependent variable can be reported as the number of occurrences or can be transformed into the number of occurrences per standard time unit (e.g., second, minute, or hour). If the observation period is variable in length, the number of occurrences per observation needs to be transformed using a standard time unit. For example, the data in Figure 8.1 could

---

FIGURE 8.1 ■ Example of Event Recording.

Number of Teacher Questions	Number of Correct Student Answers
√ √ √ √ √ √ √ √ √ √ √ √	√ √ √ √ √ √ √ √ √

√ = Occurrence of an event.

Note. The observation period was 20 minutes, and the numbers of questions asked and questions correctly answered during a classroom lecture were recorded.

be reported as 12 and 9 occurrences, respectively, or as 0.6 and 0.45, respectively, because a fixed observation time was used.

Event recording works best with discrete behaviors that have brief durations. Event recording can be used with frequency as a dimensional quantity. If a time-based element is added to event recording (i.e., time of occurrence for each event is documented), then this measurement technique can also be used to document interresponse time (IRT) or celeration.

The advantages of event recording include:

- The technique can be used to record multiple topographies of behavior and stimuli as discrete events.

- The technique is easy to use if a limited number of discrete events are being recorded. As more categories of events are added, the more complex the recording system becomes (this is true of all the measurement techniques we will discuss).

- It provides an unambiguous estimate of how often a particular behavior or stimulus occurred during an observation.

The disadvantages of event recording include:

- The technique requires continuous observation. This entails that one observer is required to monitor the setting throughout the time period being observed.

- For events that vary in length, either within a category or between categories, event recording confounds duration with frequency.

Permanent Product Recording

The *permanent product recording* measurement technique is similar to event recording, except the events of interest are recorded at the end of a period of time or after some task is completed. For example, instead of observing a child solve each of the math problems on a worksheet, the researcher can collect the worksheet at the end of the work period and record the numbers of problems attempted and correct answers. An example of this situation is shown in Figure 8.2. In this example, 25 problems were attempted and 19 solved correctly.

Permanent product data can be reported in ways similar to event recording in terms of absolute numbers versus ratios of events and time. In addition, in situations such as that presented in Figure 8.2, a percentage can be derived from the data. That is, 25 problems were attempted and 19 correctly solved, meaning that 76% of the questions were correctly answered.

Permanent product recording works best with behaviors and stimuli that have some discrete outcome that remains once the events have ended. As with event recording, this makes permanent product recording particularly useful for documenting frequency as a dimensional quantity. However, if the time at which an event is produced can be documented in some manner, it is also possible to focus on IRT or celeration.

FIGURE 8.2 ■ Example of Permanent Product Recording.	
Number of Problems Attempted	*Correct Answers*
√ √	√ √ √ √ √ √ √ √ √ √ √ √ √ √ √ √ √ √

√ = Occurrence of an event.

Note. Instead of observing a child solve each math problem on a worksheet, the researcher can collect the worksheet at the end of the work period and record the numbers of problems attempted and correct answers.

The advantages of permanent product recording include:

- It permits noncontinuous recording of behavior and stimulus events. This means that one observer can engage in other activities during the time when the experimental events are occurring.

- It allows the products to be inspected and permits an error-pattern analysis to be conducted (see Annett, 2004; Kieras & Butler, 1997). Such an analysis can be used to identify the type of mistakes that are made, in addition to an overall estimation of accurate performance.

   The disadvantage of permanent product recording is:

- Responses and stimuli must produce a tangible by-product; otherwise, the measurement technique cannot be used.

Duration Recording

The most direct measure of the dimensional quantity duration is to use the measurement technique duration. *Duration recording* documents the amount of time that elapses between the onset of an event and the end of the same event. Figure 8.3 shows an example of a completed data sheet used for duration recording. The figure represents the amount of time required to swim a single lap during a physical education class that required students to swim 10 laps each day. The duration of each of the 10 laps was recorded in Figure 8.3.

In the example from Figure 8.3, a fixed number of events was required (i.e., 10 laps), and the duration of each lap was the dependent variable of interest. These data should be summarized by the central tendency of the data (i.e., mean, mode, and/or median) and

FIGURE 8.3   ■   Example of a Completed Data Sheet used for Duration Recording.

Duration (seconds) of Each Lap Swum

Lap 1 = 48.7

Lap 2 = 49

Lap 3 = 47.1

Lap 4 = 47.3

Lap 5 = 47.8

Lap 6 = 48.2

Lap 7 = 49.3

Lap 8 = 52.8

Lap 9 = 53.7

Lap 10 = 58.6

Note. The figure represents the amount of time required to swim a single lap during a physical education class that required students to swim 10 laps each day.

some estimate of the range (i.e., absolute or relative) (see Chapter 17). For example, the mean length of a lap was 50.3 seconds (range, 47.1 to 58.6 seconds). In situations where a variable number of events can occur, it can be useful to document the base rate (i.e., the number of occurrences of the event) of events along with the average and range of durations. If an observational situation has a fixed or variable amount of time, then a percentage of the overall time an event was observed to occur can be derived. For example, talking out of turn in a mathematics class might be observed to occur during 23% of the total class time using duration recording.

The advantages of duration recording include:

- The precise estimation of the temporal extent of behaviors and stimuli can be established. This can include the amount of time each occurrence of an event lasts or the total amount of observation time a behavior occurs.

The disadvantages of duration recording include:

- The technique requires continuous observation.

- The technique also requires the use of some type of timing device (e.g., a stopwatch).

- In situations where frequent, brief events are being recorded, this technique may be cumbersome and inaccurate.

Latency Recording

Latency recording, like duration, is closely linked to a specific dimensional quantity, in this case latency. With latency recording, the time between the onset of a stimulus or behavior and the subsequent onset of the target response is recorded. An example of data reflecting latency recording is shown in Figure 8.4. The data sheet shows the number of seconds that elapsed between a teacher request and a student complying with the request. During the observation, 6 different requests were made with a median latency to compliance of 7.15 (range, 4.8 to 45.1).

In some instances the experimental situation may be arranged so that a fixed number of stimulus presentations is presented; in other cases the number may be allowed to vary under naturalistic conditions. In either situation, the central tendency and some measure of variability can be reported because the total latency in seconds can be divided by the number of stimulus presentations.

The advantages of latency recording are:

● This recording technique provides an index of the temporal relation between one event and another.

The disadvantages of latency recording are:

● If stimulus presentations are not fixed, the number of events may vary considerably from one observation to the next.

● The technique requires continuous observation.

● The technique requires the use of some type of timing device (e.g., a stopwatch).

● The response of interest may have no causal relation to the stimulus presentation, and the relation between the two variables may be only correlational.

FIGURE 8.4 ■ Example of a Completed Data Sheet used for Latency Recording.

Latency (seconds) to Student Compliance

Request 1 =   5.3

Request 2 = 45.1

Request 3 = 12.4

Request 4 =   8.1

Request 5 =   6.2

Request 6 =   4.8

Note. The data sheet shows the number of seconds that elapsed between a teacher request and a student complying with the request.

Partial-Interval Recording

Rather than recording discrete events as they occur as has been done with each of the previous four recording techniques, the remaining three techniques use sampling strategies to *estimate* the occurrence of stimuli and behaviors. That is, they divide observations into discrete intervals of time and note the occurrence or nonoccurrence of particular events. This process does not provide for an exact recording of what occurred, but instead provides an approximation of what stimuli and behaviors were observed.

In the case of *partial-interval recording*, if an event of interest is observed to occur at any time within a specific time interval, the interval is scored as an occurrence of the stimulus or response. If the same event occurs multiple times within the interval, it is still scored simply as an occurrence. If the event of interest is not observed during the interval, then it is scored as a nonoccurrence of the stimulus or response. Figure 8.5 (left-hand panel) shows an example of partial-interval recording. In this example, one behavior was recorded (e.g., hitting another student) during the observation (left side of figure). When the behavior was observed, an *X* was marked in the interval box. The figure shows that 8 out of 10 intervals were scored as occurrences of the response using partial-interval recording. Such an outcome would be summarized as the response having occurred during 80% of observation intervals.

The length of an interval is an important consideration when using partial-interval recording. Overall, the smaller the interval, the more accurate the estimate of the occurrence of the behavior will be (Kahng et al., 2021; Powell et al., 1975). To illustrate this concept, a sensitive interval would be 1 second. This would very accurately track when a behavior did, or did not, occur. This can be compared with a time interval of 1 minute. A 1-minute interval would overestimate the occurrence of an event because the event would only need to occur once in the interval to be scored as an occurrence. However, using very brief intervals (e.g., 1 second) would make the recording of events difficult, if not impossible. Therefore, by convention, researchers tend to use intervals that are 5, 10, or 15 seconds in length, with shorter intervals being preferable to minimize inflation of the estimated occurrence of behavior. In addition, there is an important interaction between the interval length and the duration of the event being recorded (Repp et al., 1976). The briefer the event being analyzed, the shorter the interval should be so as not to inflate how often the behavior is occurring.

The advantages of partial-interval recording include

- The technique can provide an estimate of the occurrence of behaviors and stimuli without requiring that every event be recorded.

- The technique does not require continuous observation.

The disadvantages of partial-interval recording include:

- It requires some type of cueing device to signal the observer when an interval begins and ends.

- If larger intervals are used, particularly with brief events, this observation technique overestimates the occurrence of the response.

FIGURE 8.5 ■ Example of Partial-Interval (Left-Hand Panel), Whole-Interval (Center Panel), and Momentary-Interval Recording (Rght-Hand Panel).

Behavior	Partial	Whole	Momentary
|	X		X
I	X		
|	X		X
|	X		X
|	X		X
|	X	X	X
|	X		
I	X		
Outcome:	*80%*	*10%*	*50%*

Note. On the far-left side of the figure is real-time onset and offset of the behavior being observed. When the behavior met the requirement for an occurrence, an "*X*" was marked in the interval box. The percentage of intervals scored is summarized at the bottom of the figure.

Whole-Interval Recording

A second approach to interval estimates of behaviors and stimuli is *whole-interval recording*. In this approach, the event of interest has to occur throughout the entire interval to be scored as an occurrence. If responding occurs for most, but not all, of the interval, the interval is scored as a nonoccurrence. An example of whole-interval recording is presented in Figure 8.5

(center panel). In relation to the behavior that occurred, the only interval in which responding was scored as occurring was for the seventh interval. Even though behaviors were observed in multiple intervals, only once was the behavior observed to occur continuously throughout an interval. The result is an estimate that behavior occurred during 10% of the intervals.

Clearly, the behavior of interest occurred more than 10% of the time during the observational period, and this discrepancy is a particular concern with whole-interval recording procedures. For behaviors that occur briefly, this approach to measurement underestimates the actual occurrence of behavior. This characteristic of the procedure is exacerbated if longer intervals are chosen. So, again, with interval measurement procedures there is an interaction between the duration of behavior and interval length (Repp et al., 1976). For this reason, whole-interval recording is typically used only when the behavior and/or stimuli being observed are of long duration. Because of these concerns, whole-interval recording procedures are rarely used by researchers (Kelly, 1977).

The advantage of whole-interval recording is:

- The technique can provide an estimate of the occurrence of behaviors and stimuli that have long durations without requiring that every event be recorded.

The disadvantages of whole-interval recording include:

- The technique requires continuous observation.

- It requires some type of cueing device to signal the observer when an interval begins and ends.

- If larger intervals are used, particularly with brief events, this observation technique underestimates the occurrence of the response.

Momentary-Interval Recording

The final type of interval recording system to be discussed is *momentary-interval recording*, which is also referred to as *time sampling* or *momentary-time sampling* (e.g., Harrop & Daniels, 1986). Using this approach, observations only occur for a subset of an interval. Hence, only a part (i.e., a moment) of the entire interval is observed. Typically, the nonobservation part of the interval is referred to as the *wait* component, and the observational part is referred to as the *record* component. For example, a researcher may select a 10-second interval in which there are 5-second wait and 5-second record components. In this instance the observer would not observe during the first 5 seconds of the interval and then record the occurrence of events for the final 5 seconds of the interval. Most often, the record component uses a strategy similar to partial-interval recording (i.e., the event need only occur once), but it is possible to use this recording technique using a whole-interval criterion.

Figure 8.5 (right-hand panel) shows the use of a 10-second momentary-interval recording procedure with 9-second wait and 1-second record components. The result was that 5 out of 10 intervals were scored as the behavior occurring, producing an estimate of 50% of the intervals. Using momentary-interval recording, intervals of 5, 10, or 15 seconds are typically used, but intervals of 30 seconds or 1 minute (or more) can be used to estimate the occurrence of behavior. Typically, the longer the overall observation time, the larger the interval can be. Interacting with this is the length of the record component, which often ranges from 1 second for shorter intervals to 15 seconds for longer intervals.

A particular advantage of momentary-interval recording is that one observer can record the behavior of multiple individuals during the same observation session. For example, if a researcher is using a 15-second interval with 10-second wait and 5-second record components, then the observer could monitor up to three different students at a time. The observer could do this by observing each student for 5 seconds, then shifting their attention to the next student for 5 seconds, then observing the third student for the same time period, and then begin the process over again.

The advantages of momentary-interval recording include:

- It allows for a potentially efficient use of observer time for simultaneously recording multiple participants.

- The technique does not require continuous observation.

The disadvantages of momentary-interval recording include:

- It requires some type of cueing device to signal the observer when an interval begins and ends.

- It can underestimate or overestimate the occurrence of events as a function of event duration and frequency and the length of wait and record components.

ADDITIONAL CONSIDERATIONS IN RECORDING SYSTEMS

Recording Medium

An issue closely related to the selection of measurement techniques is the medium used to record behavior and stimuli. After developing an observational code and selecting a measurement technique, there must be some means of capturing events in some fashion for later analysis. Typically, researchers either directly observe sessions or record them using videotape or some other digital medium. The advantage of collecting data while directly observing the session is primarily one of efficiency. Once the session is finished, the data have already been collected and are ready for the next step, data analysis (see Part V). The advantage of capturing the session on videotape is that the events are available for repeated analysis. This means that if the observational code needs to be altered, all sessions can be rescored using the revised protocol. In addition, because the sessions are captured for repeated viewing, more elaborate observational codes can be used. The primary disadvantages of recording sessions for later scoring are the time involved and the fact that not all events occurring in a setting can be captured with a video camera or related device.

A related decision is whether to use paper-and-pencil or computerized systems. Paper-and-pencil systems, as the name implies, use readily available technologies to record behavior and stimuli. Advantages of paper-and-pencil systems include the ease with which they can be created and used. An alternative is to use a computer-based data acquisition program that includes software and hardware for collecting and recording information (Kahng et al., 2021). Advantages of computer-based systems are (a) the ability to quickly summarize data, (b) downloading data onto other computers for data analysis, and (c) the ease of simultaneously recording multiple behaviors (via a keypad or keyboard). However, most instances of data collection do not require computer-based systems, and the majority of data analyses reported in published studies can be recorded using paper-and-pencil systems (see Miltenberger et al., 1999).

Sampling Settings

An important decision regarding recording systems is what settings (and the behaviors and stimuli that occur within them) will be sampled for observation. There are two general types of settings in which educational research is conducted: *natural settings* and *analogue settings*. Natural settings are those settings in which the behaviors of interest are expected to occur in a student's typical life. They include home, community, and school settings in which the person lives, works, and is educated (Kennedy, 2003). Such settings are the primary goal of any applied research endeavor because it is behavior change in a person's natural settings that is the ultimate goal of any educational research effort. However, it is often necessary to conduct a series of studies under more controlled circumstances before the findings can be extrapolated to natural settings. Such studies are often referred to as being conducted in analogue settings, although terms such as *clinic, pullout*, and *laboratory settings* are also used. In analogue settings, the goal is to reduce the number of extraneous variables that can influence behavior in order to analyze more fundamental functional relations (Wacker, 2000). If experimenters conducting research in analogue settings are successful, the end result will be a better understanding of behavior that can be used in natural settings to improve student outcomes. Currently, there is a great deal of professional and policymaker interest in extending analogue research findings to natural settings, and this process is referred to variously as *research-to-practice* or *translational research* (see Lerman, 2003; Malouf & Schiller, 1995; Nunes et al., 2002).

As can be deduced from the previous statements, what settings need to be sampled are derived from the experimental question being addressed in a single-case analysis. If the experimental question is focused on revealing basic properties of behavior, then analogue settings are likely (but not necessarily) the preferred choice. Typically, analogue settings sample limited amounts of time and are chosen for the convenience of the researchers. For example, using brief experimental designs (Chapter 15), individual sessions may last only 5 or 10 minutes, and as few as 3 or 4 sessions may be necessary to show a functional relation. Because the goal of research in analogue settings is the discovery of behavioral processes, the length and number of sessions are defined by how long it takes to reveal the behavioral process and demonstrate a functional relation.

In natural settings the issue of sampling settings is more complex, and the best solution to the problem is to base your sampling procedures on the scope of experimental question. If the experimental question focuses on learning a certain type of mathematics performance in an algebra class, then the focus of the investigation should be on solving mathematics problems in that classroom. If the experimental question addresses the generalization of mathematical problem solving, then a larger set of contexts may be appropriate. If your experimental question is one that focuses on the entire school day or behaviors that occur at home or in the community, then those environments also need to be sampled. This does not mean that these settings have to be observed all of the time; it means only that the observations that are conducted need to reflect what occurs in those settings.

A fundamental rule in selecting the setting(s) to be sampled in a study is this: What you choose to sample will define how broadly you can draw conclusions about your findings. An important issue to attend to is whether the settings being sampled match your experimental question; otherwise, what can be concluded will be limited to what settings you have sampled. For example, if you want to study mathematical problem solving during the school day but you only sample behaviors from a single classroom setting, then your conclusions will be limited to behavior change observed in that single classroom setting. Any conclusion above and beyond that would only be speculation.

In addition, the amount of time sampled in the settings that are chosen needs to adequately represent the settings of experimental interest. The optimal choice is to observe the entire time period of experimental interest. If mathematical problem solving in algebra class is the focus of a study, then observing problem solving during the entire class period might be optimal. However, for instances where resources do not permit *exhaustive sampling* (i.e., observing the entire time period of interest), then *selective sampling* is necessary. A rule of thumb is that the sampling that occurs should closely match what would be observed if exhaustive sampling were conducted. Ideally, this sampling strategy would be empirically demonstrated (i.e., a direct comparison would be conducted). However, when an empirical demonstration is not feasible, then researchers often revert to logical arguments that the sampling strategy was adequate to address the experimental question. The former is more convincing, the latter more common.

Finally, a related issue is the occurrence of the responses and stimuli of interest. The amount of time sampled needs to allow for the responses and stimuli to occur multiple times. If the observational time frame is too restricted, then the responses and stimuli of interest will not be adequately sampled. This is typically not a concern for frequently occurring behaviors (e.g., solving mathematics problems), but can be a significant procedural challenge when dealing with behaviors or stimuli that occur infrequently (e.g., refusing to accept a car ride from a stranger). Often, the only realistic solution to studying infrequently occurring responses and stimuli is to resort to analogue settings that can simulate the occurrence of these events to generate a rate of occurrence that is acceptable for analysis.

Training Observers

Observer errors, whether using computerized or paper-and-pencil recording systems, are the primary source of error in observational data. Because of this fact, researchers need to train observers to collect data on behaviors and stimuli with the greatest accuracy and fidelity possible. In this section, we will discuss steps that researchers can follow to help ensure that their data are collected with the greatest possible integrity.

The first step in training observers is fairly obvious: You need to identify and select individuals who can serve as data collectors. There is no specific rule about who can, or cannot, serve as observers, but there are some general characteristics and logistical issues that need to be considered. A general set of requirements is that each observer needs to be punctual, commit the effort to learn the observational code, accept critical feedback about the quality of observations, and show the appropriate etiquette for the settings being observed. An additional positive characteristic is that the individual is willing to stay with the research team for an extended amount of time (i.e., several years) so that effort of training novice observers is minimized. Beyond these requirements, anyone willing to serve as a research assistant can effectively collect high-quality direct observation data.

Following the selection and hiring of observers, university-approved ethics training needs to be conducted. All institutions of higher education or research institutes have an institutionally sanctioned training program for new research staff that has been approved by funding agencies (e.g., the National Institutes of Health). The training typically involves issues of confidentiality, observer etiquette, data storage and reporting, and accuracy of information.

The next step is to systematically train observers. The first requirement is that each observer memorize the observational code and the definition of each event in the code. This should be followed by discussion of examples that are positive and negative instances of events in the observational code. Once observers verbally understand the observational code, they need to be introduced to the recording system and recording medium that will be used. Often, observers practice by observing videotaped examples of the types of situations they will be observing. Typically, this entails watching a videotaped example, discussing individual occurrences of behavior and stimuli, coming to agreement on their categorization, agreeing on how the events will be physically recorded, and so on. This then proceeds into observers independently and silently scoring videos. These data are then analyzed using an index of *interobserver agreement* (see Chapter 9) to estimate the extent to which two observers are consistent with each other. Typically, training continues until a minimum of 80% interobserver agreement is reached, although the higher the agreement, the better.

At this point, observational sessions in the settings where data will be collected can be conducted. An important issue to be aware of when first entering an environment is that of *observational reactivity*. "Reactivity" stems from how people in a classroom or another educational setting change their behavior when novel observers are introduced into the situation. This change in behavior can result in spurious baseline data. Therefore, initial observations are generally considered *in vivo* training opportunities (i.e., nonexperimental data) to allow observers and those being observed to adapt to the data collection process.

An additional element of observer training is periodic retraining (or "recalibration"), typically using the original training materials. The reason for this retraining is to avoid what is referred to as *observer drift*. Observer drift occurs when, during the course of an experiment, the definitions observers are using implicitly or explicitly change. For example, in baseline, observers may score any hand-to-head contact as an instance of self-injury, but as the experiment unfolds, what is recorded might change to only hand-to-head events that look forceful. This drift in the coding criterion would likely result in a decreased number of events being recorded, which could undesirably alter the experimental outcomes and interpretation of the data. To minimize the occurrence of observer drift, periodic retraining is conducted to help ensure that the original definitions are used throughout a study.

Recording Independent Variables

Typically, data are collected only in regard to the dependent measures used in a study. This is a necessary set of procedures that allow researchers to monitor the dependent variables of interest. However, rarely do researchers collect quantitative information on their independent variables (Gresham et al., 1993; Ledford & Gast, 2014). Indeed, Gresham et al. (1993) estimated that only 9% of published studies present data on the independent variable. As was noted by Peterson et al. (1982), "a curious double standard has developed in operant technology whereby certain variables (e.g., social behavior, smiling, and attention) routinely have operational definitions and some measure of observer reliability when the observed behavior is the target response or dependent variable, but no such rigor is applied as antecedents or consequences to the target behavior, as independent variables" (pp. 478–479). This oversight is indeed strange, given the rigor and precision that is the hallmark of single-case designs. For researchers not to measure the status of their interventions relative to changes in behavior seems an important oversight. Such measures allow for an assessment of the integrity of the independent variable during the conduct of an experiment.

The primary concern when data are not collected regarding the status of the independent variable is that the researchers cannot objectively establish the degree to which an intervention is implemented with fidelity. Without this information, we can only assume that the independent variable was implemented with precision and consistency. However, given the complexities of educational settings, this is probably a fallacious assumption. In the absence of this type of information, researchers and consumers cannot assess the degree to which variation in the dependent variable covaries with the independent variable in anything other than a binomial manner. That is, we have to follow the researchers' verbal statements that the intervention is present or absent, but we do not have data that allow measurement along a continuous scale. It would seem like the collection of data regarding the independent variable would be desirable in terms of quantitatively estimating the presence and extent of the independent variable and how dependent and independent variables covary during a study.

When researchers do collect data on their independent variables, this information is often referred to as *treatment integrity, intervention fidelity,* or *implementation reliability* data. The collection of this type of information requires several steps be taken by researchers. First, the independent variable needs to be operationally defined. Second, dimensional quantities need to be selected that adequately characterize the intervention. Third, a recording system needs to be developed to gather information regarding the independent variable. Fourth, a recording medium needs to be identified. Finally, observers need to be trained in the use of the recording system and achieve a consistent level of interobserver agreement.

An example of a study where data were collected regarding dependent and independent variables is provided by Kennedy (1994). As shown in Figure 8.6, two variables were tracked in relation to student behavior: problem behavior and social affect. In addition, two variables were tracked in relation to teacher behavior: task demands and social comments. Because task demands and social comments were the two primary elements of the independent variable, this

---

FIGURE 8.6 ■ Example of Data Collection Regarding Dependent and Independent Variables.

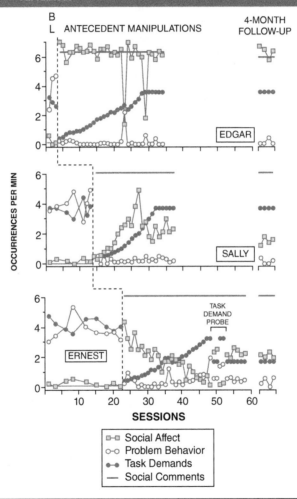

Note. Frequency of occurrence is plotted along the vertical axis and sessions along the horizontal axis for three students, Edgar, Sally, and Ernest. Two variables were tracked in relation to student behavior: problem behavior (open circles) and social affect (shaded squares). In addition, two variables were tracked in relation to teacher behavior: task demands (closed circles) and social comments (solid line). Because task demands and social comments were the two primary elements of the independent variable, this measurement arrangement constitutes a treatment integrity check. (Figure 2, p. 166 from: Kennedy, C. H. (1994). Manipulating antecedent conditions to alter the stimulus control of problem behavior. *Journal of Applied Behavior Analysis, 27,* 161–170. Copyright 1994 by the Society for the Experimental Analysis of Behavior. Reproduced by permission.)

arrangement constitutes a treatment integrity check. During baseline, task demands occurred at a consistent rate, as did the problem behaviors of Edgar, Sally, and Ernest. Positive affect (student behavior) and social comments (teacher behavior) were low during baseline. The independent variable consisted of the teacher making frequent social comments and gradually increasing the number of demands. Over time, demands were increased to baseline levels, but problem behaviors occurred at much lower rates than in baseline. This arrangement allowed for the documentation of how student and teacher behavior covaried during the study.

By documenting the degree to which an independent variable is implemented with fidelity (i.e., the degree to which it was designed to be implemented), researchers gain the ability to more closely track changes in behavior relative to implementation and withdrawal of interventions. This process allows for more definitive statements to be made regarding the interrelation between interventions and dependent measures. Not only does this allow more precise conclusions to be drawn, but it also allows for the potential analysis of parametric variations in the independent variable and how they may, or may not, influence behaviors of educational interest.

CONCLUSION

This chapter has reviewed the basics of recording systems, one element involved in the development and use of measurement systems to estimate the occurrence of experimental events. In combination with the chapters on dimensional quantities and interobserver agreement, this chapter provides the basis for gathering quantitative information regarding dependent and independent variables. Because of the importance of observational data to applied research in educational settings, the issues discussed in Part III of this book need to be carefully adhered to. Otherwise, the data being collected, no matter how elegant they may look in graphic form (see Chapter 16), will not be of interest because they will not accurately reflect the events that were of experimental interest.

REFLECTION QUESTIONS

1. What elements constitute the key aspects of an observational recording system, and why?

2. How do dimensional quantities and different approaches to recording information differ from each other? How might they be the same?

3. Which recording methods directly measure a specific dimensional quantity rather than estimate its occurrence?

4. In what situation might you want to use whole-interval recording, rather than the other two types of behavioral estimation methods, to measure responding?

5. What advantages and/or disadvantages do paper-and-pencil versus digital recording approaches have relative to each other?

9 VARIABLE INTEGRITY

LEARNING OBJECTIVES

After reading this chapter, you will be able to

9.1   Illustrate the rationale for collecting interobserver agreement in achieving variable integrity.

9.2   Utilize several methods for calculating interobserver agreement.

9.3   Determine acceptable outcome levels, frequency of agreement checks, and the interaction between levels and frequency in interobserver checks.

9.4   Evaluate three key elements in developing and implementing procedural fidelity assessments.

If all recordings of behavior could be automated, then measurement issues in single-case designs would be greatly simplified. All that would need to be done is calibrate the apparatus for accuracy, collect the data after they are recorded, and maintain the integrity of the machine. However, many of the environments and behaviors of interest in educational research do not lend themselves to automated recording. For example, most of the behaviors engaged in during recess or lunch would be difficult to mechanically record. Similarly, social interactions during class or the occurrence of challenging behaviors may not readily be mechanically recorded.

Because of this characteristic of applied settings, researchers have developed a set of procedures over the last 60 years to carefully measure behavior in real-life settings. One aspect of these measurement procedures not discussed in Chapter 8 is the issue of *variable integrity*. This term refers to monitoring the consistency with which dependent and independent variables (and extraneous variables, if warranted) are being measured during a study. The goal is to quantitatively establish the degree to which measures that are being taken of people's behavior are consistent. When measuring the integrity of dependent variable recording, synonyms for these procedures are *interobserver agreement, interrater reliability*, and simply *reliability*. In the remainder of the book, I will use *interobserver agreement* to refer to these procedures as a matter of convention, but the terms are interchangeable. We will also discuss the parallel case of measuring the integrity of the independent variable. This process is referred to as *procedural fidelity*.

In this chapter, we will first review interobserver agreement and then discuss procedural fidelity estimates.

WHY COLLECT INTEROBSERVER AGREEMENT?

When behavior cannot be automatically recorded, researchers using single-case designs rely on human beings to score when a particular behavior occurs or does not occur. By its very nature this process introduces unwanted variability into the measurement process. That variability takes the form of not recording with perfect consistency the occurrence or nonoccurrence of each of the variables of interest. The introduction of human error into the recording process requires that certain steps be taken to monitor and assess the types of errors that might be occurring.

Collecting interobserver agreement data allows researchers to monitor and assess the integrity with which information regarding dependent variables is being recorded. Typically, two trained observers *independently* record the behaviors of interest at the same time using the same measurement procedures. The independence of those observations is important because it ensures that what is being recorded is the sole product of the person producing the recording. This independence allows for an objective comparison of how two different people capture the occurrence and nonoccurrence of behavior using the measurement system. By doing this, a researcher can estimate the degree to which two separate people using the recording procedure agree on what occurred and did not occur.

Notice the careful language that is being used in the discussion of interobserver agreement data. When discussing interobserver agreement, people use words like *agreement, reliable*, and *consistent* to describe how the data are interpreted. Researchers avoid using terms like *accuracy, exactness*, and *truthfulness*. This is because even though two individuals can independently record behavior and perfectly agree on its occurrence and nonoccurrence, they both can be equally inaccurate in their recording of behavior (Deitz, 1988; Johnston et al., 2020). Hence, interobserver agreement data allow for an assessment of the consistency with which two observers agree about the recording of behavior, but it is not a measure of the accuracy of their recordings.

For interobserver agreement data to be collected, both observers should be trained on the use of the same behavioral code, recording system, and observational contexts. If this rather obvious criterion is met, then the independent recording of the same behavioral situation allows a researcher to assess the degree to which different observers agree. This is important for at least three reasons.

First, estimating interobserver agreement can be used as a training standard for new data recorders. After a new observer has been trained on an observational code and recording procedure, having that person record behavior at the same time as an experienced data collector allows for a quantitative index of their agreement. This facilitates being able to estimate the degree to which the new observer is recording behavior in a similar manner to more experienced observers. A calibration strategy such as this allows for a consistent standard to be established regarding when new observers have been adequately trained in observational techniques.

A second reason to collect interobserver agreement data—the primary reason—is to estimate how consistent data recorders are when collecting data during the experiment.

This allows for an unambiguous estimation of the degree to which various observers during a study were able to use the measurement system to record behavioral events. Presenting this information to others allows them to judge the degree to which data were collected with consistency among observers. The higher the degree of interobserver agreement, the more consistent observers were in their use of the measurement system. That is, changes in the status of a variable (e.g., a dependent variable) are likely due to changes in the experimental situation (e.g., introduction of the independent variable), rather than variability introduced by different observers. This information is typically reported in the Method section of a manuscript (see Box 9.1).

BOX 9.1: WHERE DO RESEARCHERS REPORT INTEROBSERVER AGREEMENT DATA WHEN PUBLISHING THEIR FINDINGS?

Occasionally, researchers mistakenly report interobserver agreement outcomes in the Results section of a manuscript, rather than in the Method section. Along with artificially separating the interobserver agreement procedures and formulas from the resulting data, it also mischaracterizes what these data represent. Interobserver agreement data are not the result of an experimental analysis, like the percentage of intervals of a behavior or the duration of an event. Instead, interobserver agreement data are integrity checks on how the observational system is being used to collect information. Because of this, interobserver agreement data are procedural checks on the consistency with which the measurement system was used and are, therefore, not results of the study, but an integral part of the procedures used to conduct the investigation. Given this observation, it is most accurate to report agreement procedures, formulas, and outcomes in a section at the end of the Method, titled *Interobserver Agreement*.

A third reason to collect interobserver agreement information is to avoid *observer drift*. Observer drift occurs when the original definitions used by observers in a behavioral code shift during the course of a study (Kazdin, 1977). For example, the behavior, hitting one's head against objects, might be operationally defined as contact of a person's head with any object. However, over the course of the study, observers might begin to judge *intentionality* and record precursor behaviors (e.g., moving the head toward an object) as if they were head hits (see Figure 9.1 for a visualized example of observer drift). This drift in the use of the definition could seriously threaten the integrity of data being collected. To help keep observer drift from occurring, ongoing review of observational codes by observers as a form of recalibration and the collection of interobserver agreement checks in each phase of the study are typically used. In addition, many researchers use videotapes of events for retraining of observers as a means of ensuring consistency not only among observers but within observers over time.

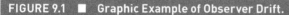

> **FIGURE 9.1** ■ **Graphic Example of Observer Drift.**

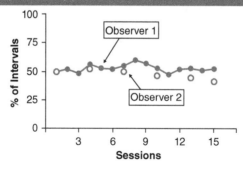

Note. The figure shows two observers (1 and 2) and their recordings of behavior represented on the *y*-axis as percentage of intervals. Initially the observers have a high level of consistency, but over time the two observers' scores separate with Observer 1 remaining constant and Observer 2 "drifting" lower. (From Figure 1, p. 74: Artman, K., Wolery, M., & Yoder, P. (2012). Embracing our visual inspection and analysis tradition: Graphing interobserver agreement data. *Remedial and Special Education, 33*(2), 71–77. Copyright 2012 by Hammill Institute on Disabilities. Reproduced by permission.)

DIFFERENT FORMULAS FOR CALCULATING INTEROBSERVER AGREEMENT

The previous sections of this chapter provided you with a general idea of what interobserver agreement is and why this type of data is collected. In this section we will discuss various approaches to summarizing and calculating interobserver agreement data (see Shoukri, 2003; Watkins & Pacheco, 2000). The review of formulas will be selective and not encompass either correlational approaches or complex statistical approaches (see Box 9.2). Instead, what we will review are approaches to estimating interobserver agreement that are currently used in single-case research—that is, approaches to calculating interobserver agreement that researchers have found useful in conducting research.

BOX 9.2: INTEROBSERVER AGREEMENT, CORRELATIONS, AND BASE RATES

Two additional approaches to calculating interobserver agreement are not discussed in this book, even though there are precedents for doing so. However, each is not discussed for a different reason. The first is the use of correlation coefficients (typically, *Pearson product-moment coefficients*) to estimate interobserver agreement. An important flaw in the use of correlation coefficients to compute interobserver agreement is that extremely high correlations can be obtained even if the observers never actually agree on an occurrence of behavior. As long as the two scores increase or decrease their estimates in a similar proportion, the correlation between what is recorded will be very high.

A second type of interobserver agreement not discussed in the text is *kappa* (*k*). The *k* statistic was initially developed by Cohen (1960) and suggested for use in calculating interobserver agreement by Hartmann (1977). The goal of using *k* in interobserver agreement calculations is an intellectually valid one: The statistic controls for some of the *base rate* issues inherent in the recording of behavior. By base rate, what is meant is the probability of occurrence associated with a particular behavior. If behaviors occur very frequently (i.e., have a high base rate), the chance that two observers will randomly agree a behavior occurred is increased relative to behaviors that occur less frequently. This statistical phenomenon inflates the estimation of interobserver agreement. The *k* statistic compensates for base rate issues by introducing a correction for random agreements. Although *k* has certain merits, it is rarely reported in the research literature relating to single-case designs. Therefore, although the goals associated with the use of this statistic are meritorious, its lack of use by researchers argues against its utility in estimating interobserver agreement.

Table 9.1 presents a hypothetical data set that will be used to illustrate the different approaches to calculating interobserver agreement. Data were recorded using a 10-second partial-interval recording procedure. There are 10 intervals of observation present in the table. Two observers (1 and 2) independently recorded the response of interest. The first time that a response was observed to occur in an interval was recorded as an *R*. In the first interval, neither observer recorded a response. In the second interval, both observers recorded the occurrence of a response. During the third interval, only Observer 1 recorded the occurrence of a response, and so on. Overall, Observer 1 recorded 5 occurrences of the response, as did Observer 2.

Total Agreement

A straightforward way of calculating interobserver agreement is to use a *total agreement* approach (also known as the *frequency-ratio* approach). Using a total agreement strategy, a researcher sums the total number of responses recorded by each observer, divides the smaller total by the larger total, and multiplies the amount by 100% (see Araujo & Born, 1985). The formula for total agreement is

$$S / L \times 100\%$$

where *S* is the smaller total and *L* is the larger total. Using the data in Table 9.1 to calculate total agreement would require the following steps: (a) Observer 1 recorded 5 responses. (b) Observer 2 recorded 5 responses. (c) Since the values are equivalent, either can serve as the numerator or

TABLE 9.1 ■ Hypothetical Data on the Occurrence and Nonoccurrence of a Single Response (R)										
	10-Second Intervals									
	1	2	3	4	5	6	7	8	9	10
Observer 1		R	R			R		R	R	
Observer 2		R		R		R		R	R	

denominator. (d) The result of dividing 5 by 5 is 1. (e) Multiplying 1 by 100% equals 100%. Therefore, using total agreement as an index of interobserver agreement for the data in Table 9.1 results in an outcome of 100% agreement.

A benefit of total agreement is that it is easy to conceptualize and calculate. A second benefit is that it can be used to calculate interobserver agreement in instances where observers have not accurately aligned their intervals (i.e., one observer began recording during the first interval, but the second did not begin until the third interval). A third advantage of using total agreement is that it is relatively sensitive to overall levels of responding.

With those benefits noted, however, *there is an important limitation to using a total agreement approach for estimating interobserver agreement.* Although this approach to interobserver agreement does provide an index of the overall occurrence of behavior, it does not provide an estimation of whether both observers agree on the occurrence of individual instances of behavior. Therefore, you can arrive at high levels of agreement but may have never agreed on the occurrence of a single behavior. For example, if the pattern of data collection shown in Table 9.1 during Intervals 3 and 4 were repeated throughout an observational session, using total agreement as an estimate of interobserver agreement, the outcome would be 100% agreement. Clearly, this is an issue of concern in terms of interpreting what the datum actually represents.

Interval Agreement

An approach to calculating interobserver agreement that takes into account when behavior occurs is *interval agreement.* This approach to estimating interobserver agreement is also referred to as *combined, point-by-point,* or *overall* agreement (Watkins & Pacheco, 2000). Interval agreement requires an interval system of measurement be used to record behavior. To calculate interval agreement, the recording of behavior is compared between the two observers on an interval-by-interval basis. Note that one observer is identified as the "primary" observer whose recordings are used as the reference standard for other observers. If both observers recorded the response as occurring or not occurring in a particular interval, it is scored as an *agreement.* If one observer recorded the occurrence of a response in an interval but the secondary observer did not, it is considered a *disagreement.* Then, the total number of agreements is divided by the total number of agreements plus disagreements, and the sum is multiplied by 100%. The formula for interval agreement is

$$A/(A + D) \times 100\%$$

where A is agreements and D is disagreements.

This approach requires the following steps: (a) Score each interval as an agreement or disagreement. (b) Sum the number of agreements. (c) Sum the number of disagreements. (d) Divide the number of agreements by the number of agreements plus disagreements. (e) Multiply the quantity from Step d by 100%. Using the data from Table 9.2 would result in the following calculations: Agreements were scored for 8 of the intervals, and disagreements were scored for 2 of the intervals. Dividing 8 by 10 results in 0.8. Multiplying this product by 100% results in an interobserver agreement score of 80%.

TABLE 9.2 ■ Hypothetical Data on the Occurrence and Nonoccurrence of a Response (R)										
	10-Second Intervals									
	1	2	3	4	5	6	7	8	9	10
Observer 1[a]		R	R			R		R	R	
Observer 2		R		R		R		R	R	
	A	A	D	D	A	A	A	A	A	A

Note. A = agreement; D = disagreement.

[a] Primary observer.

Clearly, interval agreement is more precise than total agreement for estimating interobserver agreement. That precision stems from the interval-by-interval basis for comparing the data. Such a procedure allows for overall estimation of how two observers scored behavior, but does so based on specific time units. Because of these positive features, interval agreement has become one of the most commonly used indexes of interobserver agreement.

Interval agreement does have a drawback that relates to the *base rate* of behavior (see Box 9.2). Because this approach to interobserver agreement scores agreements on an interval-by-interval basis, at very high or low occurrences of a response it may not adequately represent whether observers actually agreed on the occurrence or nonoccurrence of responding (Bijou et al., 1968). For example, if behavior was scored only once during an observation, similar to Table 9.2, and the observers disagreed on its occurrence, interval agreement would still be very high (i.e., 90%). However, in this case the observers would never have agreed on the occurrence of the response. A similar inflation of the interobserver agreement index occurs when behaviors occur very frequently. Because of this concern, researchers have developed a more stringent interobserver agreement scoring strategy called occurrence/nonoccurrence agreement.

Occurrence/Nonoccurrence Agreement

An even more stringent approach to estimating interobserver agreement is to calculate interval agreement for both the occurrence and nonoccurrence of a behavior. Referred to as *occurrence/nonoccurrence agreement*, this approach allows for the calculating of two agreement coefficients: one for the *occurrence of the response* and one for the *nonoccurrence of the response*. This strategy does not suffer from inflation by extremely high or low rates of events because the dual-reporting structure of the interobserver agreement measure allows for the separation of the occurrence and nonoccurrence of the same event (Hawkins & Dotson, 1975).

The formula for occurrence/nonoccurrence agreement is the same as interval agreement, except two separate calculations are conducted, one for the agreement and one for nonagreement. Each statistic is then reported separately (cf. Johnson & Bolstad, 1973). To calculate interval agreement, one observer is designated as the *primary observer* (e.g., Observer 1 in Table 9.3) and the other observer as the *secondary observer* (e.g., Observer 2 in table 9.3). To calculate *occurrence agreement*, each time a response was recorded by the primary observer, a check is made regarding whether the secondary observer also recorded an occurrence. If both observers scored the occurrence of a behavior, then an "occurrence agreement" is tallied (denoted as A+ in Table 9.3). If Observer 1 scored an occurrence and Observer 2 scored a nonoccurrence, then an "occurrence disagreement" is tallied (denoted as D+ in Table 9.3). The remainder of the calculation is the same as for interval agreement.

To calculate *nonoccurrence agreement*, each time a response was scored as not occurring by the primary observer, a check is made regarding whether the secondary observer scored the interval as a nonoccurrence. If both observers scored the nonoccurrence of a behavior, then an "nonoccurrence agreement" is tallied. If Observer 1 scored a nonoccurrence and Observer 2 scored an occurrence, then a "nonoccurrence disagreement" is tallied. Again, the remainder of the calculation is the same as for interval agreement.

Using this process with the data from Table 9.3, occurrence agreement would result in the following outcomes being tallied: occurrence agreement for Intervals 2, 6, 8, and 9 and occurrence disagreement for Interval 3. Using the interval agreement formula, we would calculate 4 divided by 5 (four plus one) multiplied by 100% equals 80%. Nonoccurrence agreement for Intervals 1, 5, 7, and 10 and occurrence disagreement for Interval 4. Using the interval agreement formula, we would calculate 4 divided by 5 (four plus one) multiplied by 100% equals 80%. The result would be reported as the observers obtaining 80% occurrence agreement and 80% nonoccurrence agreement for the behavior of interest.

A variation on the separate reporting of occurrence and nonoccurrence agreement outcomes was proposed by Hawkins and Dotson (1975). These authors proposed deriving a mean from the occurrence and nonoccurrence agreement outcomes (which would be 80% in our example) and using this produce as an estimate of interobserver agreement. This approach is referred to as *mean occurrence/nonoccurrence agreement*. Although mentioned here for completeness, this approach to combining interobserver coefficients is rarely reported in the contemporary research literature.

TABLE 9.3 ■ Hypothetical Data on the Occurrence and Nonoccurrence of a Response (R)										
	10-Second Intervals									
	1	2	3	4	5	6	7	8	9	10
Observer 1[a]		R	R			R		R	R	
Observer 2		R		R		R		R	R	
	A–	A+	D+	D–	A–	A+	A–	A+	A+	A–

Note. A = agreement; D = disagreement; "+" = occurrence; "–" = nonoccurrence.

[a]Primary observer.

Occurrence/nonoccurrence agreement is an increasingly common means of reporting interobserver agreement (Kelly, 1977; Watkins & Pacheco, 2000). It is the most rigorous of the commonly used approaches to interobserver agreement and, because of this characteristic, is the preferred means of calculating interobserver agreement. Sometimes, for thoroughness, researchers will report both interval agreement (as an overall index of interobserver agreement) and occurrence/nonoccurrence agreement to fully characterize the degree to which consistency was obtained by different observers during a study.

Additional Interobserver Agreement Approaches

There are several additional approaches to calculating interobserver agreement that are used by researchers depending on the characteristics of the dimensional quantities of behavior and recording systems being used.

Exact Agreement

Repp et al. (1976) proposed an approach to scoring event-by-interval data referred to as *exact agreement*. Using this approach, a researcher scores whether two observers scored the same number of behavioral events during each interval of observation. Table 9.4 shows a hypothetical data set we will use to calculate exact agreement. To calculate exact agreement we will use the A divided by A plus D multiplied by 100% formula. Using the data from Table 9.4, we will score Intervals 1, 2, 5, 7, 8, and 10 as agreements and Intervals 3, 4, 6, and 9 as disagreements. Therefore, 6 divided by 10 multiplied by 100% equals 60%.

The strength of this approach to interobserver agreement is also its greatest weakness. That is, because the criterion for an agreement is so rigorous, it is difficult to obtain a satisfactory level of interobserver agreement. (For this reason, we will *not* discuss the possibility of creating formulas for occurrence/nonoccurrence exact agreement!)

Duration or Latency Agreement

To calculate interobserver agreement for either duration or latency data, researchers use the total agreement approach we discussed previously (i.e., $S/L \times 100\%$). For example, the total duration of behavior recorded might equal 300 seconds for Observer 1 and 264 seconds for Observer 2, which would result in 88% interobserver agreement. Similarly, if the total latency of behavior

TABLE 9.4 ■ Hypothetical Data for the Event-by-Interval Recording of a Single Response (the Number Within Each Interval Is the Frequency of Occurrence)										
	10-Second Intervals									
	1	2	3	4	5	6	7	8	9	10
Observer 1		3	1			6		1	2	
Observer 2		3		1		4		1	1	

recorded was 75 seconds for Observer 1 and 84 seconds for Observer 2, the result would be 89% interobserver agreement. Whether calculating duration or latency agreement using this method, the same limitations discussed previously apply and need to be taken into account when interpreting the interobserver agreement outcomes.

Event or Permanent Product Agreement

As with duration or latency, when calculating event or permanent product agreement, the total agreement approach is warranted. For example, if 42 behavioral products were scored by Observer 1 and 40 were scored by Observer 2, then 95% interobserver agreement would be obtained. Even with its liabilities, total agreement is the most appropriate statistic to use with event or permanent product data.

LEVELS AND FREQUENCIES OF INTEROBSERVER AGREEMENT

So far we have been discussing why to collect interobserver agreement data and methods for calculating the estimates. At this point, it is time to talk about what outcome levels are *acceptable for interobserver agreement* and *how frequently this information needs to be gathered*. We will initially discuss each of these concepts separately, but by their nature an appropriate treatment of this topic requires an elaboration of how they interrelate.

Acceptable Interobserver Agreement Outcomes

Given the formulas we have just discussed and the various numbers that were derived from our calculations, the question of how high these levels need to be is raised. Or, said another way, how high do the percentages have to be to be considered as acceptable levels of observer consistency? The *convention* used in applied research is that a minimum of 80% interobserver agreement needs to be achieved. However, this is only a convention. There is no scientific justification for why 80% is necessary, only a long history of researchers using this percentage as a benchmark of acceptability and being successful in their research activities (see Hausman et al., 2022).

There are, of course, factors that make the 80% standard either too high or too low. When using an observational code with multiple behaviors that have complex definitions, researchers often accept slightly lower interobserver agreement outcomes. Similarly, if the environments in which observations are conducted are very complex or challenging to collect data, lower estimates might be acceptable. The base rate of each behavior is also very important. High levels of agreement on behaviors that occur nearly continuously are not as impressive as when the same level of agreement is achieved for behaviors that occur at moderate or low rates. Each of these factors needs to be considered when weighing the acceptability of a particular interobserver agreement outcome.

Two additional factors need to be considered: (a) the type of interobserver agreement formula being used and (b) the sensitivity of behavior change relative to the independent variable. Obviously, if the same data set is considered and two agreement formulas are used that differ in the degree of stringency, different interobserver agreement estimates will be arrived at.

For example, in the previous section, for the data presented in Table 9.1, an outcome of 100% was obtained using total agreement and 80% using interval agreement. Therefore, it is critical that, when reporting interobserver agreement data, the specific formula be reported in the text so other researchers can judge the level that was obtained in relation to the statistic used to make the calculations. A final issue that requires consideration is the degree to which behavior changes from baseline to intervention. If there is a high degree of variability from one condition to the next or the level of behavior change is small across conditions, interobserver agreement outcomes will need to be higher. This is because the variability produced by the inconsistencies of observation may become greater than the effect of the independent variable.

Percentage of Observations

How many observational sessions need to have interobserver agreement data collected to adequately assess the consistency of measurement? *Again, there is no scientifically defensible standard that has been arrived at.* There are, however, conventions that have evolved over the last 40 years of applied research using single-case designs. In general, when discussing or reporting interobserver agreement data, the overall number of sessions included for agreement checks is expressed as a percentage. The current convention is that 20% of observations is a minimal percentage and 33% is preferable.

Interactions Between Levels and Frequencies of Interobserver Agreement

As should be clear by now, the collection of interobserver agreement data is a necessary and integral aspect of single-case research, and the interpretation of these data is largely based on convention. Along with the previously mentioned variables that influence how often to collect interobserver agreement data and what level should be achieved, there is one more consideration. In general, the higher the level of agreement obtained by observers, the lower the overall percentage of sessions that need to have agreement checks included. Or, stated conversely, the lower the level of agreement, the more sessions that need to be included in agreement checks. Overall, it is best to keep the purpose of interobserver agreement in mind when making decisions about how high and how often. That is, this type of data is collected to allow the researcher to estimate the consistency with which data are being collected and to use this information to arrive at an appropriate interpretation of the data that emerge from an investigation.

PROCEDURAL FIDELITY

A second broad form of variable integrity is *the measurement of how consistently the independent variable is administered.* As noted earlier in this chapter, the preferred term for this type of measurement is *procedural fidelity.* However, there are other terms that have been used in the literature such as *treatment integrity, treatment fidelity, procedural reliability, implementation fidelity,* and *independent variable integrity.* The current preferred term is *procedural fidelity* because not all independent variables in single-case designs are interventions or treatments, so *procedure* seems to be the most descriptive although *independent variable* is equally descriptive (if somewhat longer as a term). The word *fidelity* seems to have been adopted largely by convention.

The first articles presenting procedural fidelity as a means of documenting the independent variable were in the fields of neurodevelopmental disabilities (Billingsley et al., 1980) and clinical psychology (Yeaton & Sechrest, 1981) (see also Peterson et al., 1982). Since the early 1980s there has been an increasing trend in the use of procedural fidelity. An article by Ledford and Wolery (2013) showed a steady increase in the use of this measurement approach with approximately 70% of articles surveyed using procedural fidelity as part of their experimental methods in recent years (see Figure 9.2; see also DiGennaro Reed & Codding, 2014). There have also been calls for procedural fidelity to be *required* in single-case design studies (Horner et al., 2005).

Given the increasing use of procedural fidelity, it is safe to say that it has become a standard measure in single-case research studies. The importance of procedural fidelity is obvious. Documenting the degree to which the independent variable is accurately and consistently implemented is a procedural necessity for estimating the status of the intervention or procedure. Without such measures, one has no empirical evidence that the independent variable was implemented as described in the Procedures section of an experiment.

There are *three key elements* in developing and implementing procedural fidelity assessments. First, the intervention needs to be task analyzed to identify the critical steps that are used in the intervention (see Gresham et al., 1993; Strain et al., 2021). An example of this process is provided by Pennington and McComas (2017). The authors studied a well-established intervention referred as the good-behavior game (GBG) (Barrish et al., 1969). The GBG intervention

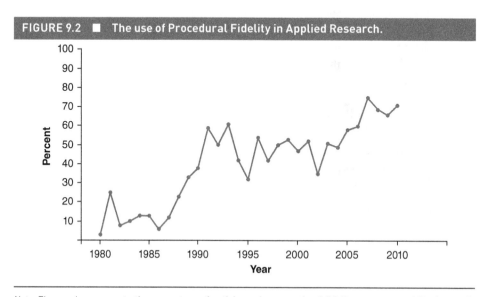

FIGURE 9.2 ■ The use of Procedural Fidelity in Applied Research.

Note. The *y*-axis represents the percentage of articles using procedural fidelity measures, while the *x*-axis shows the years that were assessed. (From Figure 1, p. 182: Ledford, J. R., & Wolery, M. (2013). Procedural fidelity: An analysis of measurement and reporting practices. *Journal of Early Intervention, 35*(2), 173–193. Copyright 2013 by Sage Publications. Reproduced by permission.)

was broken down into six steps: (a) "telling students the game was beginning, (b) only awarding points during the specified game time, (c) awarding points when the whole team or all team members within a group were on task, (d) not awarding points when team members were off task, (e) informing students when the game was finished, and (f) delivering prizes to the winning team" (Pennington & McComas, 2017, p. 178). These steps in the task analysis were the basis for defining key components of the independent variable using a checklist for recording each element of the intervention.

The second key element involves training the instructors in the implementation of the interventions. Using the task analysis from the previous key element, support providers are taught how to deliver the intervention as prescribed and to do so in a consistent manner. The third key element in assessing procedural fidelity is monitoring intervention delivery. Initially, observers are trained on examples and nonexamples of each step in the task analysis typically using in situ or videotaped sessions of exemplary instruction. Once trained, observers then collect data during baseline and independent variable conditions to assess the degree to which components of the interventions are being utilized. This approach allows for the documentation of what intervention components are and are not being delivered during various phases of an investigation.

As with interobserver agreement, the percentage of sessions subjected to procedural fidelity checks is between 20% and 33%. However, this is only a convention. There is also the need to conduct observer consistency checks when measuring the independent variable just as there is for the dependent variable (see Essig et al., 2023). The formulas used to calculate these assessments are the same as those used for interobserver agreement. Again, there seems to be a convention in the existing literature of $\geq$ 80% agreement between observers, but this too is a convention. One area still in need of development is the interrelation between the fidelity with which the independent variable is implemented and the resulting effect on the dependent variable(s). While it is intuitive that the higher the level of procedural fidelity, the greater the effect on the dependent variable(s), this is only an assumption and requires research to validate/invalidate the accuracy of this hypothesis (Baer et al., 1987).

CONCLUSION

Variable integrity data provides an important means of assessing the consistency with which the dependent and independent variables analyzed in a study are measured. Although variable integrity data do not establish whether observers' recordings are veridical, interobserver agreement and procedural fidelity information does allow for an estimate of whether different individuals could use a measurement system to collect consistent information. A variety of formulas can be used to collect this information, each of which varies in its level of rigor. In addition, there are a number of conventions that have developed regarding how often variable integrity data are gathered and what level of agreement should be obtained. However, there is no scientifically defensible standard other than to observe that the conventions allow researchers to effectively engage in research activities that are replicated by others.

REFLECTION QUESTIONS

1. Explain why correlations are considered poor estimates of interobserver agreement.

2. What are techniques for minimizing the occurrence of "observer drift"?

3. Why would using event-by-interval recording be considered more challenging than total agreement or similar measures?

4. Measuring the fidelity of treatment has become a very popular approach to estimating variable integrity. Why do you think this is the case?

5. Why do you think researchers use a fixed percentage of sessions and a fixed threshold of agreement when assessing interobserver agreement? Is this the best way?

DESIGN TACTICS

10 A-B-A-B DESIGNS

LEARNING OBJECTIVES

After reading this chapter, you will be able to

10.1 Apply an A-B-A-B design in an experimental inquiry, and determine when reversibility of behavior might present a concern.

10.2 Apply a B-A-B design.

10.3 Apply an A-B-C and associated designs.

10.4 Apply changing-criterion designs.

10.5 Compare and contrast A-B-A, A-B-A-B, A-B-A-B-A-B, B-A-B, and A-B-C and associated designs.

In the previous three sections, we have discussed general approaches to experimentation, the use of single-case designs, establishing functional relations, replication, and how to define and measure behavior. At this point we will turn our attention to design tactics used in single-case research to establish experimental control over the dependent variable by the independent variable. To review our previous definition, single-case designs are used to demonstrate experimental control over the behavior of a single participant. That individual participant serves as both the "control" and "experimental" participant to borrow phraseology from experimental and quasi-experimental group designs (Shadish et al., 2002). In addition, repeated sampling of the dependent variable occurs over time to establish patterns of behavior in baseline and intervention phases.

One design tactic that is at the heart of single-case designs in both frequency of use by researchers and how experimental control is established over behavior is the *A-B-A-B design*. This design tactic is at the core of single-case design logic and how experimental control is demonstrated. Before we discuss in detail the A-B-A-B design and its many variants, a review of more rudimentary designs discussed previously in Chapter 4 may be helpful. The central logic for all experimentation, whether single-case design or some other experimental approach, is the logic of planned comparisons (see Chapter 1). In general, planned comparisons take the form of two experimental conditions being compared to each other. Implicit in this definition is that some type of dependent variable is established and, at a minimum, is assessed in the presence and absence of an independent variable. Differences between the two phases can be attributed to the independent variable if certain preconditions are met.

In single-case designs, these preconditions are concisely referred to as the establishment of a *functional relation*. For single-case designs, all planned comparisons fall into the logic of how to arrange baseline (A) and intervention (B) conditions. In its most elemental form, all single-case designs are arrangements of *A-B conditions*. For example, establishing a baseline of reading fluency provides the opportunity to compare the same student's reading when the student is receiving some type of intervention. However, with an A-B arrangement, attributing any differences between the two conditions to the influence of the independent variable is premature. This interpretative limitation is necessary because of possible threats to internal validity (see Chapter 4).

To control for threats to internal validity, or at least minimize the possibility that extraneous variables are influencing experimental outcomes, researchers using single-case designs use the concept of *replication*. In this instance, to be precise, they use within-participant direct replication (see Chapter 5). That is, following an A-B sequence of experimental conditions, the researcher then reverts to the A condition to see if the original baseline pattern of behavior can be reestablished with the removal of the independent variable. If this is indeed the case, then our confidence increases that a functional relation is being established between independent and dependent variables. This type of experimental sequence is referred to as an *A-B-A design*.

A-B-A-B DESIGNS

An A-B-A design is the minimal type of experimental arrangement that can establish experimental control in single-case research. However, if the experimental situation permits, researchers prefer to reintroduce the independent variable at least once. Such an arrangement constitutes an *A-B-A-B design*. Thus, when using an A-B-A-B design the researcher begins with a baseline, introduces an intervention, returns to baseline, and then reintroduces the same intervention. If levels of the dependent variable(s) covary with the presence and absence of the independent variable, then a high degree of experimental control has been established over responding.

Researchers prefer to use A-B-A-B designs instead of A-B-A designs for at least two reasons. First, the A-B-A-B design allows for two separate instances of replication. The first possible replication occurs when the baseline is reintroduced (i.e., A-B-A). If successful, the baseline pattern of responding is reestablished following the removal of the independent variable. The second replication occurs when the intervention is reintroduced (i.e., A-B-A-B). Again, if successful, the initial experimental effect is reestablished for a second time. This A-B-A-B arrangement allows for the replication of both baseline patterns of behavior and intervention effects.

A second reason that researchers prefer using A-B-A-B designs to A-B-A designs is the applied nature of educational research. By its definition, applied behavior analysis focuses on "applications of the experimental analysis of behavior to problems of social importance" (*Journal of Applied Behavior Analysis* [*JABA*], 1968–present). Implicit in this statement is that researchers are focusing on instances in which a person is faced with a situation they and/or others are distressed by because of the occurrence of too many or too few behaviors. Therefore, if an intervention improves this problematic situation, it is ethically appropriate to end a study in a manner that permits the participant to receive the most beneficial intervention (i.e., A-B-A-B).

An example of an A-B-A-B design that appeared in the first issue of *JABA* is presented in Figure 10.1. In this study by Hall et al. (1968), the effect of contingent teacher praise on the task engagement of elementary school students was analyzed. The dependent variable was the percentage of intervals in which students were engaged with class activities. Baseline consisted of the teacher's typical instructional practices in the classroom. Students whose baseline levels of task engagement were the lowest in the class were selected for participation in the study. One such student was Robbie, who was noted as "a particularly disruptive student" (Hall et al., 1968, p. 3). The independent variable was comprised of training the teacher to provide contingent verbal praise to Robbie when he was engaged with class activities.

During the initial baseline, the student engaged in study behavior during approximately 30% of the observation intervals. When contingent teacher attention was provided to Robbie during the "reinforcement" phase, his task engagement increased over successive days. The teacher then reversed back to their baseline teaching strategies, and the student's engagement immediately decreased, generally replicating the previous baseline (see Box 10.1). Then, when

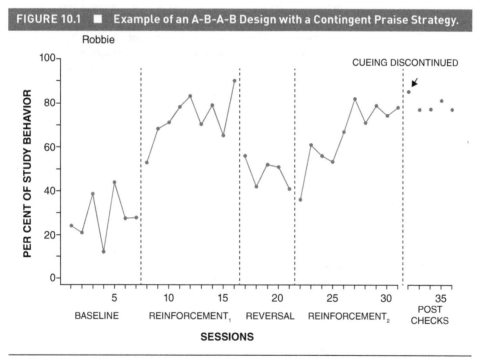

FIGURE 10.1 ■ Example of an A-B-A-B Design with a Contingent Praise Strategy.

Note. This graph highlights the effects of a teacher's contingent praise on the task engagement of a student with behavioral challenges, using an A-B-A-B design. The vertical axis represents the percentage of intervals in which Robbie was engaged in classroom learning activities. The intervention was the first demonstration of what later would evolve into the *good-behavior game*, an intervention that has become a common intervention for improving student performance in school settings. (Figure 1, p. 3, from: Hall, R. V., Lund, D., & Jackson, D. (1968). Effects of teacher attention on study behavior. *Journal of Applied Behavior Analysis, 1*(1), 1–12. Copyright 1968 by the Society for the Experimental Analysis of Behavior. Reproduced by permission.)

the independent variable was reintroduced, his performance improved a second time. The result was the establishment of a functional relation between the teacher's contingent praise and the student's task engagement using an A-B-A-B design.

BOX 10.1: DO WE REVERSE OR WITHDRAW INDEPENDENT VARIABLES?

A recurrent theme in this book is the precise use of language to minimize ambiguity or mis-communication. Using words that imply something that is not present can be misleading and result in the misinterpretation of research findings. However, adding to the difficulty in language use is that multiple terms are often used synonymously in a particular field of research, even though their dictionary meanings imply different things. Such is the case with the language relating to A-B-A-B designs. In particular, two terms are often used synonymously to refer to the act of moving from the B to A phases of the design. Those terms are *reversal* and *withdrawal*. It is common to read a passage such as "a reversal of the intervention to baseline was conducted." Equally common are phrases such as "the intervention was withdrawn and the procedures returned to baseline." There is a historical distinction in the use of the two terms in relation to A-B-A-B designs. The term *reversal* was initially used by Baer et al. (1968) in reference to the effect on behavior that occurs when the independent variable is removed. That is, levels of the behavior should reverse to baseline patterns of responding. However, Leitenberg (1973) noted that the term *withdrawal* was more accurate, because it describes the procedural act of removing the intervention without presuming that a change in behavior will occur. Whatever their histories and distinctions are, currently, both terms are used interchangeably when describing A-B-A-B designs, even though they imply slightly different meanings. Apparently, this distinction is more academic than practical for researchers.

A second example of an A-B-A-B design is provided by Angell et al. (2011) and is shown in Figure 10.2. In this instance, the investigators chose additional replications of the A-B format to conduct an A-B-A-B-A-B analysis. The study focused on a Power Card strategy to decrease the latency (in seconds) of initiating transitions during the school day. The students were preteens who had extensive support needs and were receiving special education services. Figure 10.2 shows the data for one participant (Quincy) across different school days and the effects of the Power Card strategy. During the initial baseline (labeled A_1), the student had a mean latency to comply of 29 seconds. When the intervention was introduced (labeled B_1), Quincy's compliance time dropped to 11 seconds. The authors then shifted back to baseline, recorded an increase in response latency replicating the previous baseline phase, and proceeded to conduct multiple replications of the Power Card effect in comparison to the baseline condition. Angell et al. replicated the effect shown in Figure 10.2 with two additional students.

Reversibility of Behavior

An important design issue when using A-B-A-B designs is whether the behavior change produced during the initial B phase will return to baseline levels during the second A phase. This

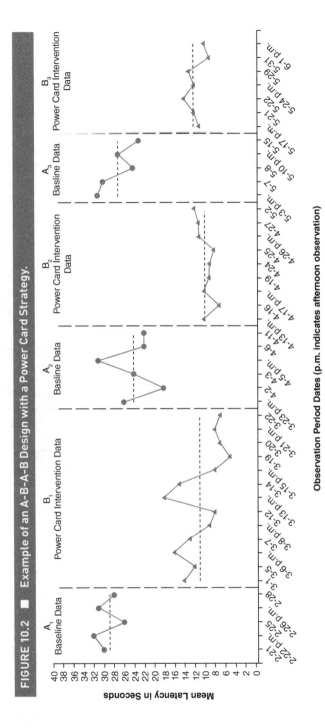

FIGURE 10.2 ■ Example of an A-B-A-B Design with a Power Card Strategy.

Observation Period Dates (p.m. indicates afternoon observation)

Note. The behavior of interest was the initiation of transition routines by a preteen with autism who often refused transition requests. The intervention used a Power Card strategy to initiate changes in routines. Observations were made across successive days labeled as the month-day on the x-axis. (Figure 2, p. 211, from: Angell, M. E., Nicholson, J. K., Watts, E. H., & Blum, C. (2011). Using a multicomponent adapted power card strategy to decrease latency during interactivity transitions for three children with developmental disabilities. *Focus on Autism and Other Developmental Disabilities, 26*(4), 206–217. Copyright 2011 by the Hammill Institute on Disabilities. Reproduced by permission.)

issue has been referred to the *reversibility of behavior* (Sidman, 1960). Because the logic of an A-B-A-B design is predicated on behavior changing from the first baseline to the first intervention phase and then changing back to baseline levels during the second baseline, reversibility of behavior is critical to the integrity of this experimental design. If no reversal back to baseline occurs during the second baseline phase, experimental control may be lost, and no functional relation has been demonstrated.

Such an effect is not unusual, particularly when the intervention introduces a new skill into the person's repertoire. Once a skill is learned, it is hard to reverse the effects of instruction. For example, once a student has learned that the written words *dog* and *hund* both refer to canines in English and Swedish, respectively, it is difficult to unlearn this information. Or, to be more precise, once a behavior is brought under *stimulus control*, such discriminative control over responding is difficult to disrupt (see Maguire & Allen, 2022; Sidman, 1994). Hence, when dealing with newly learned behaviors, the reversibility of what is learned has important implications for how you design your study. (Box 10.2 introduces a general type of single-case design that is particularly well suited for analyzing nonreversible behavior.)

BOX 10.2: CAN SINGLE-CASE DESIGNS BE USED TO ANALYZE NONREVERSIBLE BEHAVIOR?

An "urban legend" or "meme" researchers using single-case designs hear repeatedly from other researchers is that this approach to experimental design cannot be used to study nonreversible behavior. Examples provided often include learning sight words, addition, multiplication, and word definitions. This type of knowledge is often referred to as *cognitive processes* in educational research, but among behavior analysts the term *stimulus control* is typically used. In fact, researchers using $N = 1$ designs began developing experimental methods to study nonreversible behaviors beginning in the 1950s and have developed a range of experimental methods for studying such behavior. The most commonly used experimental approaches for studying these types of cognitive phenomena include repeated-acquisition designs. They were developed specifically for the analysis of nonreversible behavior and are a great resource for researchers using single-case designs. We will have a more in-depth discussion of these designs in Chapter 13.

An example of problems with reversibility of behavior using A-B-A-B designs is illustrated in Figure 10.3. In this analysis, De Prey and Sugai (2002) studied the effects of a supervision and precorrection intervention on the problem behaviors of a class of sixth graders. The classroom management strategy was studied in relation to the percentage of intervals in which minor behavioral infractions occurred during the social studies class. During the initial baseline phase, De Prey and Sugai documented consistently high levels of minor behavior problems (range, 89% to 100% of sessions). The intervention reduced these occurrences to approximately 50% of intervals by the 10th through 13th sessions. When the intervention was withdrawn, behavior problems in the classroom became more variable than during the final sessions of the first intervention phase, but the behaviors did not return to baseline levels and substantially overlapped with the previous intervention phase. However, when the classroom management techniques were reintroduced, clear decreases in minor behavior problems were observed.

The data in Figure 10.3 highlight two issues that should be considered in the use of A-B-A-B designs. First is the issue of reversibility. In the De Prey and Sugai (2002) study, the reversal in the pattern of behavior during the second baseline was weak. In fact, their experimental control relies primarily on the changes in behavior that occurred during the first intervention and the precipitous drop in behavior that occurred during the second intervention phase. This means that two data points (Sessions 17 and 18) are the primary basis for claiming experimental control. This observation raises the second consideration. When behaviors only partially reverse in an A-B-A-B experiment, it is often more convincing if additional baseline and intervention phases are conducted. Given the experimental results displayed in Figure 10.3, additional repeats would have added to the believability that the intervention was the primary source of behavioral control.

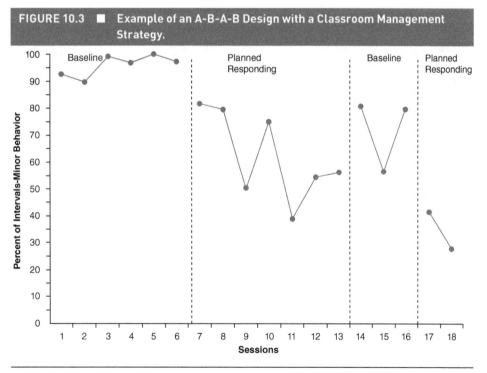

FIGURE 10.3 ■ Example of an A-B-A-B Design with a Classroom Management Strategy.

Note. This figure illustrates the effects of a supervision and precorrection intervention on the problem behaviors of a class of sixth graders. The classroom management strategy was studied in relation to the percentage of intervals in which minor behavioral infractions occurred during the social studies class. (Figure 1, p. 261, from: De Prey, R. L., & Sugai, G. (2002). The effect of active supervision and pre-correction on minor behavioral incidents in a sixth-grade general education classroom. *Journal of Behavioral Education, 11,* 255–262. Copyright 2002 by Human Sciences Press, Inc. Reproduced with permission from Springer Nature Customer Service Center.)

B-A-B DESIGNS

In some instances when a researcher seeks to conduct an experiment in educational settings, an intervention may already be in place. This might occur because an innovative teacher has developed their own intervention that appears to be effective and wants to test this hypothesis following the initial intervention. In other instances, an intervention may have been implemented prematurely with the establishment of experimental control only possible by using a variant of the A-B-A-B design type. A single-case design that is particularly effective in instances such as these is the *B-A-B design*.

B-A-B designs begin when an intervention has already been implemented. Experimental control using this type of design relies on the dependent variable being sensitive to the withdrawal or reversal of the independent variable during the B to A phase change. In addition, behavioral levels need to change again when the intervention is reintroduced in the second B phase. In this sense, the B-A-B is the inverse of the A-B-A design.

Use of a B-A-B design is illustrated in a study by McHugh et al. (2022) (see Figure 10.4). McHugh et al. began their analysis of mask wearing by adults with intellectual disabilities during the COVID-19 pandemic. The first participant they worked with, Ethan, began the experiment with an intervention in place (labeled SSR) that prompted and positively reinforced him for wearing a face covering. They observed a pattern in which he wore the mask for approximately

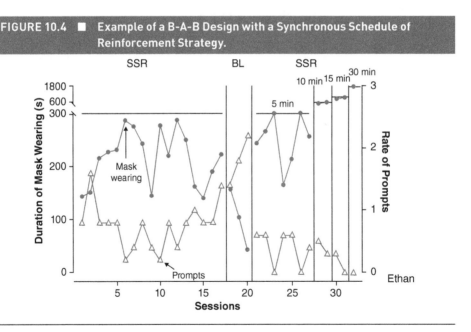

FIGURE 10.4 ■ Example of a B-A-B Design with a Synchronous Schedule of Reinforcement Strategy.

Note. This graph portrays the effects of a synchronous schedule of reinforcement on the mask wearing of an adult with intellectual disabilities. The duration of mask wearing (closed circles) and the number of staff prompts (open triangles) are arrayed along the vertical axes. (Figure 1, p. 1165, from: McHugh, C. L., Dozier, C. L., Diaz de Villegas, S. C., & Kanaman, N. A. (2022). Using synchronous reinforcement to increase mask wearing in adults with intellectual and developmental disabilities. *Journal of Applied Behavior Analysis, 55*(4), 1157–1171. Copyright 2022 by the Society for the Experimental Analysis of Behavior. Reproduced by permission.)

5 minutes per session. On Session 16 they removed the SSR intervention and observed mask wearing rapidly decrease across sessions. On Session 21 they reintroduced the independent variable and saw an immediate increase in mask wearing. Following this phase of the investigation, the authors gradually increased the time requirements for wearing the mask, which resulted in Ethan wearing his mask for 30-minute intervals with minimal staff prompting.

A second example of using a B-A-B design comes from the work of Pace and Toyer (2000). In this outpatient clinic example, the authors were presented with the case of a girl with severe disabilities whose parents had started her on an iron and multivitamin nutritional supplement (see Figure 10.5). The girl's case was referred to the behavioral clinic because she engaged in pica (i.e., eating indigestible objects), which can be life threatening. Her parents reported significant improvements in the girl's pica since they had begun the vitamin therapy. When Pace and Toyer assessed the occurrence of pica during the initial B phase, very few instances of pica were observed. When the multivitamin component of the intervention was removed and the girl

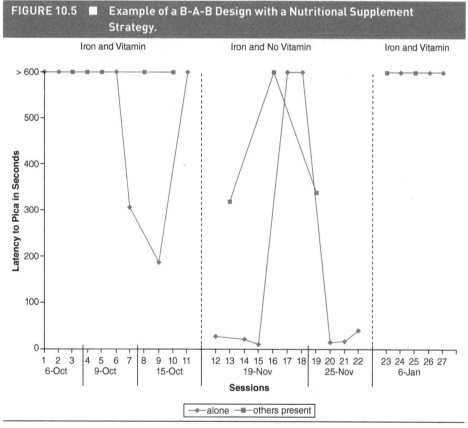

FIGURE 10.5 ■ Example of a B-A-B Design with a Nutritional Supplement Strategy.

This graph illustrates the effects of a multivitamin nutritional supplement on the occurrence of pica. The dependent variable was the latency to the first occurrence of pica, which was studied when an adult was present (closed square) or absent (closed diamond). (Figure 1, p. 621, from: Pace, G. M., & Toyer, E. A. (2000). The effects of a vitamin supplement on the pica of a child with severe mental retardation. *Journal of Applied Behavior Analysis, 33,* 619–622. Copyright 2000 by the Society for the Experimental Analysis of Behavior. Reproduced by permission.)

again was assessed in the clinic, she engaged in more instances of pica. This effect was reversed when the multivitamin was again given to her on a regular basis. Using a B-A-B design, Pace and Toyer provided provocative evidence that nutrition may be related to some cases of pica.

When using B-A-B designs, an additional baseline can be added to further replicate findings (i.e., B-A-B-A). Such direct replications can further increase the believability that a functional relation has been established between dependent and independent variables. If this pattern of direct replication is continued (e.g., B-A-B-A-B), then the B-A-B design begins to acquire many of the properties of the A-B-A-B design. A primary limitation of the B-A-B design is that there is no initial baseline pattern of behavior. This limits a researcher's ability to make statements about how the intervention impacted the initial pattern of behavior. That is, there is no evidence that the behavior was problematic prior to intervention, although if experimental control is demonstrated, behavior is worsened during the subsequent baseline phase. With this interpretative limitation of B-A-B designs noted, they are useful in situations when the analysis of previously implemented interventions is of interest to educational researchers.

A-B-C AND ASSOCIATED DESIGNS

An important variation of the A-B-A-B design is the *A-B-C and associated designs*. In the A-B-C design, an additional condition is added to the A-B-A-B analysis. That is, the "C" element in the A-B-C design provides the researcher with an additional opportunity to analyze how various conditions influence behavior. What makes A-B-C-B designs of particular interest to researchers is the opportunity to move beyond demonstration experiments (Chapter 5), which are typically the focus of A-B-A-B designs. That is, contrasting a baseline with an intervention phase allows a researcher to assess the degree to which the intervention alters the previously established baseline. However, with the addition of a C phase, a researcher has the possibility of conducing component, parametric, or comparative analysis. Not only can a single person be used as the experimental and control participant, but that person can also be used as a contrast participant. These types of experimental arrangements provide single-case researchers with a high degree of tactical flexibility when conducting analyses.

An example of an A-B-C design is provided by Goldstein et al. (1992). Figure 10.6 shows the results of a peer-mediated intervention analysis by Goldstein and colleagues. The frequency with which communicative acts and social behaviors occurred were the dependent variables. The participants were five inner-city preschool children with autism. Initially, a baseline condition (A phase) was contrasted with peer-mediated intervention (B phase) to improve social and communicative behavior. This intervention phase was then contrasted with a C phase in which the peers without disabilities interacted in a less structured manner with the child with autism. This reversal in social initiation contingencies was then compared with the effects of the previous peer-mediated instruction strategy (B phase). This arrangement constituted an A-B-C-B single-case design and showed that the peer-mediated intervention was effective in teaching social/communicative skills and that unstructured social interaction in groups was not enough to produce these results.

FIGURE 10.6 ■ Example of an A-B-C Design.

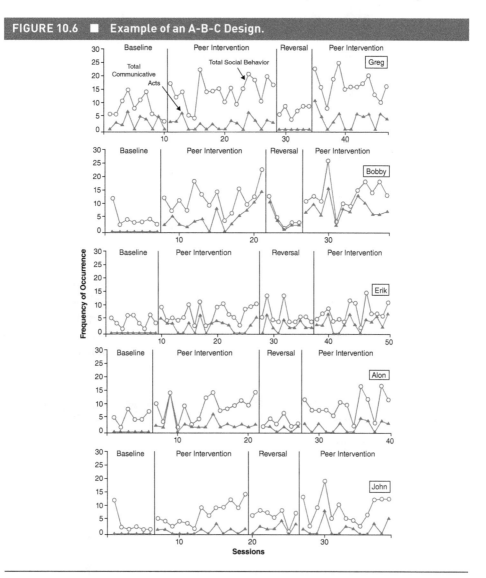

Note. The frequency with which communicative acts and social behaviors occurred were the dependent variables. The participants were five preschool children with autism. Initially, a baseline condition (A phase) was contrasted with peer-mediated intervention (B phase) to improve social and communicative behavior. This intervention phase was then contrasted with a C phase in which the peers without disabilities interacted in a less structured manner with the child with autism (Figure 2, p. 297, from: Goldstein, H., Kaczmarek, L., Pennington, R., & Shafer, K. (1992). Peer-mediated intervention: Attending to, commenting on, and acknowledging the behavior of preschoolers with autism. *Journal of Applied Behavior Analysis, 25*(2), 289–305. Copyright 1992 by the Society for the Experimental Analysis of Behavior. Reproduced by permission.)

Such an A-B-C-B arrangement of experimental conditions allows certain conclusions to be drawn, but also limits the ability to draw other conclusions. The A-B-C-B design permits strong statements about possible functional relations between the B-C-B components of the study. This is because the effects that might occur from changing from the B to C phase are replicated by returning to the B phase. The general logic is the same as an A-B-A or B-A-B design. However, less can be said about the relation between A and B phases, since no replication of the A phase occurs. In addition, the ability to draw conclusions between the A and C phases is severely constrained. Neither the A nor the C phases were replicated, nor were they directly contrasted with each other. Therefore, when using an A-B-C-B design—or its associated designs, which we will discuss momentarily—a great deal of thought needs to be employed when interpreting the results of the study. In the Goldstein et al. example, the primary comparison is between peer-mediated and reversal conditions, with less interpretative emphasis placed on other possible juxtapositions.

There are multiple variations on the A-B-C design. Depending on the variation produced, a different set of interpretative possibilities occur. For example, adding an additional comparison between A and B phases, such as in an A-B-C-B-A-B design, permits clearer statements to be made regarding baseline and the B intervention. Similarly, adding additional A and C phases, such as in an A-B-C-B-A-C-A design, allows for more interpretation of the relation between the baseline and C phases.

An example of how the A-B-C design can be elaborated upon is provided by Kennedy and Souza (1995) and shown in Figure 10.7. The authors studied how various conditions influenced the self-injurious eye poking of a young man with severe disabilities. Their dependent variable was the number of eye pokes per hour, measured across successive school days. Three phases were compared: (a) baseline with no additional stimulation, (b) music as a stimulus to interact

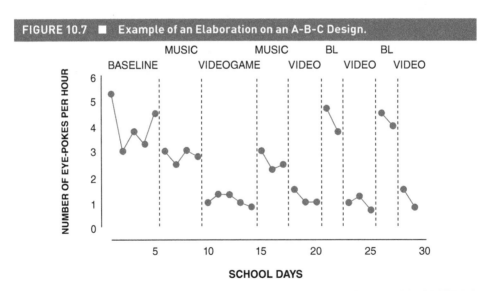

FIGURE 10.7 ■ Example of an Elaboration on an A-B-C Design.

Note. The dependent variable was the number of eye pokes per hour, measured across successive school days. Three phases were compared: (a) baseline with no additional stimulation, (b) music as a stimulus to interact with, and (c) a video game as a stimulus to interact with. The experimental design was an A-B-C-B-C-A-C-A-C arrangement. (Figure 3, p. 33, from: Kennedy, C. H., & Souza, G. (1995). Functional analysis and treatment of eye poking. *Journal of Applied Behavior Analysis, 28,* 27–37. Copyright 1995 by the Society for the Experimental Analysis of Behavior. Reproduced by permission.)

with, and (c) a video game as a stimulus to interact with. The experimental design was an A-B-C-B-C-A-C-A-C arrangement. Eye poking was highest in baseline, was lowest in the video game condition, and occurred at a moderate level in the music condition. Because replicated comparisons were conducted for various pairings of phases (i.e., B versus C, and A versus C), statements could be made about functional relations between each of the first two phases analyzed and the C phase.

In addition to the many permutations of A, B, and C phases that can be arranged, additional phases can be added to the A-B-A-B design logic. For example, D and E phases can be added to extend the analytical scope of a study, permitting even more comparisons among independent variables. However, there is a limit to how elaborate such a design can be. For meaningful comparisons to be made among all conditions, the addition of each new phase produces a multiplicative effect on the number of comparisons that can be conducted. Because of this feature of A-B-C-B designs, the use of too many additional phases to the analysis can render the experimental design intractable. As a design alternative for analyzing multiple conditions, the reader should see Chapter 11, which introduces the *multielement design*.

CHANGING-CRITERION DESIGN

An important variation of the A-B-A-B design family is the *changing-criterion design*. This analytical approach uses a sequential phase change tactic to systematically increase or decrease some quantitative dimension of the independent variable to assess potential corresponding changes in the dependent measure. Originally presented as a conceptual approach by Hall (1971) with an experimental demonstration provided by Weis and Hall (1971), the changing-criterion design was formally described in 1976 by Hartmann and Hall. Going further back in time, the articles just cited noted that their inspiration for the design type was derived from Sidman's (1960, Chapter 7) discussion of parametric variations in baseline conditions in order to establish functional relations.

Although Hartmann and Hall (1976) initially described changing-criterion designs as a variant of the multiple-baseline design (see Chapter 12), this design is more appropriately considered a variant of the A-B-A-B design type. This is because, as we will see in the following section, it does not establish multiple, independent baselines upon which to analyze parametric changes in the intervention but, rather, establishes a single baseline upon which to study the effects of an independent variable (see also Cooper et al., 2020). Therefore, the changing-criterion design is included as a subsection in this chapter.

As noted by Hartmann and Hall (1976) and refined by Klein et al. (2017), there are at least three critical elements in this experimental approach that distinguish it from other $N = 1$ designs. First, a baseline is created and continues until a stable or steady-state pattern is established in which the trend is essentially flat (see Chapter 16 for quantitative approaches to assessing slope stability). This requirement is also needed in each of the subsequent changes to a quantitative parameter of the independent variable. Second, after establishing a steady baseline, the initial (and subsequent) changes in the independent variable need to produce a clear change in the level of the dependent variable that itself stabilizes into a consistent stable pattern. Finally, as the parametric variation in the intervention is systematically increased or decreased across subsequent phases, the strength of the functional relation is established and built by repeated changes in the independent variable. As is illustrated with examples as follows, these are not minor design requirements for the relation between independent and dependent variables.

This design approach best qualifies for the designation of A-B-C-D-E or A-B1-B2-B3-B4 in single-case nomenclature. An example of the sequential phase change logic in the changing-criterion design is shown in the original formulation presented by Hartmann and Hall (1976). Figure 10.8 shows the number of correctly solved mathematical problems by a young man with behavioral disorders. The intervention was contingent access to playing basketball upon success-fully completing a fixed number of division problems. After establishing a baseline with a low performance level, the treatment was implemented requiring the student to complete two math-ematics problems to earn recess. Correct responding immediately adjusted to this performance criterion (labeled *B* in the graph). The independent variable was then incrementally increased by one for each sequent phase with a stability criterion for correct responding of at least three consecutive sessions at the new contingency level (labeled *C* through *K*). Experimental control was demonstrated because each change in the parametric level of the intervention tracked to a corresponding change in the number of division problems solved correctly.

FIGURE 10.8 ■ Example of a Changing Criterion Design.

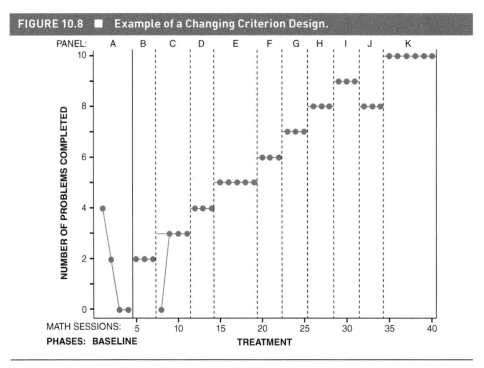

Note. The graph shows the number of correctly solved mathematical problems by a young man with behavioral disorders. The intervention was contingent access to playing basketball upon successfully completing a fixed number of division problems. After a baseline phase (Phase A), the criteria for earning basketball time was increased over successive phases of the study (labeled *B–K*). (Figure 1, p. 538, from: Hartmann, D. P., & Hall, R. V. (1976). The changing criterion design. *Journal of Applied Behavior Analysis, 9*(4), 527–532. Copyright 1976 by the Society for the Experimental Analysis of Behavior. Reproduced by permission.)

A second example from the field of kinesiology is shown in Figure 10.9. In this study employing a changing-criterion design, Furlonger et al. (2017) analyzed the effect of a self-management intervention on the rock-climbing performance of young adults. Several discrete rock-climbing skills were targeted for intervention: powerball grip, one-handed pull-ups, and multistage fitness. Figure 10.9 shows the effects of parametric changes in the performance criteria for multistage fitness. Furlonger et al. established a consistent baseline on a multistage fitness test and then increased the performance criteria by 15% above baseline performance. Once a stable change in the dependent measure was established, two additional changes in performance criteria were sequentially layered into the self-management goals with test improvements of 30% and the 45% above the original baseline being achieved. As with the previous example, experimental control was established through the close relation between intervention criteria and performance levels over the three successive phase changes.

It should be noted that the changing-criterion design is vulnerable to several classic threats to internal validity that can limit its utility as an experimental tactic. The first threat is *history effects*.

FIGURE 10.9 ■ **Example of a Changing Criterion Design with Layered Parametric Changes.**

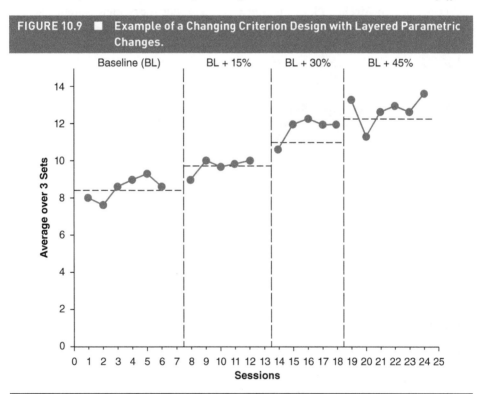

Note. The figure shows the effect of a self-management intervention on the rock-climbing performance of young adults. A consistent baseline was established on a multistage fitness test, and then the performance criteria was increased by 15% parametric increases above baseline performance. (Figure 1, p. 9, from: Furlonger, B. E., Oey, A., Moore, D., Busacca, M., & Scott, D. (2017). Improving amateur indoor rock climbing performance using a changing criterion design within a self-management program. *The Sport Journal, 19*(1), 1–16 (https://thespor tjournal.org/article/improving-amateur-indoor-rock-climbing-performance-using-a-changing-criterion-des ign-within-a-self-management-program/). Copyright 2017 by the United States Sports Academy. Reproduced with permission from *The Sport Journal.*)

Because the design specifies consistent increases (or decreases) over time, it is possible that another variable not being tracked by investigators is causing or interacting with the presumed independent variable. Possible examples would include a physician prescribing and adjusting a psychotropic medication for treating behavioral symptoms of attention deficit hyperactivity disorder (ADHD) or out-of-school tutoring provided by a child's parents influencing mathematics performance. Relatedly, *maturation effects* can influence developmental issues such as communication complexity or social skills acquisition, and *measurement threats* such as "observer drift" can potentially influence results in a manner that mimics an intervention.

To address these well-known threats to internal validity, refinements in this design type have been suggested. First, McDougall (2005) has introduced the *range-bound technique* to improve the design integrity of changing-criteria designs. In this design variant the criterion after each phase change includes not only a specific goal (e.g., three division problems solved correctly; see Hartmann and Hall, 1976), but an upper and lower range within which the dependent measure should vary before a subsequent phase change is implemented. An example of this design refinement is from McDougall, who presented data regarding the running performance of an individual and a systematic self-monitoring program for improving the number of minutes ran each week (see Figure 10.10). The weekly bounded criteria were met throughout the study and allowed for a systematic increase in the targeted behavior over time.

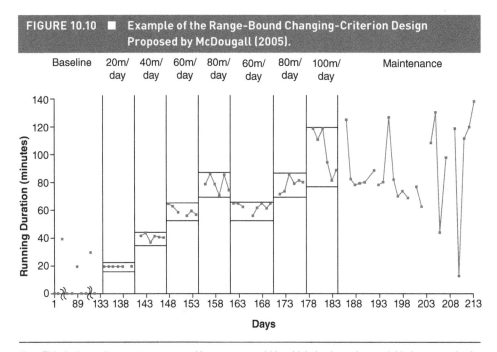

FIGURE 10.10 ■ Example of the Range-Bound Changing-Criterion Design Proposed by McDougall (2005).

Note. This design variant creates upper and lower ranges within which the dependent variable is expected to be bounded before phase changes are introduced. In this example the design type was used to analyze the duration of running across weeks. (Figure 1, p. 132, from: McDougall, D. (2005). The range-bound changing criterion design. *Behavioral Interventions: Theory and Practice in Residential and Community-Based Clinical Programs, 20*(2), 129–137. Copyright 2005 by John Wiley & Sons, Ltd. Reproduced by permission.)

However, it should be noted that the previous example is still susceptible to history, maturation, and measurement threats to internal validity. An alternative approach, which was originally used by Hartmann and Hall (1976), is to embed a reversal or "reverse titration" within the sequence of increasing (or decreasing) criteria for the behavior(s) of interest. This approach allows for a change in the level of the dependent variable that is opposite of the changing-criterion design sequence and helps rule out confounding variables. An example of this technique is provided by McDaniel and Bruhn (2016). The authors used a check-in/check-out intervention to improve the challenging behavior of middle school students. Figure 10.11 shows the embedding of the return to baseline during Sessions 15–17 of the changing-criterion design, which helped increase the internal validity of the findings.

STRENGTHS AND LIMITATIONS

A-B-A-B designs are an extension of A-B-A designs. A-B-A-B designs allow researchers to compare two conditions within a single individual. The number of replications conducted is primarily a function of the clarity of the data. In some instances, an A-B-A-B sequence is sufficient;

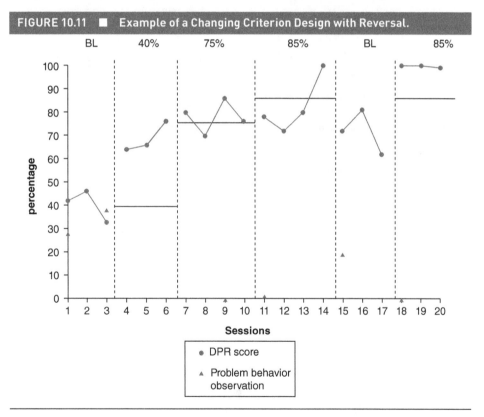

FIGURE 10.11   ■   Example of a Changing Criterion Design with Reversal.

Note. Perhaps the best approach to increasing internal validity using changing-criterion designs is to embed a reversal to baseline (BL) or a previously established criterion level (see also Figure 10.1). This study shows the use of such a design to improve the performance of a middle school student named Kaiya. (Figure 1, p. 202, from: McDaniel, S. C., & Bruhn, A. L. (2016). Using a changing-criterion design to evaluate the effects of check-in/check-out with goal modification. *Journal of Positive Behavior Interventions, 18*(4), 197–208. Copyright 2015 by the Hammill Institute on Disabilities. Reproduced by permission.)

in other conditions, an A-B-A-B-A-B sequence (or more repeats) may be necessary to demonstrate a functional relation. B-A-B designs, a variant of the A-B-A-B design, can be used to demonstrate the effects of a previously established intervention. In addition, this design type allows for the comparison of additional phases using A-B-C and associated designs, allowing for more complex analytical comparisons. Because of this flexibility, the A-B-A-B single-case design is a tactic frequently used by researchers.

There are, however, some limitations of this design type. First, if a behavior is not reversible, an A-B-A-B design is not appropriate (see Box 10.1). For instances in which behavior change is not reversible, researchers typically opt for another single-case design, such as the repeated-acquisition design (Chapter 13). Second, if reversal of the behavior to baseline levels is deemed unacceptable because of the risks involved, a multiple-baseline design (Chapter 12) is preferred over an A-B-A-B design or other types of single-case designs. Finally, if a large number of conditions need to be compared or multiple repeats of a smaller number of conditions are necessary, then A-B-A-B designs may become intractable, particularly in educational settings. In these instances, researchers typically use multielement (Chapter 11) or brief experimental designs (Chapter 14).

REFLECTION QUESTIONS

1. Can you describe how an A-B-A-B design shows if an independent variable influences the measures of behavior used in an experiment?

2. Why are behavioral effects that are not reversible not appropriate for withdrawal designs?

3. What role does direct replication serve in establishing experimental control using A-B-A-B designs?

4. Describe why some researchers differentiate between "withdrawal" and "reversal" experimental designs.

5. Can you think of examples when a changing-criterion design might be used with multiplicative increases or decreases for the dependent variable level rather than the standard additive approach?

11 MULTIELEMENT DESIGNS

In this chapter we will discuss the use of *multielement designs* in single-case research. The term *multielement design* was coined by Sidman (1960) and introduced to single-case researchers by Ulman and Sulzer-Azaroff (1975). More than any other type of single-case design tactic, the multielement design has had a diverse set of nomenclature associated with it. Terms referring to this design type have included *alternating-treatments design* (Barlow & Hayes, 1979; Barlow & Hersen, 1984; Ledford & Gast, 2018), *multiple-schedule design* (Agras et al., 1969; Hersen & Barlow, 1976; Leitenberg, 1973), *multitreatment design* (Kazdin, 2020), and *simultaneous-treatment design* (Browning, 1967; Kazdin & Geesey, 1977). As is discussed in Box 11.1, most of these terms are not accurate or only refer to a subset of multielement designs we will discuss in this chapter. Therefore, we will use *multielement designs* to refer to this design tactic because of its historical precedence, technical accuracy, and inclusiveness.

BOX 11.1: VARIOUS NAMES AND MEANINGS FOR MULTIELEMENT DESIGNS

Multielement designs have been referred to using a variety of terms, some more accurate than others. The term *multielement design* was actually coined by basic researchers working in operant laboratories during the 1950s, and the term was codified in Sidman's *Tactics of Scientific Research* (1960), which described research practices in the experimental analysis of behavior. Because of this history, Ulman and Sulzer-Azaroff (1975) used the term *multielement design* to introduce applied researchers to this novel experimental tactic. However, at the same time, other applied researchers were developing new designs, some very similar to multielement designs, and naming them within the contexts of their own research efforts. This resulted in terms such as *alternating-treatments designs, multiple-schedule designs, multitreatment designs*, and *simultaneous-treatment designs*. However, *multielement designs* has persisted in use and is the preferred term in contemporary single-case research because it is more encompassing and accurate than the other terms. For example, multiple-schedule designs actually refer to the use of multiple schedules of reinforcement that require alternation between distinct reinforcement contingencies and discriminative stimuli (see Ferster & Skinner, 1957), something that does not apply to all multielement designs. Similarly, simultaneous-treatment designs refer to choice procedures that allow a participant to select which intervention they experience. In contemporary parlance, such designs are part of what is referred to as concurrent operant designs (see Chapter 15). Because a range of single-case designs can be used to compare multiple treatments, the term *multitreatment design* has been viewed as too vague. The term *alternating-treatments design* has a somewhat more complex history and will be discussed in a later subsection of this chapter. So, although some readers may disagree, this text has adopted the use of *multielement designs* as the preferred term for this type of single-case design.

In the previous chapter we discussed the gradual alternation between A and B phases of a study as a means of establishing experimental control. These A-B-A-B designs can be used to develop functional relations under a range of circumstances. However, one limitation of the A-B-A-B design and its variants makes other single-case designs, such as the multielement design, a desirable alternative. Specifically, A-B-A-B designs become intractable when a range of conditions are experimentally analyzed. However, multielement designs make the comparison of multiple conditions feasible.

MULTIELEMENT DESIGNS

Multielement designs alternate between various conditions as a means of demonstrating experimental control. In particular, these designs rely on *response differentiation* between or among conditions to establish a functional relation. That is, in at least two of the conditions being analyzed, responding needs to occur at distinctly different levels to demonstrate a functional relation. In its most simplified arrangement, a multielement design could be used to study the effects of two conditions: baseline (A) and intervention (B). Using this design approach, a researcher alternates between the A and B conditions from session to session. This rapid switching between conditions is then analyzed to assess whether levels of behavior under each of the two conditions are different. If response differentiation occurs between the A and B conditions, then a functional relation has been demonstrated.

An example of the use of the multielement design is provided by Stevens and Burns (2021). The authors compared a reading intervention to a "baseline" condition on the reading comprehension of 3 fourth-grade students with mild to moderate intellectual disabilities. The intervention was comprised of practicing keywords using an incremental rehearsal (IR) technique.

Baseline was the "business as usual" instructional approach specified on the students' individualized education plans. The results shown in Figure 11.1 indicate that the IR intervention resulted in consistently higher rates of correct word read per minute for all three students. Such a design allows for multiple direct replications of the experimental effect within a participant over a brief time period.

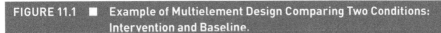

FIGURE 11.1 ■ Example of Multielement Design Comparing Two Conditions: Intervention and Baseline.

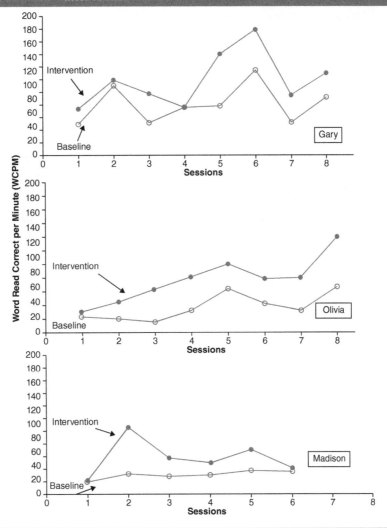

Note. The intervention was composed of a keywords strategy intended to increase word recognition, reading fluency, and comprehension. The figure shows the effects of the intervention on words read correctly per minute (a measure of reading fluency) for three students. (Figure 3, p. 239, from: Stevens, M. A., & Burns, M. K. (2021). Practicing keywords to increase reading performance of students with intellectual disability. *American Journal on Intellectual and Developmental Disabilities, 126*(3), 230–248. Copyright by American Association on Intellectual and Developmental Disabilities. Reproduced by permission.)

Figure 11.2 shows a more elaborate multielement design. In this study by Taylor et al. (2002), three different conditions were analyzed. The dependent variable of interest was the reading comprehension of students with learning disabilities. The first condition, "self-questioning," required students to answer a set of prescribed questions after reading a passage. The second condition, "story mapping," had students draw a graphic representation of what they had just read in a passage. The third condition, "no intervention," required the students to read the passage with no supplemental aids. These different reading conditions were alternated across days. The data show that the highest number of test questions answered correctly occurred in the self-questioning condition, followed by the story mapping condition and no intervention condition, respectively.

Another example of a multielement design is shown in Figure 11.3. In this classic study by Iwata et al. (1982/1994), the self-injurious behavior (SIB) of children with neurodevelopmental disabilities was studied to identify possible reinforcers maintaining the behavior. Four distinct conditions were analyzed: (a) removal of task demands contingent on self-injury (Academic), (b) no interaction or other stimulation (Alone), (c) adult attention contingent on self-injury (Social Disapproval), and (d) an enriched environment with toys and adult attention (Play). Figure 11.3 shows that each of the four children's self-injury displayed a different pattern across conditions. For Child 1, self-injury occurred only in the Academic condition. For Child 2, the pattern of

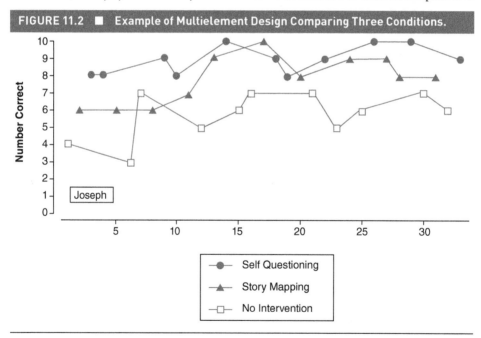

FIGURE 11.2 ■ Example of Multielement Design Comparing Three Conditions.

Note. The dependent variable of interest was the reading comprehension of students with learning disabilities (vertical axis). The first condition, "self-questioning," required students to answer a set of prescribed questions after reading a passage (closed circles). The second condition, "story mapping," had students draw a graphic representation of what they had just read in a passage (closed triangles). The third condition, "no intervention," required the student to read the passage with no supplemental aids (open squares). These different reading conditions were alternated across days (horizontal axis). (Figure 1, p. 79, from: Taylor, L. K., Alber, S. R., & Walker, D. W. (2002). The comparative effects of a modified self-questioning strategy and story mapping on the reading comprehension of elementary students with learning disabilities. *Journal of Behavioral Education, 11,* 69–87. Copyright 2002 by Human Sciences Press, Inc. Reproduced with permission from Springer Nature Customer Service Center.)

FIGURE 11.3 ■ Example of Multielement Design Comparing Four Conditions.

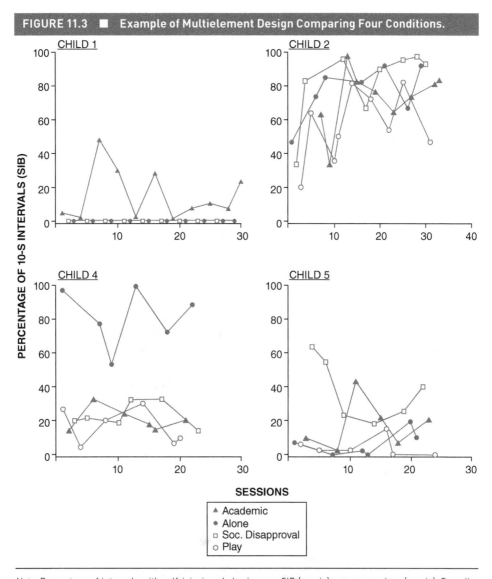

Note. Percentage of intervals with self-injurious behaviors, or SIB (*y*-axis), across sessions (*x*-axis). Four distinct conditions were analyzed: (a) removal of task demands contingent on self-injury (Academic; closed triangles), (b) no interaction or other stimulation (Alone; closed circles), (c) adult attention contingent on self-injury (Social Disapproval; open squares), and (d) an enriched environment with toys and adult attention (Play; open circles). (Figure 2, p. 205, from: Iwata, B. A., Dorsey, M. F., Slifer, K. J., Bauman, K. E., & Richman, G. S. (1994). Toward a functional analysis of self-injury. *Journal of Applied Behavior Analysis, 27,* 197–209. [Reprinted from *Analysis and Intervention in Developmental Disabilities,* 1982, Vol. 2, pp. 3–20.] Copyright 1994 by the Society for the Experimental Analysis of Behavior. Reproduced by permission.)

self-injury is largely undifferentiated. The self-injury of Child 4 was highest during the Alone condition, and the behavior of Child 5 was highest during the Social Disapproval condition. Using this multielement design, Iwata et al. were able to demonstrate that each child's self-injury had a distinct set of conditions under which it occurred, suggesting that each child's behavior might need an individually tailored intervention plan.

Each of the experiments just reviewed used a multielement design to establish a functional relation within a single participant. Although each experiment used different dependent measures and studied different experimental conditions, all shared features common to multielement designs. Each set of authors identified distinct experimental conditions, alternating among them from session to session, and observed the degree of response differentiation that resulted. This general set of requirements forms the basis of multielement designs.

TACTICAL ISSUES AND MULTIELEMENT DESIGNS

There are a number of issues that come into play when using multielement designs that require elaboration. What constitutes an appropriate set of conditions for analysis, how to identify interactions among conditions, and specific variants of the multiple-baseline design all deserve discussion. In the following sections, we will discuss each of these issues as they relate to this particular design tactic and the establishment of functional relations.

Baseline Versus Independent Variables

Most single-case researchers would agree that some type of baseline condition needs to be established in order to establish experimental control. But, as was discussed in Chapters 3 and 5, what constitutes a "baseline" is open for discussion. In the sense that Sidman (1960) used the term, a baseline is an initial experimental condition. The experimenter explicitly defines its characteristics, particularly in reference to the independent variable with which the baseline will be compared. Hence, a baseline is a procedural arrangement defined in relation to the experimental design that will be used to study the functional properties of an independent variable. For example, a researcher might establish behavior on a variable-ratio (VR) schedule of positive reinforcement to compare its effects relative to a variable-interval (VI) schedule of positive reinforcement (see Catania et al., 1977). In this instance, the VR schedule is the baseline, and the VI schedule is the independent variable. The *variable* aspect of the reinforcement contingency was chosen by the experimenter to be held constant across phases so the response-dependent nature of the contingency could be analyzed. *The rationale for choosing the baseline condition rests entirely on the nature of the experimental question.*

However, in educational research, and applied psychology more generally, baselines are sometimes equated with currently existing educational conditions. This in part reflects the applied nature of these types of analyses where problematic circumstances are often the starting point to test an intervention (sometimes referred to as the "business as usual" condition). Nonetheless, this does not imply that baselines are a priori the currently existing situation. Instead, what constitutes an appropriate baseline is directly referenced to the experimental question and the hypothesis being studied. If a demonstration question (Chapter 5) is of experimental interest, then a preexisting baseline (e.g., typical classroom teaching practices) may be appropriate to show that the intervention improves behavior. If other types of experimental questions are being asked (e.g., comparative, component, or parametric), an appropriate baseline condition may be constituted by some other arrangement in relation to the independent variable.

An example of what is an appropriate baseline can be illustrated by a study focusing on the on-task behavior of three students with attention deficit hyperactivity disorder (ADHD). Flood et al.

(2002) used six different conditions in a multielement design to better understand what conditions increased or decreased on-task behavior (see Figure 11.4). None of the conditions selected by Flood et al. was a "typical" classroom arrangement. Instead, these authors selected a set of conditions that they hypothesized might contribute to challenging behaviors (e.g., Difficult Demand, Alone, Adult Attention, or Peer Attention conditions) and contrasted them with conditions not hypothesized to contribute to challenging behaviors (e.g., Easy Demand or Control conditions). These latter two

FIGURE 11.4 ■ Example of Determining Baseline.

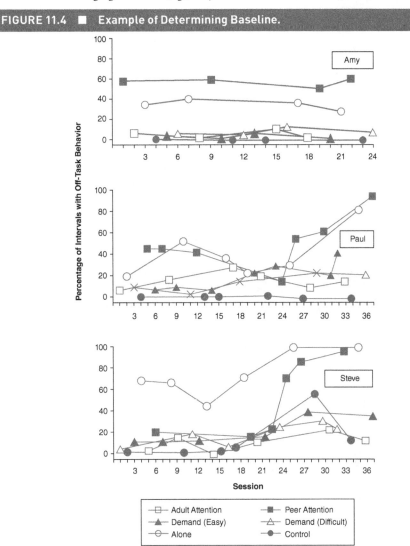

Note. The figure shows an analysis of off-task behavior for three students with ADHD (Amy, Paul, and Steve). The dependent variable was the percentage of intervals with off-task behavior. Six independent variables were included in the analysis (i.e., Adult Attention, Being Alone, Control, Difficult Demand, Easy Demand, and Peer Attention conditions). (Figure 1, p. 202, from: Flood, W. A., Wilder, D. A., Flood, A. L., & Masuda, A. (2002). Peer-mediated reinforcement plus prompting as treatment for off-task behavior in children with attention deficit hyperactivity disorder. *Journal of Applied Behavior Analysis, 35,* 199–204. Copyright 2002 by the Society for the Experimental Analysis of Behavior. Reproduced by permission.)

conditions were selected because they were likely to produce low levels of off-task behavior and could serve as comparisons for the conditions that were more likely to produce off-task behavior. In a sense, the Easy Demand and Control conditions could be considered a baseline for comparison with the other conditions. More importantly, the constitution and selection of these conditions followed from the experimental question, not preexisting conditions.

Flood et al.'s (2002) inclusion of the Easy Demand and Control conditions also served to produce response differentiation among conditions, an outcome necessary for establishing a functional relation. In a multielement design (or any experimental design, for that matter), differences between conditions are necessary to show experimental control. An example of an instance in which a multielement design did not produce response differentiation is presented in Figure 11.5. In this example, Wunderlich et al. (2020) studied the vocal stereotypies of children with autism spectrum disorder (ASD). The dependent variable was the percentage of intervals of stereotypy during an assessment session. Independent variables included Attention, Demand, No Interaction, and Play conditions. Figure 11.5 shows that for one child (Jake) his behavior was similar across all experimental conditions and no response differentiation occurred. The authors then repeated a single condition over time but again found no difference from the original multielement analysis, suggesting no interaction effects were occurring. For Jake's stereotypical behavior, no experimental control was demonstrated in the analysis because no differences were observed across conditions.

What constitutes a baseline in a multielement design (or any single-case design) depends on the experimental question. What you choose to study depends on what you want to learn from

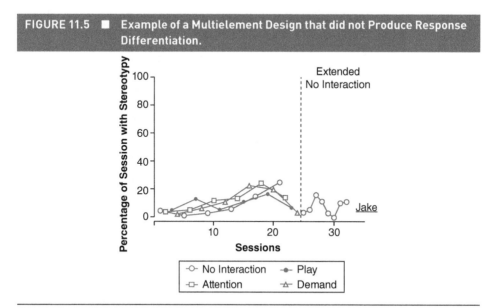

FIGURE 11.5 ■ Example of a Multielement Design that did not Produce Response Differentiation.

Note. A functional analysis of stereotypical behavior using a multielement design with four conditions: Attention, Demand, No Interaction, and Play. The multielement analysis was then followed up with a single condition (No Interaction) to assess for possible interaction effects. The dependent variable is arrayed along the ordinate as the percentage of intervals with stereotypy. (Figure 3, p. 686, from: Wunderlich, K. L., Vollmer, T. R., Mehrkam, L. R., Feuerbacher, E. N., Slocum, S. K., Kronfli, F. R., & Pizarro, E. (2020). The stability of function of automatically reinforced vocal stereotypy over time. *Journal of Applied Behavior Analysis, 53*(2), 678–689. Copyright 2000 by the Society for the Experimental Analysis of Behavior. Reproduced by permission.)

the experimental analysis. However, what is critical is the conditions be chosen to produce some degree of response differentiation.

Interactions Among Conditions

Because of the rapid alternation between conditions in multielement designs, there is always the possibility that the effects on behavior in one condition may influence behavior in another condition. Several terms have been used to describe this phenomenon, including *sequence effects, carryover effects, alternation effects*, and *multiple-treatment interference* (see Barlow & Hersen, 1984). Because each of these terms refers to some instance of an interaction among conditions, we will refer to these effects by a generic term, suggested by Hains and Baer (1989), *interaction effects*.

A hypothetical example of an interaction effect can be derived from the experiment depicted in Figure 11.3. It is possible that in such an experimental sequence exposure to the Academic condition prior to the Play condition will influence behavior in the latter condition if high levels of responding are seen in the former condition. This might occur because of behavioral momentum from the Academic to the Play condition or a disruption in stimulus control exerted by the Play condition (Podlesnik et al., 2021; Trump et al., 2021). The net result might be that the level of behavior observed in the Play condition is partly an artifact of the sequence of conditions (i.e., Academic, then Play), rather than an absolute product of the Play condition itself.

Schematically, we can model this phenomenon using the following symbols: A = Academic condition; B = Alone condition; C = Social Disapproval condition; D = Play condition; - = movement from one condition to another with no interaction effect; and * = the occurrence of an interaction effect. In the experimental sequence just discussed, the following events occurred:

B-C-A*D

Thus, the condition sequence Alone, Social Disapproval, Academic, and Play occurred, with an interaction effect occurring from the Academic to the Play condition. However, in this example, if the Play and Academic conditions are reversed, no interaction effect is observed:

B-C-D-A

Such an arrangement shows that the effects of one condition on another are due to the sequence in which they occur, in addition to the absolute effects the individual condition has on behavior. Or, we might find that anytime a condition is preceded by the Academic condition, there is an interaction effect:

C-B-A*D or A*C-D-B or D-A*B-C

In many areas of psychology the traditional approach to "controlling" for interaction effects has been to use randomization or counterbalancing techniques (Campbell & Stanley, 1963; Shadish et al., 2002). Randomization refers to using some stochastic process to assign a sequence to events that is independent of the events themselves. Examples of how to do this include using a random numbers table, using an app-based algorithm, and rolling dice. The logic is that, on average, each condition is equally likely to occur before and after each other condition, with no experimenter bias in sequencing being introduced. So, for instance, the following sequence might be randomly generated:

C-B-A-D-A-C-D-B-D-A-B-C

In this sequence, each condition is presented three times in a multielement design. Therefore, the influence of a possible interaction effect is randomly distributed across the experiment. However, a researcher versed in single-case design methodology would quickly point out that no control of the sequence effect has been established. *Randomization in single-case designs is not a control technique* like it is in nomothetically based experimental designs. Instead, what has occurred is that from a statistical perspective, the change in behavior produced by the interaction effect has been equally distributed across conditions. If the "A" condition always produced an interaction with the condition that followed it, the following interaction sequence would occur:

C-B-A*D-A*C-D-B-D-A*B-C

Counterbalancing takes a more direct approach to equally distributing possible interaction effects across conditions. Counterbalancing is a technique that has the same goal as randomization but arranges the sequence of conditions in a *planned manner*. For example, a researcher might choose to use a Latin square counterbalancing technique (e.g., Masson, n.d.) in which each condition appears in each ordinal position once and each condition precedes and follows each condition once. Using our example from Figure 11.3, the following sequence could be generated:

A-D-B-C-D-C-A-B-B-A-C-D-C-B-D-A

However, like the randomization technique, if interaction effects are present, the interaction effects shown as follows will still occur:

A*D-B-C-D-C-A*B-B-A*C-D-C-B-D-A

Hence, although randomization and counterbalancing techniques equally distribute the interaction effect across conditions, *there is no control for this effect from an experimental standpoint* (see Box 11.2). All that is accomplished is the statistical averaging of the effect across conditions. In instances where interaction effects might occur, single-case researchers (cf. Hains & Baer, 1989) have suggested that the appropriate approach to understanding these effects is to conduct an experimental analysis of the phenomenon causing the interaction. That is, when interaction effects are suspected in an experiment, that effect then becomes the serendipitous focus of the analysis (even though such an analysis was not initially the experimental question). One of the more elegant aspects of single-case designs is that they permit such experimental flexibility, allowing the researcher to explore a phenomenon as it is revealed rather than having to rigidly follow a planned experimental sequence (e.g., Johnston et al., 2020; McGonigle et al., 1987; Shapiro et al., 1982).

BOX 11.2: ARE RANDOMIZATION OR COUNTERBALANCING CONTROL TECHNIQUES IN MULTIELEMENT DESIGNS?

Any introductory course in experimental psychology will teach you the importance of randomization and counterbalancing when designing an experiment. In fact, these techniques are often referred to as control techniques in such contexts. However, this is a logic based on group-comparison designs and the statistical analyses associated with their use (i.e., nomothetic conceptualizations of data). If interaction effects occur, then randomizing or counterbalancing will evenly distribute those effects across conditions so that their mathematical presence will equally influence the data in all other conditions. However, in single-case designs, or any idiographic approach to experimentation, such an experimental tactic is not a control technique in the sense that experimental control is established. For researchers using single-case designs, control techniques are associated with the establishment of a functional relation between variables to explain why some behavioral effect occurs. If an interaction effect occurs, it is the result of a behavioral process that is uncontrolled within the existing experimental arrangement. In single-case designs, such instances are invitations for further experimental analysis and discovery. Or, as Murray Sidman wrote in *Tactics of Scientific Research* (1960), "variability is not mere noise in the system. It is the major datum" (pp. 197–198).

Interestingly, single-case researchers have adopted the convention of randomizing the sequence of experimental conditions when using multielement designs. Presumably, the benefit of doing this is that a researcher is attempting to distribute possible interaction effects evenly across the experimental analysis. If interaction effects are present and robust, then the sequence of events should be revealed through visual analysis of the data. However, some researchers, particularly in behavioral pharmacology (which, by definition, is the study of interaction effects), have adopted the convention of using fixed sequences of conditions and reversing the sequence to assess for the presence of interaction effects. Which approach is more scientifically useful in educational settings remains to be seen.

An example of this process of following your data is exemplified by Berg et al. (2000). Berg and colleagues conducted a functional analysis of problem behavior for a young child with multiple disabilities and problem behavior. During previous analyses, these authors had noticed possible interaction effects for the child's problem behavior. In particular, they had noticed that in some assessments adult attention was a positive reinforcer for problem behavior but in other assessments the same attention was a neutral stimulus. Berg et al. hypothesized that exposure to adult attention before an assessment session might decrease the value of adult attention as a reinforcer (this behavioral process is referred as a motivating operation; see Laraway et al., 2003; McGill, 1999). To test this hypothesis the authors systematically manipulated the amount of adult attention prior to sessions analyzing whether adult attention functioned as a positive reinforcer for problem behavior. Figure 11.6 shows the percentage of intervals in which self-injury was observed during sessions testing whether adult attention influenced this behavior. Two types of conditions were analyzed: (a) The child was alone before the attention assessment, or (b) the child played with an adult before the attention assessment. The results showed that prior exposure to adult attention decreased the reinforcing value of adult attention during the functional analysis. Berg et al. not only noticed an interaction effect but were able to successfully analyze the interaction and explain why it occurred.

One strategy that can assist in identifying interaction effects involves the graphic analysis of data (see Chapter 16). When plotting data from a multielement design in a graph so the data can be visually analyzed, a researcher has two options. The data points can be plotted so separate sessions overlap (see Figure 11.1), or the data can be arrayed to show each session in sequence

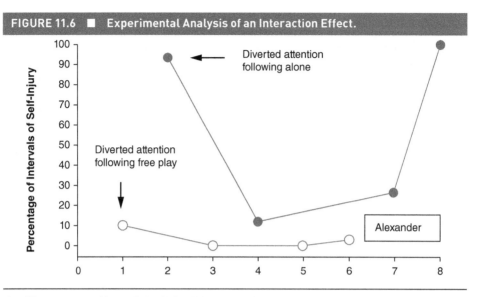

FIGURE 11.6 ■ **Experimental Analysis of an Interaction Effect.**

Note. The percentage of intervals in which self-injury was observed during sessions that tested whether adult attention influenced this behavior. Two types of conditions were analyzed: (a) The child was alone before the attention assessment, or (b) the child played with an adult before the attention assessment. (Figure 2, p. 469, from: Berg, W. K., Peck, S., Wacker, D. P., Harding, J., McComas, J., Richman, D., & Brown, K. (2000). The effects of presession exposure to attention on the results of assessments of attention as a reinforcer. *Journal of Applied Behavior Analysis, 33,* 463–477. Copyright 2000 by the Society for the Experimental Analysis of Behavior. Reproduced by permission.)

(see Figure 11.2). One value of plotting the data in sequence is that you can see which sessions preceded or followed other sessions. This approach to visualizing information allows for easier detection of interaction effects when using multielement designs.

Alternating-Treatments Design

The alternating-treatments design (ATD) is a variant of the multielement design. As introduced in the late 1970s (Barlow & Hayes, 1979), the ATD is a special instance of the broader set of designs discussed in this chapter. As noted by Barlow and Hayes (1979), "in the typical design [i.e., ATD], after a baseline period, two treatments (A and B) are administered, alternating with each other, and the effects on one behavior are observed" (p. 200). This description of an ATD was accompanied by Figure 11.7. In the figure, a baseline period (Phase One) was followed by a second phase in which two independent variables were administered in a multielement design, with the more effective intervention continuing into Phase Three. Interestingly, Barlow and Hersen (1984), in their influential single-case design text, included a chapter titled "Alternating Treatments Design" that expanded the scope of the original ATD to encompass what had previously been referred to as multielement designs (the chapter and terminology had not been present in their earlier edition, Hersen & Barlow, 1976). Also of historical interest, in a contemporaneous and similarly influential text on single-case designs, Kazdin (1982) included a similar chapter but titled it "Multi-Treatment Designs."

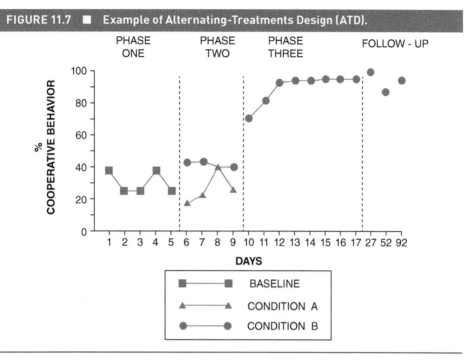

FIGURE 11.7 ■ Example of Alternating-Treatments Design (ATD).

Note. In this ATD design, a baseline period (Phase One) was followed by a second phase in which two independent variables were administered in a multielement design, with the more effective intervention continuing into Phase Three. (Figure 1, p. 201, from: Barlow, D. H., & Hayes, S. C. (1979). Alternating treatments design: One strategy for comparing the effects of two treatments in a single subject. *Journal of Applied Behavior Analysis, 12,* 199–210. Copyright 1979 by the Society for the Experimental Analysis of Behavior. Reproduced by permission.)

Clearly, such a procedural arrangement is consistent with the multielement design logic, but the inclusion of a baseline and final phase using a single intervention allows for conditions that limit the scope of the design. In fact, these conditions present substantial interpretative limitations when using the ATD. First, the instigation of an experiment with a baseline that is not replicated in subsequent phases of the study makes the pattern of behavior difficult to interpret. Since the only analysis of behavior under baseline conditions is during the start of the study and is not repeated, there is no attempt to return to baseline conditions. Second, the inclusion of the final phase in which the more effective intervention is in place is a positive aspect of the design from an applied standpoint, but, as in baseline, these data are somewhat difficult to interpret because of the lack of any additional experimental manipulations. However, the second phase of the ATD design is a classic multielement design and can be used to demonstrate experimental control.

An augmentation to the ATD that improves at least the first concern previously mentioned is shown in Figure 11.8. In this figure, Kennedy and Souza (1995) used a modified ATD to analyze the eye poking of a young man with severe disabilities. In keeping with the ATD tactic, these authors established a baseline and then introduced two interventions. However, in this design, the baseline phase of the investigation was extended into the second phase, allowing

FIGURE 11.8 ■ Example of Augmented Alternating-Treatments Design (ATD).

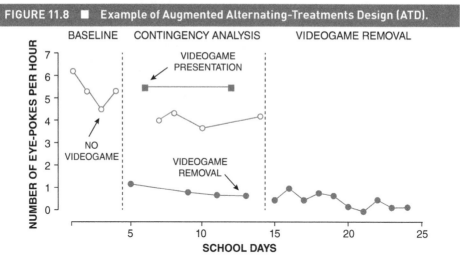

Note. In this figure, a modified ATD was used to analyze the eye poking of a young man with severe disabilities. In keeping with the ATD tactic, these authors established a baseline and then introduced two interventions. However, in this design, the baseline phase of the investigation was extended into the second phase, allowing comparisons among the independent variables and baseline. The study ended with an extended phase in which the most effective intervention was assessed. (Figure 4, p. 34, from: Kennedy, C. H., & Souza, G. (1995). Functional analysis and treatment of eye-poking. *Journal of Applied Behavior Analysis, 28,* 27–37. Copyright 1995 by the Society for the Experimental Analysis of Behavior. Reproduced by permission.)

comparisons among the independent variables and baseline. The study ended with an extended phase in which the most effective intervention was assessed. This design arrangement allowed for a comparison of baseline and interventions, although the extended third phase was largely nonanalytical.

STRENGTHS AND LIMITATIONS

Multielement designs have a long and distinguished history in the experimental analysis of behavior (Sidman, 1960). Relatively early in the development of applied behavior analysis, this design tactic was introduced to researchers (Ulman & Sulzer-Azaroff, 1975). The use of multielement designs provides researchers with a powerful analytical tool for exploring behavioral processes. As long as response differentiation occurs across at least one condition, then experimental control can be readily demonstrated.

Multielement designs allow researchers to analyze two or more experimental conditions using a single participant. In recently published reports, it is not unusual for authors to compare five or six different experimental conditions. Such flexibility allows a researcher to build in high levels of experimental control and contrast conditions that are not permitted by other single-case designs. For this reason alone, multielement designs are an important analytical tool. However, not only is this design type encompassing a large number of experimental comparisons, but the rapid alternation between or among conditions allows for this analytical process to unfold rapidly when compared with other design tactics.

There are, of course, limiting factors to the use of multielement designs. The primary limitation of multielement designs rests on the issue of behavioral reversibility. If a change in behavior produced by an independent variable cannot be reversed by the withdrawal of the intervention, then multielement designs are not a suitable design alternative (see Chapter 13). A second limitation in using multielement designs is the potential for interaction effects, where the effect on behavior of baseline and/or independent variable conditions is influenced by the presence or juxtaposition of other conditions. But, as argued by Hains and Baer (1989), the inducement of interaction effects can provide for the opportunity for additional analyses of the behavioral processes that cause interaction effects (which may be scientifically useful). However, in instances where interaction effects may be a concern, then A-B-A-B (Chapter 10), multiple-baseline (Chapter 12), or combined designs (Chapter 15) might be preferable alternatives.

REFLECTION QUESTIONS

1. Can you describe how a multielement design shows if an independent variable influences the measures of behavior used in an experiment?

2. Why are there so many different names for multielement designs, and to what degree is one term more or less accurate than the other terms?

3. Is there a limit to the number of independent variable conditions that can be included in a multielement design? Explain your answer.

4. When thinking about multielement designs, why would some researchers consider interaction effects experimental "confounds," while others view them as "opportunities"?

5. Is randomization a control technique applicable to multielement designs?

12 MULTIPLE-BASELINE DESIGNS

LEARNING OBJECTIVES

After reading this chapter, you will be able to

12.1 Differentiate the tiers of experimental control that may exist in a multiple-baseline design.

12.2 Discuss two distinct variations of multiple-baseline design.

12.3 Evaluate the strengths and limitations of a multiple-baseline experimental design.

Unlike the use of A-B-A-B or multielement designs, the use of a *multiple-baseline design* does not require the withdrawal, reversal, or repeated alternation of conditions. Instead, as the name implies, *two or more baselines* are concurrently established, and the independent variable is sequentially introduced across the baselines. This means that once an intervention is introduced, it is not removed. For instances in which the effects of the independent variable cannot be reversed once behavior is exposed to it, then multiple-baseline designs are an important alternative to the single-case designs we have discussed so far. In addition, because the design logic is based on an A-B sequence for each baseline, such designs have the logistical advantage of requiring fewer changes in an educational setting than other $N = 1$ designs. Because of this characteristic, some researchers consider the absence of a return to baseline as ethically more desirable (see Box 12.1).

BOX 12.1: ARE MULTIPLE-BASELINE DESIGNS ETHICALLY PREFERABLE TO OTHER SINGLE-CASE DESIGNS?

A concern that has been noted about A-B-A-B and multielement designs is that the return to baseline may not be ethically desirable. This is because the baseline condition may have exposed the person to some undesirable situation, such as bullying by peers or the occurrence of self-injurious behavior. Following a successful intervention that improves the problematic situation, a return to the undesirable situation could be considered ethically unacceptable since it would reexpose the person to negative circumstances. This has led some researchers to prefer multiple-baseline designs to other types of single-case designs. However, this preference is relative, not absolute. One of the drawbacks of a multiple-baseline design, by definition, is the prolongation of baseline conditions for the lower tiers of the design. For the behaviors, people, and so on that are exposed to the lower tiers of a multiple-baseline design, an extended exposure to the problematic situation is required. For instances that may expose a participant to prolonged baseline conditions, an A-B-A-B or multielement design may minimize the person's exposure to the undesirable situation. Indeed, if exposure to a baseline condition is a clear ethical concern, then single-case designs, such as multielement or brief designs, that minimize the number of baseline sessions may be the most desirable alternative.

An example of a multiple-baseline design is provided in Figure 12.1. This study, by Clark et al. (2004), used an intensive onsite technical assistance intervention to improve the teaching practices of a special educator, Sally. The dependent variable was the percentage of components correctly completed for each of three teaching skills: (a) informal assessments, (b) quality individualized education plans (IEPs), and (c) adaptations to the general education curriculum. Each of these teaching skills comprised an individual *tier* of the multiple-baseline design, making this a *multiple-baseline across-behaviors design*.

In a multiple-baseline design, as previously noted, the independent variable is sequentially administered across different tiers or baselines. The design logic requires researchers to simultaneously evaluate different patterns of behavior as the design is implemented. For instance, in Figure 12.1, the first baseline (i.e., informal assessments) was stable over two weeks. When the intervention was implemented, there was an immediate increase in the educator's correct use of informal assessment. However, there was no change in the level of behaviors on the other two tiers of the multiple-baseline design at the same point in time. This shows that only behaviors directly receiving the intervention were influenced by the treatment. On Week 6, the intervention was implemented for the second baseline (i.e., quality IEPs), and this dependent variable increased over several weeks. In addition, behavior on the first baseline continued to maintain at high levels with the independent variable in place, but behaviors on the third tier (i.e., adaptations) remained at low levels while still in baseline. Hence, only behaviors that had received intervention improved. Finally, on Week 13, the intervention was applied to the behaviors represented on the third tier of the multiple-baseline design, and improvements were immediately observed.

Figure 12.1 illustrates the basic logic of a multiple-baseline design. Individual baselines are established, consistent response patterns are observed, and then the independent variable is systematically introduced to one baseline at a time. The researcher waits until a clear change in the pattern of behavior occurs for the baseline receiving the intervention, with the other tier(s) remaining stable. The process is then repeated with the second tier, and so on. If changes in the dependent variable occur only when the independent variable is introduced, then a functional relation is demonstrated.

FIGURE 12.1 ■ Example of A Multiple-baseline Across-behaviors Design.

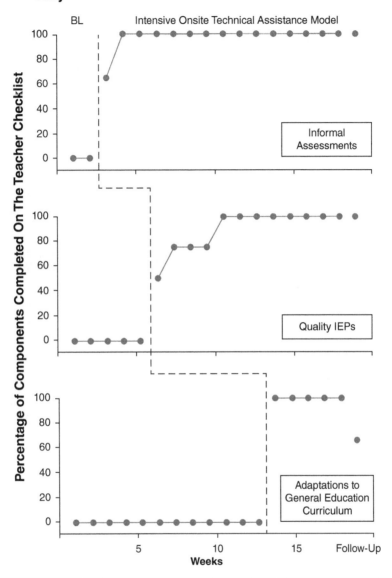

Note: The dependent variable was the percentage of components correctly completed for each of three teaching skills: (a) informal assessments, (b) quality IEPs, and (c) adaptations to the general education curriculum. The intervention was an intensive onsite technical assistance intervention to improve the teaching practices of a special educator, Sally, from baseline (BL). (Figure 1, p. 258, from: Clark, N. M., Cushing, L. S., & Kennedy, C. H. (2004). An intensive onsite technical assistance model to promote inclusive educational practices for students with disabilities in middle school and high school. *Research and Practice for Persons With Severe Disabilities, 29*(4), 253–262. Copyright 2004 by TASH. Reproduced by permission.)

BASIC MULTIPLE-BASELINE DESIGNS

Traditionally, multiple-baseline designs have been described as occurring across *behaviors, people, settings, stimuli, or times* (Baer et al., 1968). That is, the tiers of the multiple-baseline design can be comprised of a range of events that might be associated with a particular experimental question. A multiple-baseline design across behaviors was previously shown in Figure 12.1. An example of a multiple-baseline design across people is presented in Figure 12.2. "People" can refer to students, educators, administrators, family members, related services professionals, and so on. In this study by Chen et al. (2005), they sought to improve the correct facial/emotional labeling of three adolescents with autism spectrum disorder (ASD). The three students—Zhu, Lin, and Lai—were taught to correctly label facial expressions using augmented-reality 3-D presentations. Baselines were established concurrently for each of the three students' behaviors, and the intervention was sequentially introduced one tier at a time and only after a change in the pattern of behavior from baseline had been demonstrated. This experimental design represents an initial experimental effect in an A-B sequence for Zhu that was replicated once for Lin and once for Lai (see Box 12.2 for discussion of how this design approach deviates from an $N = 1$ design logic).

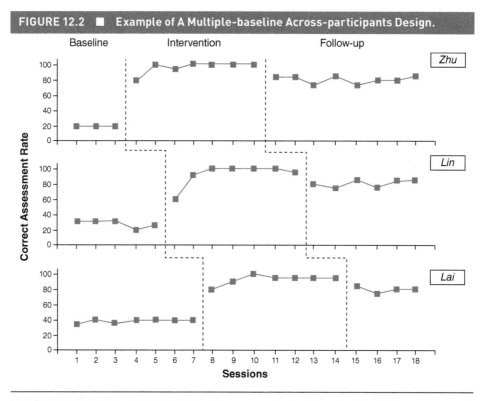

FIGURE 12.2 ■ Example of A Multiple-baseline Across-participants Design.

Note: The y-axis shows the correct labeling of facial expressions by Zhu, Lin, and Lai. The individuals were taught to label facial expressions using augmented-reality 3-D avatar simulations. (Figure 4, p. 401, from: Chen, C. H., Lee, I. J., & Lin, L. Y. (2015). Augmented reality-based self-facial modeling to promote the emotional expression and social skills of adolescents with autism spectrum disorders. *Research in Developmental Disabilities, 36,* 396–403. Copyright 2014 by Elsevier Ltd. Reproduced by permission.)

BOX 12.2: IS A MULTIPLE-BASELINE ACROSS-PARTICIPANTS DESIGN A SINGLE-CASE DESIGN?

Perhaps the most frequently used single-case design is the multiple-baseline across-participants design. However, this design, by definition, requires the intervention to be staggered across different people. Demonstrating experimental control with such a design requires a minimum of two, and often more, participants. Such an arrangement violates the logic of single-case designs, which focuses on experimental control being established with an *N* = 1. However, although the multiple-baseline across-participants design is not technically an *N* = 1 experimental design, it has been used effectively for over 50 years to analyze educationally relevant behavior and has yielded a variety of important experimental findings. Apparently, for researchers, the utility of the multiple-baseline across-participants design outweighs the logical contradiction this design presents.

Another example of a multiple-baseline design is shown in Figure 12.3. This figure shows a multiple-baseline across-settings design. The study by Kennedy et al. (1997) analyzed the effects of a peer support program on the social contacts between a student with extensive support needs (Max) and his peers without disabilities in two general education classes. This experimental design represents the *minimal number* of tiers a multiple baseline can have and still show a replicated effect (i.e., two) (see Chapter 3). In the Kennedy et al. study, stable baselines were established, and the independent variable was introduced sequentially across the class periods. In each instance, the intervention was associated with an increase in the number of social contacts and the number of peers interacted with. Hence, a functional relation was established.

When multiple-baseline across-stimuli designs are used, anything that might serve as an event for interaction could be incorporated into the design (e.g., toys or game apps). If a multiple-baseline across-time design is used, then other factors, such as setting, people, and behaviors, are held constant, while the intervention is sequentially implemented across different times of the day (e.g., morning versus afternoon). In general, any event that is of experimental interest can be incorporated into a multiple-baseline design. As long as the event meets the requirements for operationalization we discussed in Chapter 7, then it can be used as a tier in a multiple-baseline design. In addition, as was shown in Figure 4.3 from Chapter 4, multiple-baseline designs can also incorporate combinations of behaviors, people, settings, stimuli, or times into the tiers of the design.

Although there is a minimal number of tiers that are required for replication when using multiple-baseline designs (i.e., two), there is no upper limit to the number of tiers that can be incorporated into the design (other than the tractability of too many tiers). An important issue with any multiple-baseline design is the *functional independence* of each tier. That is, when an intervention is introduced for one tier, the effect on the dependent variable should not "spill over" to other tiers in the design. If this occurs, then experimental control may not be achieved.

Another issue with establishing experimental control via multiple-baseline designs relates to *delayed intervention effects*. Because introducing the intervention across tiers of the multiple

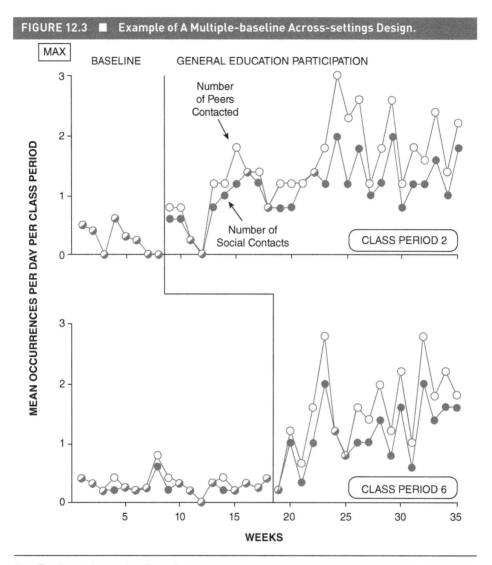

FIGURE 12.3 ■ Example of A Multiple-baseline Across-settings Design.

Note: This figure pictures the effects of a peer support program on the social contacts between a student with severe disabilities (Max) and his peers without disabilities in two classes. This experimental design represents the minimal number of tiers a multiple baseline can have and still show a replicated effect. (Figure 2, p. 178, from: Kennedy, C. H., Cushing, L., & Itkonen, T. (1997). General education participation increases the social contacts and friendship networks of students with severe disabilities. *Journal of Behavioral Education, 7*, 167–189. Copyright 1997 by Human Sciences Press, Inc. Reproduced with permission from Springer Nature Customer Service Center.)

baseline design requires the dependent variable to change its pattern of occurrence, delayed intervention effects can be a concern. If the next intervention is intervened upon too soon, a functional relation will not be demonstrated. Conversely, if the effect of the independent variable is sufficiently delayed, then in some instances *maturational processes* (i.e., a threat to internal validity) may change the behaviors in other tiers of the design. If this occurs, then baselines

FIGURE 12.4 ■ Example of A Multiprobe Multiple-baseline Design.

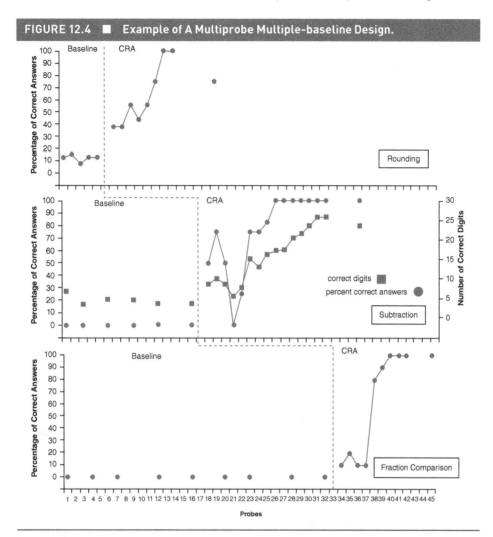

Note: The dependent variables included rounding, subtraction, and fraction comparison skills shown as the percentage of correct answers on the left vertical axis (closed circles) and the number of correct digits on the right vertical axis (closed squares). The independent variable was use of a CRA instructional sequencing intervention. (Figure 5, p. 510, from: Hinton, V. M., & Flores, M. M. (2019). The effects of the concrete-representational-abstract sequence for students at risk for mathematics failure. *Journal of Behavioral Education, 28*(4), 493–516. Copyright 2019 by Human Sciences Press, Inc. Reproduced with permission from Springer Nature Customer Service Center.)

would begin showing improvements in the absence of the independent variable and, again, experimental control would be compromised.

MULTIPLE-BASELINE DESIGN VARIANTS

Variants of the multiple-baseline design have emerged since the design was first used in the 1960s. We will discuss two general variations of the multiple-baseline design in this section: (a) *multiprobe multiple-baseline designs* and (b) *nonconcurrent multiple-baseline designs*.

Multiprobe Multiple-Baseline Designs

Horner and Baer (1978) introduced the multiprobe multiple-baseline design as a way of making the multiple-baseline design more efficient for researchers. In the standard multiple-baseline design we discussed in the previous section, data points are taken for each session in each tier of the multiple-baseline design. So, for tiers that receive intervention later in the experimental sequence, a large number of data points are typically collected. The multiprobe multiple baseline design takes advantage of this situation by only intermittently collecting data during the execution of the experimental series. Because data are only collected intermittently, this saves the amount of effort required to record and score observational sessions.

Importantly, data are collected only intermittently during the experiment at times that are required for estimating trends and related patterns in the data within and between the tiers. An example of this design is presented in Figure 12.4. Hinton and Flores (2019) used a multiprobe multiple-baseline design across mathematical skills to study how to increase children's understanding of number and mathematical concepts using a concrete-representational-abstract (CRA) instructional sequence. The dependent variables included the percentage of correct answers for rounding, subtraction, and fraction comparison.

In this investigation, Hinton and Flores (2019) used the multiprobe technique only for baseline assessments. Several facets of this experimental design deserve comment. First, the baseline and intervention sessions were conducted on a regular basis, but data were collected only intermittently on behavior during baseline. Therefore, the data represent a sampling of the overall performance of the mathematics skills in the baseline conditions. Second, data probes were taken intermittently, but consistently. Third, probe data were collected at strategic time points including before the start of phases and as the intervention was introduced on other tiers of the multiple-baseline design. This allowed the researchers to estimate levels of the dependent variable at each time point surrounding when the intervention was introduced. These characteristics are critical for demonstrating a functional relation with this type of design.

As can be seen in Figure 12.4, Hinton and Flores (2019) met these design requirements.

Discrete mathematics skills only increased following the introduction of the CRA intervention. At each time point that data probes were collected during baseline across the tiers, low levels of correct answers were observed. However, each time the intervention was introduced, the specific mathematics skill increased while the others remained in the baseline range of performance. Thus, experimental control was demonstrated even though less than 50% of the baseline sessions had data collected on child behaviors.

A second type of multiprobe multiple-baseline design was introduced by Tawney and Gast (1984). The design is also referred to as a *multiple-probe design*. This type of design is particularly useful for studying *generalization processes* (Carnett et al., 2022; Stokes & Baer, 1977). In this type of single-case design, data probes are collected at multiple time points for each tier of the multiple-baseline design: (a) baseline and (b) instructional sessions. In addition, two types of behavioral variables are included in each tier of the design: (1) target and (2) generalization behaviors. Baseline probes are collected on all target and generalization behaviors across tiers; then an intervention is introduced to the first-tier target behaviors. When behavior change has occurred (e.g., response acquisition), probes are taken across all target and generalization behaviors to assess their status. This process is then repeated, in sequence, for the remaining tiers in the design.

An example of this design tactic was used in a study by Barton (2015). Figure 12.5 shows the data from a child with ASD named Casey. The treatment was comprised of a system of least prompts and teacher praise. Of interest were the acquisition of three behaviors (pretend play, symbolic play, and social interaction) and generalization probes for each of these behaviors in an unprompted context. Data were initially collected across all behaviors of interest to estimate levels of social and imitative behavior. The prompting intervention was then introduced that directly taught Casey how to engage in pretend play. Once the instructional criteria were met for pretend play, probes across behaviors were again conducted in an unprompted generalization context. In this instance, only pretend play was acquired, and the other behaviors remained at baseline levels. This process was subsequently repeated on each set of behaviors, with symbolic play and social interaction only occurring after receiving instruction.

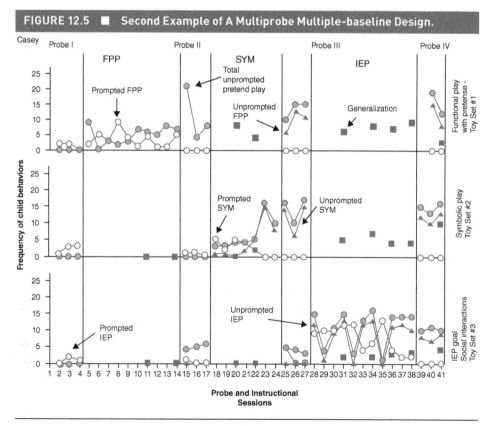

FIGURE 12.5 ■ Second Example of A Multiprobe Multiple-baseline Design.

Note: Data from a child with ASD named Casey. The behaviors of interest were the acquisition of three behaviors (pretend play, symbolic play, and social interaction) and three generalization probes. (Figure 3, p. 500, from: Barton, E. E. (2015). Teaching generalized pretend play and related behaviors to young children with disabilities. *Exceptional Children, 81*(4), 489–506. Copyright 2015 by Sage Publications. Reproduced by permission.)

Multiprobe multiple-baseline designs can be efficient experimental tools as shown by the Hinton and Flores (2019) and Barton (2015) studies. Because data are intermittently collected at strategic time points within the multiple-baseline design, the amount of effort required for data collection and scoring is minimized. A primary drawback to the use of these designs is that because of the intermittent nature of data collection, this design type is less sensitive to abrupt changes in the level of behavior that might occur during baseline. In addition, if cyclical patterns of behavior are present, the intermittent sampling technique may not capture the occurrence of these patterns (see Fisher et al., 2002).

Nonconcurrent Multiple-Baseline Designs

A second variant of the multiple-baseline design is the nonconcurrent multiple baseline design. As previously noted, all single-case designs are differing configurations of A-B conditions. In the multiple-baseline design, the A-B conditions are staggered on different tiers of the experimental arrangement. The design controls for several possible threats to internal validity by staggering the introduction of the independent variable on different tiers and assessing for consistent effects.

A variation on this logic is the temporal separation of the different A-B tiers. That is, instead of all the tiers being conducted concurrently, each of the tiers can be conducted at different time points. The differing A-B tiers can be completely separated in time (e.g., different days, months, semesters, or years), there can be partial overlap, or some tiers can be time-linked while others are temporally distant. Because of this temporal feature, such designs are referred to as *nonconcurrent* (Hayes, 1981; Watson & Workman, 1981).

An example of this design type is presented in Figure 12.6. Rincón et al. (2023) studied rejection sensitivity in gay men who were experiencing anxiety relating to emotional intimacy. The dependent variable was the frequency of clinically relevant behaviors by three men (Charlie, Michel, and Danny). The independent variable was the use of functional analytic psychotherapy (FAP) designed to improve interpersonal interactions. Figure 12.6 shows the sequential improvement in clinically relevant behaviors after introducing the independent variable (see CRB2s). The data are arrayed concurrently by session number, even though each A-B analysis occurred separately.

A second example of the utility of nonconcurrent multiple-baseline designs is presented in a hypothetical case by Harvey et al. (2004). In this instance, shown in Figure 12.7, a nonconcurrent multiple-baseline design was used to analyze a larger aggregate than is usually the focus of single-case research (i.e., each "individual" was a local education agency or school district). In this instance, the intervention focused on increasing teachers' use of effective instructional practices and a consistent general education curriculum. Each tier in this design was conducted in different school semesters. In addition, in this instance, the authors labeled the tiers with the calendar dates when each A-B analysis was conducted.

Another way of graphing data from a nonconcurrent multiple-baseline design was presented by Watson and Workman (1981). In this paper, which originally introduced this design variant, the authors suggested graphing the data in a manner that reflects the temporal relation between each tier in the design. Figure 12.8 shows an example of this graphic

FIGURE 12.6 ■ Example of A Nonconcurrent Multiple-baseline Design.

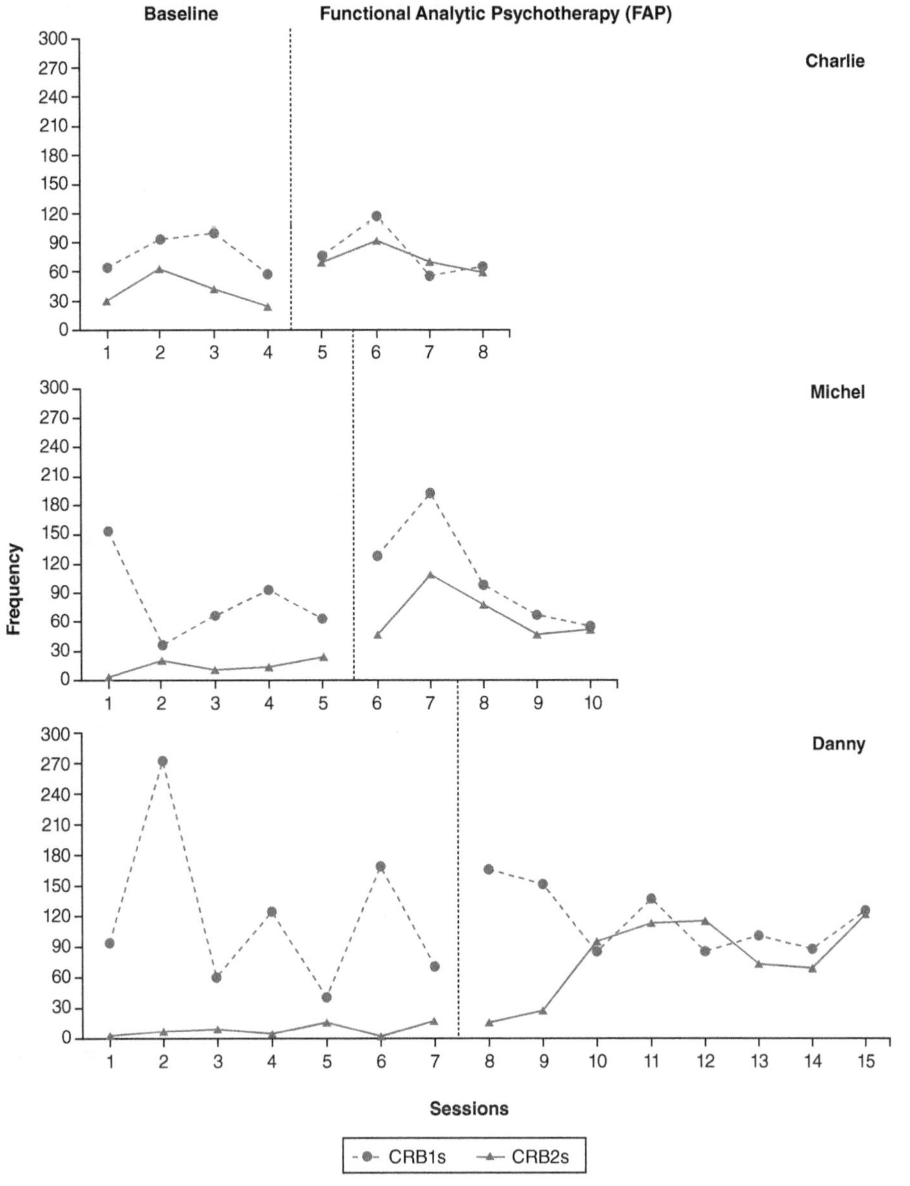

Note: The dependent variable was frequency of clinically relevant behaviors (see CRB2s in the graph) in three gay men with rejection sensitivity. The independent variable was the use of FAP to facilitate positive interpersonal interactions. (Figure 1, p. 92, from: Rincón, C. L., Muñoz-Martínez, A. M., Hoeflein, B., & Skinta, M. D. (2023). Enhancing interpersonal intimacy in Colombian gay men using functional analytic psychotherapy: An experimental nonconcurrent multiple baseline design. *Cognitive and Behavioral Practice, 30*(1), 82–95. Copyright 2023 by the Association for Behavioral and Cognitive Therapies. Reproduced by permission.)

approach using hypothetical data. Three participants were included in the analysis, with Subject 1 receiving the first baseline and intervention series, then Subject 2, and finally Subject 3. There is some overlap between the three cases, but with differing baseline lengths. Whether the graphic approach shown in Figure 12.6, 12.7, or 12.8 is used, it is important that the researchers specify in the reporting of their data when each set of A-B conditions was conducted so the reader can judge possible temporal relations between or among the various tiers of the design.

A benefit of the nonconcurrent multiple-baseline design is the ability for researchers to systematically study topics that might not otherwise be amenable to an experimental analysis (Harvey et al., 2004; Slocum et al., 2022). This includes rare cases, limited research resources, and the incorporation of larger individual units (e.g., schools, local education agencies, or state educational agencies) into single-case experimental studies. This design variant controls for most threats to internal validity (e.g., maturation, test–retest sensitivity, and instrumentation changes), with the exception of history effects (see Box 12.3). Therefore, use of this design needs to be considered within the larger context of establishing experimental control and gaining access to experimental opportunities not typically considered amenable to single-case design analysis (or other types of experimental designs).

BOX 12.3: CAN NONCONCURRENT MULTIPLE-BASELINE DESIGNS BE USED TO CONTROL FOR HISTORY EFFECTS?

With their many positive characteristics as an approach to demonstrating experimental control, nonconcurrent multiple-baseline designs have tremendous potential as an analytical tool. The primary limitation noted with this design logic is the caveat that this experimental approach has inherent limitations in controlling for *history effects*. The reason for this concern regarding internal validity is that nonconcurrent multiple-baseline designs by their nature separate in time each tier of the baseline. Therefore, idiosyncratic history effects can occur for individual tiers of the multiple-baseline tactic and introduce confounds to the interpretation of the results. However, Slocum et al. (2022) have presented a reconceptualization of the nonconcurrent version of this design type and noted that under certain conditions (i.e., temporally proximal alignment of the tiers in the design), history effects may be allayed. Therefore, researchers can under certain circumstances use nonconcurrent multiple-baseline designs with the same level of confidence as concurrent approaches (cf. Kennedy, 2022; Smith et al., 2022, for qualifications to this observation).

STRENGTHS AND LIMITATIONS

Multiple-baseline designs are probably the most used type of single-case design (Coon & Rapp, 2018). This is in part due to the simplicity of the design and its flexibility. Early on in the development of applied behavior analysis an emphasis was placed on developing experimental

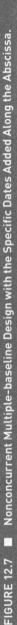

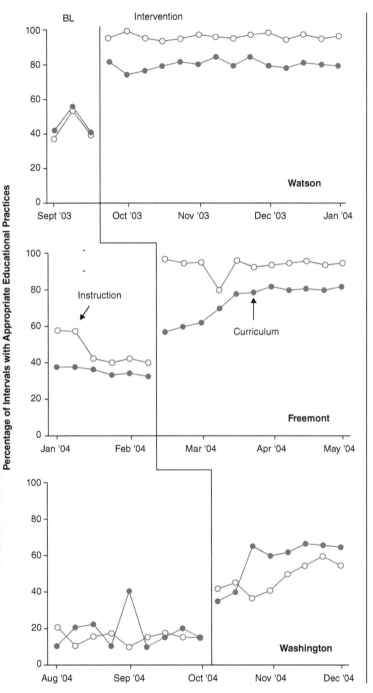

Note: In this hypothetical study, the intervention focused on increasing from baseline (BL) teachers' use of effective instructional practices and a consistent general education curriculum. Each tier n this design was conducted in different school semesters. (Figure 1, p. 271, from: Harvey, M. T., May, M. E., & Kennedy, C. H. (2004). Nonconcurrent *N* = 1 experimental designs for educational program evaluation. *Journal of Behavioral Education, 13*(4), 267–276. Copyright 2004 by Human Sciences Press, Inc. Reproduced with permission from Springer Nature Customer Service Center.)

FIGURE 12.8 ■ Method For Plotting Nonconcurrent Multiple-baseline Design Presented by Watson and Workman (1981).

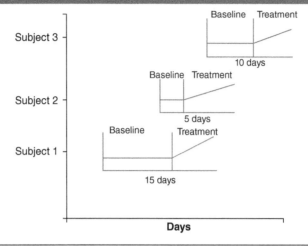

Note: Data were plotted within the temporal framework within which the A-B conditions were conducted. (Figure 1, p. 258, from: Watson, P. J., & Workman, E. A. (1981). The non-concurrent multiple baseline across-individuals design: An extension of the traditional multiple baseline design. *Journal of Behavior Therapy and Experimental Psychiatry, 12,* 257–259. Copyright 1981 by Elsevier Ltd. Reproduced by permission.)

designs that could be used by practitioners in the settings where they worked. The multiple-baseline design, whether across students, settings, behaviors, stimuli, or times, was an ideal analytical tool for such a situation (see Baer et al., 1968; Barlow et al., 1984). In addition, because of the inherent flexibility in the timing of interventions and the ability to conduct analyses in a multiprobe or nonconcurrent fashion, this tactic is easily adapted to applied settings.

Another strength of the multiple-baseline design is its utility. In situations where behavior cannot be reversed, logistical constraints do not allow the removal of the intervention, or ethical concerns make removal of the intervention unacceptable, then multiple-baseline designs are the experimental tactic of choice. However, this strength is also the primary weakness of the design. Because of its structure, it is difficult to conduct *comparative, component,* or *parametric* analyses of independent variables using the multiple-baseline design. In general, its status as an analytical tool is limited to demonstrating the general effects of an independent variable on behavior. This means that multiple-baseline designs are not very useful for exploring basic mechanisms underlying behavioral change (i.e., translational research; see Chapter 2). So, as with all the other analytical tactics we are discussing in Part IV of this book, *the utility of any particular design depends on the experimental question.*

REFLECTION QUESTIONS

1. What are the prerequisite data patterns that need to be established before an intervention can be introduced to a new tier in a multiple-baseline design?

2. How many tiers of a multiple-baseline design are needed to show experimental control if there is a clear effect on each tier?

3. Explain the logic behind the use of multiprobe, multiple-baseline designs.

4. Identify three elements in the debate over whether a nonconcurrent multiple-baseline design can control for a broad range of history effects.

5. Why would an investigator say that a multiple-baseline design across participants is not a true single-case design?

13 REPEATED-ACQUISITION DESIGNS

The difficulty of reversing some types of learned behavior is an important issue in single-case designs. Because many $N = 1$ designs rely on the manipulation of reinforcement contingencies or withdrawal of interventions, the reversal of behavior to baseline patterns is necessary to demonstrate response differentiation and experimental control. Multiple-baseline designs are used to deal with the issue of reversibility by establishing two or more baselines and then sequentially introducing the independent variable one tier at a time. Such a design tactic amounts to a staggered set of A-B experimental conditions, which is a relatively modest level of experimental control from a within-participant (ideographic) perspective.

REPEATED-ACQUISITION DESIGNS

When the reversibility of behavior is a question, an alternative design to the multiple-baseline design is the *repeated-acquisition design*. Initially introduced by Boren (1963) for basic research on learning processes, the repeated-acquisition design allows for the analysis of skill acquisition under different experimental conditions (see also Boren & Devine, 1968). The three defining characteristics of a repeated acquisition design are the (a) use of multiple equivalent learning tasks (b) in which acquisition can be studied repeatedly from one task to another (c) under at least two different experimental conditions. The participant is exposed to a particular learning task, their rate of acquisition is documented, and then the participant learns a new, equivalent task under different experimental conditions. This process is continued with new tasks until a clear difference is demonstrated between or among experimental conditions. The result is an opportunity to study the effects of various experimental conditions on learning processes, such as reading, mathematics, social studies, science, or movement skills.

An example of a repeated-acquisition design is presented in Figure 13.1. The experiment, by Dennis and Whalon (2021), analyzed the teacher- versus application-delivered instruction intended to improve children's expressive vocabulary. The students were preschoolers attending a Head Start program who were at risk for developmental delays. The stimuli were expressive verbs from storybooks. A collection of verbs was identified and ranked according to utility and complexity by a group of experts. Equivalent words were then randomly assigned to conditions. Stimuli were presented in a bascline (labeled as "pretest"), intervention sessions were delivered for four days, and then "posttests" were conducted. This process was repeated across seven or eight sets of equivalent stimuli. A total of six participants were included in the study, but for exposition brevity, only the data from Participants 4 and 5 are presented in Figure 13.1.

FIGURE 13.1 ■ Example of A Repeated-Acquisition Design.

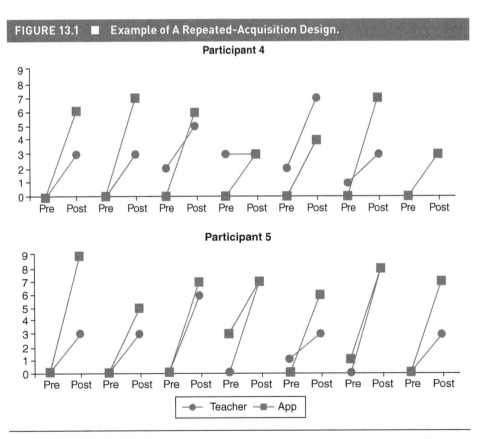

Note. This figure shows a study of expressive verb acquisition for two preschoolers attending a Head Start program and at risk for developmental disabilities (Participants 4 and 5). The dependent variable was the number of opportunities during storybook reading when targeted verbs were used correctly. The two interventions were teacher- versus application-delivered instruction. (Figure 1, p. 201, from: Dennis, L. R., & Whalon, K. J. (2021). Effects of teacher- versus application-delivered instruction on the expressive vocabulary of at-risk preschool children. *Remedial and Special Education, 42*(4), 195–206. Copyright 2021 by the Hammill Institute on Disabilities. Reprinted by permission.)

The initial pretest conditions served to empirically demonstrate whether the stimuli were of equivalent difficulty (i.e., percent correct). The posttest data points reflected the degree of expressive word acquisition from the teacher-delivered instruction (closed circles) and application-delivered instruction (closed squares). Figure 13.1 shows that Participant 4 acquired a greater percentage of expressive verbs during application-delivered instruction during the first two comparisons (and the sixth stimulus set). However, the student showed similar acquisition between conditions during comparison sets 3, 4, and 7 and a higher percentage for the teacher-delivered instruction in set 5. Participant 5 showed a more consistent pattern of higher expressive word acquisition under the application-delivered instruction condition. Given the degree of within- and between-participant direct replication, it is judicious to say that the application-delivered instruction typically resulted in better expressive verb usage for Participant 5 and the two conditions were similar for Participant 4. Across all six students in the study, there was a general pattern favoring the application-delivered instruction condition.

A second example of a repeated-acquisition design—from a study conducted by Danforth et al. (1990)—is presented in Figure 13.2. The four participants, labeled Subjects 1 through 4, were undergraduate university students. This laboratory experiment required students to learn a new sequence of arbitrary responses presented on a computer screen during each experimental session. Under one condition participants were given trial-and-error feedback (labeled Contingency Learning), and under a second condition they were verbally told what the sequence was (labeled Instructed Learning). The dependent measure for the study was the number of errors that were made before a response sequence was learned. Which condition the participants were exposed to as they acquired the sequence varied from session to session (left-hand panel of graph). After four hours had elapsed, the students were again tested to see if they remembered the sequence of responses (right-hand panel of graph). The data show that instructed learning resulted in almost error-free response acquisition, whereas contingency learning resulted in approximately 20 errors being made before a new response sequence was acquired. However, during the follow-up tests, both contingency and instructed learning resulted in a similar number of errors, showing that the pattern of acquisition did not influence remembering.

Another example of a repeated-acquisition design is presented in Figure 13.3. This figure shows a study of sight word acquisition for a 6-year-old student (Zane) who had attention deficit hyperactivity disorder (ADHD) (see Carroll et al., 2015). The dependent variable was the percentage of sight words read correctly. Four different interventions plus a control procedure were compared. The error-correction procedures included (a) multiple-response repetition; (b) removal and re-presentation of the word; (c) re-presentation of the word until independent, correct performance; and (d) single-response repetition. The authors used a variation of the classic repeated-acquisition design noted in previous studies. Carroll et al. assigned equivalent sight words to each of the intervention and control conditions and established with the baseline that words were not known by the student. They then repeated each of the conditions and matched sight words once a day until the acquisition pattern emerged. In this case, the re-presentation of the word until independent, correct performance condition resulted in the fastest acquisition for this student.

FIGURE 13.2　■　A Second Example of A Repeated-Acquisition Design.

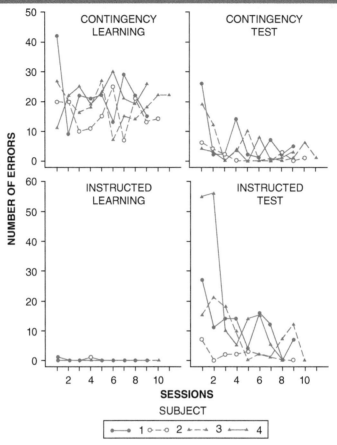

Note. The four participants, labeled Subjects 1 through 4, were undergraduate university students. This labora-tory experiment required students to learn a new sequence of arbitrary responses presented on a computer screen during each experimental session. Under one condition participants were given trial-and-error feedback (labeled Contingency Learning), and under a second condition they were verbally told what the sequence was (labeled Instructed Learning). The dependent measure for the study was the number of errors that were made until a response sequence was acquired. Which condition the participants were exposed to as they acquired the sequence varied from session to session (left-hand panel of graph). After four hours had elapsed, the students were again tested to see if they remembered the sequence of responses (right-hand panel of graph). (Figure 2, p. 101, from: Danforth, J. S., Chase, P. N., Dolan, M., & Joyce, J. H. (1990). The establishment of stimulus control by instructions and by differential reinforcement. *Journal of the Experimental Analysis of Behavior, 54*, 97–112. Copyright 1990 by the Society for the Experimental Analysis of Behavior. Reprinted by permission.)

METHODOLOGICAL ISSUES IN REPEATED-ACQUISITION DESIGNS

There are several methodological issues that need to be considered when using repeated-acquisi-tion designs (see Kirby et al., 2021, for additional criteria that can be considered). Critical issues include (a) *task comparability*, (b) *condition sequence*, and (c) *the number of conditions*. Each will be discussed in turn.

FIGURE 13.3 ■ Variation of the Repeated-Acquisition Design that Incorporates A Baseline Condition Demonstrating Stimulus Similarity.

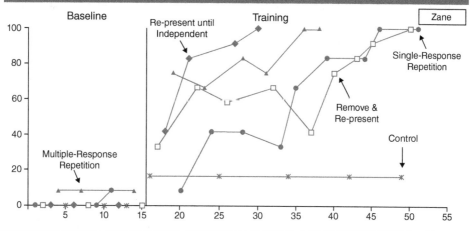

Note. Multiple error-correction procedures were compared against a control condition to teach a child with ADHD sight word reading. (Figure 3, p. 267, from: Carroll, R. A., Joachim, B. T., St. Peter, C. C., & Robinson, N. (2015). A comparison of error-correction procedures on skill acquisition during discrete-trial instruction. *Journal of Applied Behavior Analysis, 48*(2), 257–273. Copyright 1990 by the Society for the Experimental Analysis of Behavior. Reprinted by permission.)

Task Comparability

A potential methodological flaw when using repeated-acquisition designs is a bias in the tasks that are assigned to particular conditions. A key aspect of these designs is the development of a pool of equivalent stimuli that can be learned. The stimulus pool needs to be large enough that new items can be drawn upon to constitute a novel set of stimuli for each new acquisition phase. However, this process brings into light the critical need for all stimuli to be equally difficult to acquire. If one set of stimuli is more easily learned than another set, the differences in conditions may be a result of stimuli themselves and not the independent variable(s) under analysis. This would introduce an obvious confound.

The prototypical strategy for dealing with this methodological concern was used in the Danforth et al. (1990) study. In this study, Danforth et al. were able to use a stimulus pool that had a set number of elements (response keys) that could be reconstituted for each acquisition phase in a novel arrangement. Using this technique, the first acquisition phase may compare the sequence 1-5-2-4-3 for Contingency Learning and 3-2-4-5-1 for Instructional Learning. The next acquisition phase might compare the sequence 4-5-3-1-2 for Contingency Learning and 2-1-3-5-4 for Instructional Learning, and so on. For as long as novel patterns can be generated, there is no reason to believe that any one order is more difficult than another, and, therefore, task comparability is a reasonable assumption.

An approach that can be used in educational research is to develop a large enough pool of stimuli so that they can be randomly assigned to conditions. For example, if the acquisition task is successfully reading sight words, then a stimulus pool can be established that contains items of equivalent difficulty (e.g., the number of letters per word and/or the consonant–vowel combinations). When task comparability is not a reasonable assumption, then stimuli need to be empirically demonstrated to be equivalent. One means of doing this is to establish a pool of stimuli and then test acquisition of the stimuli under equivalent conditions with a few participants. This "pretesting" of the stimuli can be used to show that the stimuli are of equal difficulty and, just as importantly, show the investigator what items are outliers that need to be removed from the stimulus pool prior to conducting a study using a repeated-acquisition design.

Condition Sequence

When using repeated-acquisition designs, a similar set of issues emerges regarding condition sequencing as was discussed for multielement designs (Chapter 11). It is possible that exposure to one condition may influence performance on a subsequent task. Two procedural possibilities exist for addressing this issue. One approach is to hold the sequence of conditions fixed so that influence cannot be randomly spread between or among conditions (see Chapter 3 for a discussion of nomothetic versus idiographic conceptualizations of randomization). If interaction effects are a concern, then they can be experimentally analyzed by systematically altering the sequence of conditions and studying whether any particular condition sequence produces an altered pattern of acquisition (see Hains & Baer, 1989). A second option is the randomization approach. That is, during each acquisition phase, the experimenter can randomly assign one condition or another as first, second, and so on. Again, as was noted in Box 11.2, *randomization of conditions is not a control technique in single-case designs*; it only distributes variability evenly across conditions if a large enough sample is conducted.

Number of Conditions

How many distinct conditions can be included in a repeated-acquisition design is *an issue of tractability*. In the examples that have been presented so far, only two conditions were compared. Such a comparison between conditions is an easily executed experimental arrangement. In Figure 13.4, a study by Higgins et al. (1989) compared four conditions in a repeated-acquisition design. Participants were seven adults. The dependent variable shown in the figure is the number of errors that were made each time a new skill was learned. The independent variable was the parametric analysis of the drug atropine at various dosages (i.e., placebo, 1.5, 3, or 6 mg/kg). In addition, a time course analysis was conducted (x-axis) to analyze the temporal effect of the independent variable on behavior (i.e., prior to drug administration, 0.5, 1.5, 3, 5, 7, 9, or 24 hours post dosing). Higgins and colleagues' results show that the greater the drug dosage, the more errors participants made during acquisition, but less effect was seen when the individuals were asked to repeat a previously learned response sequence.

The data in Figure 13.4 illustrate the use of multiple conditions in repeated-acquisition designs. As with other experimental arrangements used to conduct comparative, component, or parametric analyses, the number of conditions included is a function of two issues. First, what is the minimal number of conditions that need to be included, given a particular experimental question? Second, do the number of conditions to be included in an experiment permit the successful completion of the study in a time frame that is consistent with available resources?

FIGURE 13.4 ■ Example of use of Multiple Conditions within a Repeated-Acquisition Design.

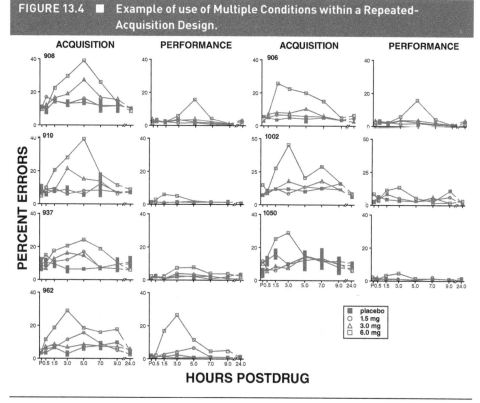

Note. Participants were seven adult males. The dependent variable shown in the figure is the number of errors that were made each time a new skill was learned. The independent variable was the parametric analysis of a drug called atropine at various dosages (i.e., placebo, 1.5, 3, or 6 mg/kg). In addition, a time course analysis was conducted (x-axis) to analyze the temporal effect of the independent variable on behavior (i.e., prior to drug administration, 0.5, 1.5, 3, 5, 7, 9, or 24 hours post dosing). (Figure 2, p. 10, from: Higgins, S. T., Woodward, B. M., & Henningfield, J. E. (1989). Effects of atropine on the repeated acquisition and performance of response sequences in humans. *Journal of the Experimental Analysis of Behavior, 51*, 5–15. Copyright 1989 by the Society for the Experimental Analysis of Behavior. Reprinted by permission.)

STRENGTHS AND LIMITATIONS

Although repeated-acquisition designs have been used in basic research since the 1960s, their use in single-case educational research has been less frequent and delayed. This follows a well-known pattern of transfer of new experimental techniques from basic laboratory settings to applied settings. Interestingly, use of such designs in applied behavioral research seems to be increasing (Tanious & Onghena, 2021). This may be in part because of increased attention to translational research integrating basic mechanisms into applied studies (see Chapter 2 and Kennedy et al., 2001).

The use of repeated-acquisition designs allows single-case researchers to study behaviors that cannot be reversed. This includes such educationally relevant behaviors as spelling, addition/subtraction, reading comprehension, and motor skill development, to name only a few.

The repeated-acquisition design is used to accomplish this analytical feat by establishing a stimulus pool of equivalent items and studying their acquisition under different experimental conditions. A primary limitation of this design is the establishment and demonstration of item substitutability (or equivalence) among the stimuli. If some type of asymmetry in task difficulty is established in the original pool of items, it may serve as an important threat to internal validity. However, if this challenge can be met, repeated-acquisition designs are an efficient means of studying learning processes, from both a basic behavioral perspective and an applied teaching orientation.

REFLECTION QUESTIONS

1. Explain the logic of using repeated-acquisition designs to demonstrate experimental control.

2. Can repeated-acquisition designs be used to analyze nonreversible behaviors?

3. What is a key source of equivalence that needs to be established when conducting a repeated-acquisition analysis?

4. Repeated-acquisition designs can be used to study cognitive tasks like sight word reading, but can they also be used to study sequences of behavior?

5. Is there a limit to the number of conditions that can be incorporated into a repeated-acquisition design?

14 BRIEF EXPERIMENTAL DESIGNS

LEARNING OBJECTIVES

After reading this chapter, you will be able to

14.1 Identify the situations in which a brief experimental design would be appropriate.

14.2 Differentiate two variants of brief experimental designs.

14.3 Evaluate the strengths and limitations of brief experimental designs.

One concern with any type of experimental design used in educational settings is the amount of time required to complete the analysis. Schools are busy settings with a large number of logistical challenges, and the sooner that an analysis can be completed, the more likely the setting can tolerate the necessary exceptions to business as usual. However, because single-case designs require repeated measures both prior to and following an intervention, the time scope of analyses is often a challenge for researchers and educators alike. Indeed, educational settings are not the only environments with time restrictions. Outpatient clinics, related-service therapies, and standardized testing all require specific tasks be accomplished in a limited amount of time.

BRIEF EXPERIMENTAL DESIGNS

Because of these logistical constraints, researchers working in educational or related settings have developed an approach to experimental design referred to as *brief experimental designs* (Wacker et al., 2004). First introduced by Cooper et al. (1990), brief experimental designs are variants of the A-B-A-B and multielement design types. They were explicitly developed for use in situations where internal validity was necessary to assess some behavioral outcome but the amount of time in which to accomplish the task was extremely limited. In the initial Cooper et al. study, parent–child interactions in an outpatient hospital setting were analyzed to establish the source of behavior problems engaged in by typically developing children. Because the researchers had only 90 minutes to complete their analysis and make treatment recommendations, they adapted currently existing single-case designs to the needs of the setting. Since this initial demonstration, dozens of studies have been published using this approach to single-case design.

Using brief experimental designs, a researcher conducts a single session under one set of conditions, conducts another type of session, and then reverses back to the initial condition if a change in behavior is observed. If no experimental influence is detected in the initial conditions, an additional condition might be tested, and then, if an effect is observed, the researcher will revert to an earlier condition to reverse the observed effect on behavior. Typically, one session is conducted before switching to another condition, and each session lasts from 5 to 15 minutes—hence the name *brief experimental design*.

VARIANTS OF BRIEF EXPERIMENTAL DESIGNS

There are two primary variants of brief experimental designs that integrate features of A-B-A-B or multielement designs.

A-B-A-B Variants

This approach to brief experimental designs follows the logic of withdrawal or reversal designs discussed in Chapter 10. An initial baseline session is conducted, and then a second condition is tested. If there is a change in the level of behavior, then the researcher returns to the initial condition. Such an arrangement constitutes a brief A-B-A design. If logistical constraints permit, additional replications can be conducted within and/or between participants, increasing the believability of the results.

An example of an A-B-A-B-A brief experimental design is presented in Figure 14.1. In this study by Richman et al. (2001), children's ability to respond to adult demands of varying complexity was analyzed. The number of directives accurately completed by four children (Brad, Eric, Brandon, and Tabitha) constituted the dependent variable. At the top of each graph are labels for each demand condition tested: (a) one-step demand with modeling prompt (1-M), (b) one-step demand with verbal prompt (1-V), (c) three-step demand with verbal prompt (3-V), (d) three-step demand with verbal prompt plus an additional discrimination (3-V Group Discrim.), and (e) three-step demand with verbal prompt plus a conjunctive discrimination (3-V Conj.). For Brad, he was able to respond to demands with response modeled by the adult (1-M), but not to demands with verbal prompts from the adult (1-V). Each session contained five demand opportunities, and the effects of demand complexity were replicated in an A-B-A-B-A sequence. Similar analyses were conducted for the other three children with sequences individualized based on each participant's response to the independent variables.

A more complex variant of the A-B-A-B brief experimental design is shown in Figure 14.2. Boyajian et al. (2001) studied the aggression, engagement, and requests ("mands") of children with attention deficit hyperactivity disorder (ADHD). Each session lasted 10 minutes in length and tested different hypotheses about why the children might be aggressive. The initial experimental conditions that each child was exposed to included play (a control condition), attention for aggression, tangible objects for aggression, and reduction in demands for aggression. Figure 14.2 shows data for Terry. Aggression during the initial four sessions was only elevated in the Tangible condition, suggesting his aggression occurred to obtain preferred objects (e.g., toys).

FIGURE 14.1 ■ Example of An A-b-a-b-a Brief Experimental Design.

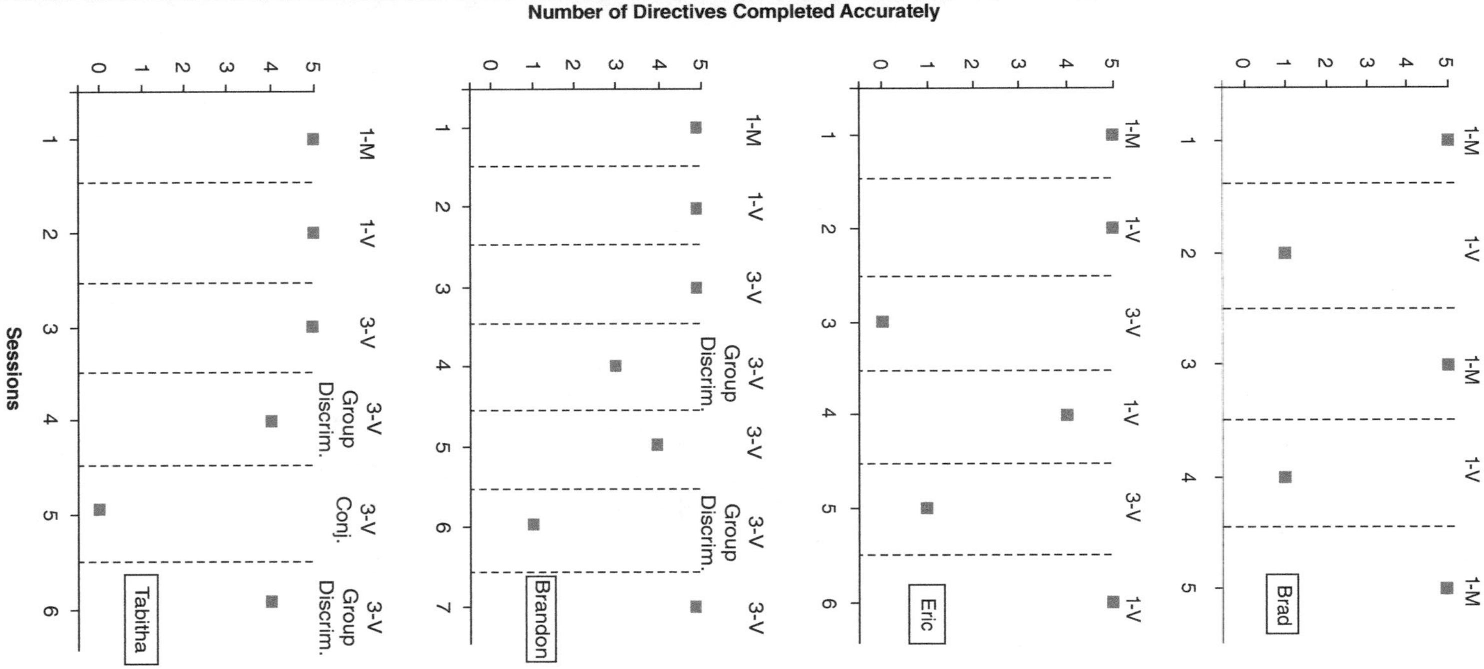

Number of Directives Completed Accurately

Sessions

Note. In this study, children's ability to respond to adult demands of varying complexity was analyzed. The number of directives accurately completed by four children (Brad, Eric, Brandon, and Tabitha) constituted the dependent variable. Each session contained five demand opportunities. At the top of each graph are labels for each demand condition tested: (a) one-step demand with modeling prompt (1-M), (b) one-step demand with verbal prompt (1-V), (c) three-step demand with verbal prompt (3-V), (d) three-step demand with verbal prompt plus an additional discrimination (3-V Group Discrim.), and (e) three-step demand with verbal prompt plus a conjunctive discrimination (3-V Conj.). (Figure 1, p. 298, from: Richman, D. M., Wacker, D. P., Brown, L. J. C., Kayser, K., Crosland, K., Stephens, T. J., & Asmus, J. (2001). Stimulus characteristics within directives: Effects on accuracy of task completion. *Journal of Applied Behavior Analysis, 34*, 289–312. Copyright 2001 by the Society for the Experimental Analysis of Behavior. Reprinted by permission.)

FIGURE 14.2 ■ Example of A Brief Experimental Design with Three Phases of Conditions.

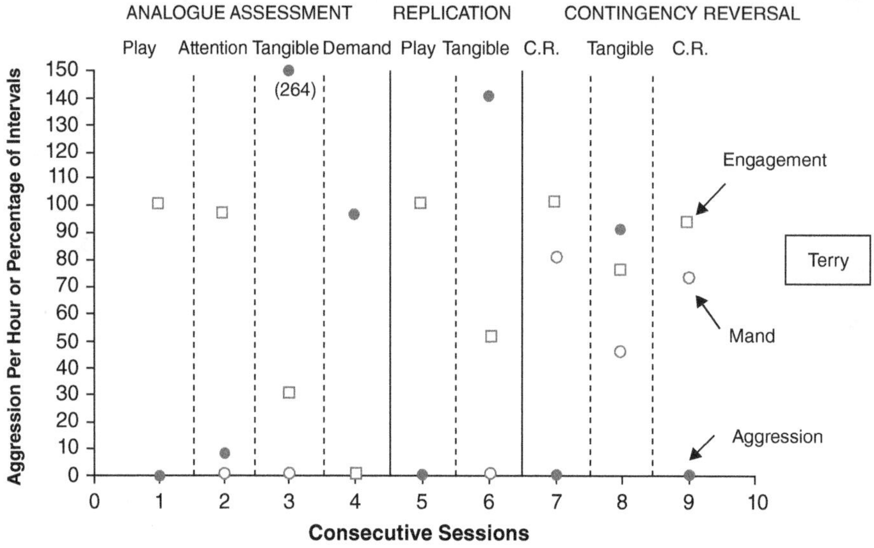

Note. The study analyzed the aggression, engagement, and requests ("mands") of Terry, a child with ADHD. Each session lasted 10 minutes in length and tested different hypotheses about why the children might be aggressive. The initial experimental conditions that Terry was exposed to included Play (a control condition), Attention for aggression, Tangible objects for aggression, and reduction in Demand for aggression. Play and Tangible conditions were then replicated in a second phase. A final phase reversed the reinforcement contingency (C.R.) to conclusively show that access to tangible items functions as a positive reinforcer. (Figure 2, p. 286, from: Boyajian, A. E., DuPaul, G. J., Handler, M. W., Eckert, T. L., & McGoey, K. E. (2001). The use of classroom-based brief functional analyses with preschoolers at-risk for attention deficit hyperactivity disorder. *School Psychology Review, 30,* 278–293 (https://doi.org/10.1080/02796015.2001.12086116). Copyright 2001 by Taylor & Francis Ltd. (http://www.tandfonline.com). Reprinted by permission.)

Two sessions were then conducted to replicate the initial finding (Sessions 5 and 6). Again, aggression was reduced during the Play condition but increased in the Tangible condition. The authors then conducted a third phase of experimental manipulations. Having already demonstrated and replicated the effect of the tangible reinforcement condition, a reversal of the reinforcement contingency was conducted (Sessions 7–9). During Sessions 7 and 9 tangible objects were provided for the absence of aggression, and during Session 8 tangible objects were provided contingent upon aggression. Consistent with the previous effects on behavior, reversal of the reinforcement contingency decreased behavior.

The experimental tactic used in Figure 14.2 highlights the degree of flexibility that is possible when using brief experimental designs. Because the design permits rapid alternation between or among conditions, the possibility for conducting comparative, component, or parametric analyses across a variety of conditions is made possible. In the case of the Boyajian et al. (2001) analysis, individual conditions were embedded within three general experimental designs (see also Baer et al., 1987). Along with a high degree of flexibility, because this design type can be used very quickly, it allows for creating and altering experimental designs in real time. By doing this type of analysis, researchers can literally follow their data and create an experimental design as patterns in behavior unfold during observations.

Multielement Variants

A second general variant of the brief experimental design uses a multielement orientation. In these designs there is an emphasis on replicating each experimental condition once or twice. The rationale for this is to assess the effect each set of experimental procedures has on the behavior(s) of interest. In addition, the sequence of conditions is not based on the presence or absence of an experimental effect in the previous condition. Instead, as was discussed in Chapter 11, conditions are either block randomized or assigned a fixed sequence.

An example of a multielement brief design is shown in Figure 14.3. In this study by Eckert et al. (2002), the oral reading fluency of six elementary school students was studied. The dependent variable was the number of words read correctly per minute. Baseline (BL) consisted of a child reading aloud with no other intervention. The Antecedent Intervention (AI) condition had the child listen to an adult read the passage and then practice the passage for three repetitions. The AI plus Contingent Reinforcement (AI+CR) condition added a reinforcement contingency for increasing reading fluency by 5% from the first to third reading repetition. The AI plus Performance Feedback (AI+PF) condition had the adult provide the child with information regarding their performance after each reading of the passage. The AI+PF+CR condition combined the previously described independent variables. This analytic approach allowed for the study of the separate and combined effects of the AI, PF, and CR interventions and qualifies as a component analysis of the AI+PF+CR intervention. The results of the Eckert et al. investigation showed that for all students the AI component increased reading fluency relative to BL and for four students combining the AI with either the PF or CR procedure further improved reading.

Another example of a multielement brief experimental design is provided by Wacker and colleagues (2004). In this study a child with developmental disabilities named Jim initially underwent an analogue functional analysis (top panel of Figure 14.4). The dependent measure was the percentage of intervals of problem behavior. The experimental conditions lasted 5 minutes and used standard analogue functional analysis procedures: Attention, Escape, Free Play, and Tangible (see Iwata et al., 1982). The results showed that problem behaviors were multiply determined, occurring in the Escape and Tangible conditions. A second analysis was then conducted under Escape and Differential Reinforcement of Communication (DRC) conditions (bottom panel). The dependent variable was the same as the previous analysis, as was the Escape condition. The DRC intervention taught the child to use language rather than problem behavior to communicate his needs. The DRC intervention was shown to be effective in reducing Jim's problem behavior in comparison to the Escape condition.

Both the Eckert et al. (2002) and Wacker et al. (2004) studies highlight how quickly and efficiently multielement brief designs can be used to establish a functional relation. Although the multielement strategy requires more sessions to be conducted than the A-B-A-B variant of the brief experimental design, it allows for replication of the effects of each condition. These additional data facilitate the estimation of patterns resulting from each experimental manipulation, if time and resources permit.

FIGURE 14.3 ■ Example of a Multielement Brief Experimental Design.

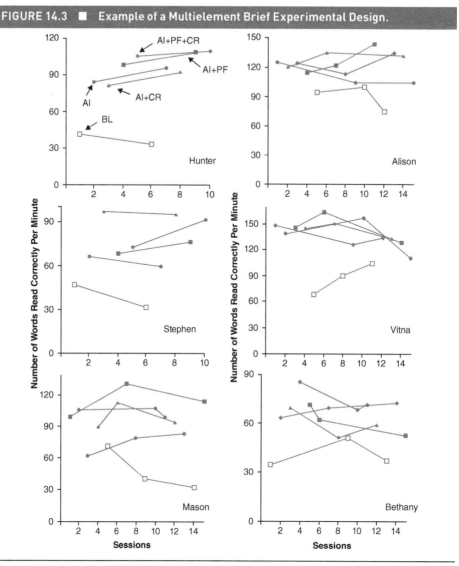

Note. The study analyzed the oral reading fluency of six elementary school students. The dependent variable was the number of words read correctly per minute. Baseline (BL) consisted of a child reading aloud with no other intervention. The Antecedent Intervention (AI) condition had the child listen to an adult read the passage and then practice the passage for three repetitions. The AI plus Contingent Reinforcement (AI+CR) condition added a reinforcement contingency for increasing reading fluency by 5% from the first to third reading repetition. The AI plus Performance Feedback (AI+PF) condition had the adult provide the child with information regarding their performance after each reading of the passage. The AI+PF+CR condition combined the previously described independent variables. (Figure 1, p. 277, from: Eckert, T. L., Ardoin, S. P., Daly, E. J., III, & Martens, B. K. (2002). Improving oral reading fluency: A brief experimental analysis of combining an antecedent intervention with consequences. *Journal of Applied Behavior Analysis, 35*, 271–281. Copyright 2002 by the Society for the Experimental Analysis of Behavior. Reprinted by permission.)

FIGURE 14.4 ■ Another Example of a Multielement Brief Experimental Design.

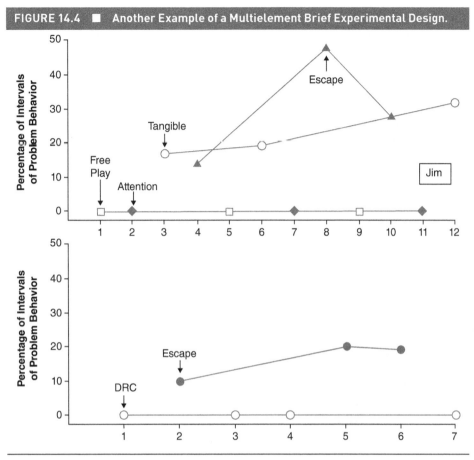

Note. In this study a child with developmental disabilities named Jim initially underwent an analogue functional analysis (top panel). The dependent measure was the percentage of intervals of problem behavior. The experimental conditions lasted 5 minutes and were standard analogue functional analysis procedures: Attention, Escape, Free Play, and Tangible (see Iwata et al., 1982). A second analysis was then conducted under Escape and Differential Reinforcement of Communication (DRC) conditions (bottom panel). The dependent variable was the same as the previous analysis, as was the Escape condition. The DRC intervention taught the child to use language rather than problem behavior to communicate his needs. (Figure 2, p. 222, from: Wacker, D., Berg, W., Harding, J., & Cooper-Brown, L. (2004). Use of brief experimental analyses in outpatient clinic and home settings. *Journal of Behavioral Education, 13*, 213–226. Copyright 2004 by Human Sciences Press, Inc. Reprinted with permission from Springer Nature Customer Service Center.)

STRENGTHS AND LIMITATIONS

Brief experimental designs emerged in response to the logistical requirements of educational and outpatient clinical settings. A perusal of the leading research journals publishing single-case design research suggests these designs are becoming increasingly common (Henry et al., 2021). The primary strength of brief experimental designs is that they can be used to demonstrate a functional relation in a limited time frame. This characteristic allows single-case designs to be used in situations where A-B or B-only approaches to intervention could be used. In addition, it allows behavior intervention plans or reading interventions, as an example, to be based on assessment data, rather than teacher or therapist intuition.

Currently, brief experimental designs use procedures consistent with A-B-A-B and multielement designs. Such arrangements provide a great deal of efficiency, as well as the requisite analytical power. That is, the A-B-A-B and multielement variants permit the demonstration of a functional relation but also allow for comparative, component, and parametric analyses. It is conceivable that multiple-baseline, repeated-acquisition, or combined designs could be integrated into a brief experimental design format, although this has yet to occur.

A primary limitation of brief experimental designs is the lack of within-condition replication. Or, said another way, because only individual data points are obtained within a particular condition, the assessment of trends or variability within a condition is often not possible. This raises the concern that the internal validity of a study might be compromised, resulting in *false-positive findings* (Bartlett et al., 2011).

Figure 14.5 shows a two-by-two matrix of possible outcomes from an experiment. A primary goal of an analysis is to arrive at a *correct-positive finding*. That is, an effect is found, and it is consistent with how the behavior–environment relations function. The inability to establish a functional relation should result in a *correct-negative finding*. That is, no effect is found because the experimental conditions were not consistent with how the behavior–environment relations function. However, another possible outcome, a false-positive finding, can occur. False-positive findings occur when an experimental effect is obtained but it is the result of some extraneous variable other than the independent variable (e.g., an interaction effect between two conditions).

False-positive findings are always a concern in any research domain. For example, setting the probability value of an inferential statistic in group-comparison research at $p < .05$, by definition, guarantees that 1 in 20 positive findings is due to chance and is a false positive. Because single-case research follows an inductive approach, false-positive findings resulting from chance are not

FIGURE 14.5 ■ Two-By-Two Matrix of Possible Outcomes from an Experiment.

Veridical Result	Experimental Result: Effect	Experimental Result: No Effect
Effect	Correct positive finding	False negative result
No Effect	False positive result	Correct negative result

Note. Experimental results are the outcomes of an experimental analysis. *Veridical results* are what should have occurred if the analysis was accurate. A primary goal of an analysis is to arrive at a *correct-positive finding*. That is, an effect is identified and is consistent with how the behavior–environment relations function. The inability to establish a functional relation should result in a *correct-negative finding*. That is, no effect is found because the experimental conditions were not consistent with how the behavior–environment relations function. A *false-negative finding* occurs when some type of behavioral phenomenon exists but the experimental procedures fail to identify it as a functional relation. *False-positive findings* occur when an experimental effect is obtained, but it is the result of some extraneous variable other than the independent variable (e.g., an interaction effect between two conditions).

an issue (see Chapter 3). However, false-positive findings resulting from inadequate experimental procedures or the influence of extraneous variables are always a concern. Because brief experimental designs base the demonstration of experimental control on the minimal amount of information possible, they are probably more susceptible to producing false-positive findings than extended experimental analyses. However, this differential sensitivity to producing false positives has yet to be empirically demonstrated and is, therefore, only an argument based on logic (see Chapter 1).

A second concern with brief experimental designs is that they may be more likely to produce *false negative findings*. A false negative finding occurs when some type of behavioral phenomenon exists but the experimental procedures fail to identify it as a functional relation. For example, a child's problem behavior may be due to an idiosyncratic event (e.g., the sound of an ambulance) that is not analyzed in a functional behavioral assessment, and, therefore, the researchers may not observe the behaviors of concern and conclude that no problem exists (see Wacker et al., 2004). The identification of false-negative findings is a particularly difficult task because of the absence of a finding. Because brief experimental designs occur during a limited amount of time, they may not sample enough behavioral situations to identify variables that occur infrequently.

A related concern is the use of short session lengths. This is not a concern particular to brief experimental designs and applies to any experimental analysis. However, because the use of brief experimental designs is primarily based on limited availability of research participants, it is probably most germane to this design tactic. As discussed in Chapter 7, the length of an observational session should be determined by criteria that focus on the adequacy of the time being sampled to represent accurately the activities of an educational context and the behavioral processes being studied. Research has shown that reducing session lengths can result in increased false-positive and false-negative findings (Wallace & Iwata, 1999). Therefore, the use of brief sessions may produce behavioral effects that are transient (i.e., false-positive findings) or not allow the expression of behavioral processes that take longer to unfold (i.e., false-negative findings). As with any experimental question, if the researcher suspects that session length is influencing the results of a study, they should make a point of analyzing this effect to understand its influence on behavior.

REFLECTION QUESTIONS

1. If brief experimental designs are adaptations of other single-case designs, are there any design types that cannot be implemented in an abbreviated format?

2. How might brief experimental designs be viewed as particularly useful in clinical or education contexts?

3. Because brief experimental designs contain so few data points, can these designs be used to study behavioral mechanisms in the absence of steady behavioral states?

4. Explain why there is increased attention to false-positive results when using brief experimental designs.

5. Describe the variables within a brief experimental design that might produce false-negative results.

15 COMBINED DESIGNS

LEARNING OBJECTIVES

After reading this chapter, you will be able to

15.1   Explain the purpose of combined designs.

15.2   Demonstrate tactics used in creating combined designs.

15.3   Evaluate the strengths and limitations of combined designs.

In previous chapters in this section, we have discussed individual approaches to design tactics. That is, I have attempted to discuss each approach to design within a single-case logic as if it were a distinct and separate approach to experimental design. This perspective to using individual design tactics is an introduction to single-case designs. Many of the most exciting and innovative uses of these designs derive from a synthetic approach to experimental design—that is, the combining of individual single-case designs to explore mechanisms of action that have yet to yield to experimental analysis. In this section, we will introduce these designs and refer to them as *combined designs*.

COMBINED DESIGNS

By merging two or more different single-case design tactics, combined designs provide the researcher with multiple ways of demonstrating a functional relation. There are several benefits to using combined designs. First, and perhaps most importantly, combined designs can be used to study more complex behavioral processes than an individual single-case design might permit. For example, a researcher may want to simultaneously compare two different conditions via a multielement design while also analyzing the effect of a third variable on each of the two conditions using an A-B-A-B design. Second, if one aspect of a combined design, say a multiple-baseline design, fails to show a functional relation, another aspect of the design, for example an A-B-A-B design, may be used to demonstrate experimental control. Third, combined designs, because they can be used to demonstrate experimental control in multiple ways, provide stronger demonstrations of functional relations. That is, these designs can be used to show multiple replications within an experimental analysis. Given these positive attributes, it is not surprising that in recent years there has been an increase in the use of combined designs by single-case researchers.

Early methodology textbooks on single-case designs either did not mention combined designs (e.g., Barlow & Hersen, 1984) or mentioned them briefly (e.g., Kazdin, 1982). When combined designs were discussed, it was typically in the context of adding an additional design element to an experiment if initial attempts at demonstrating experimental control were unsuccessful. However, since the 1980s the field of behavior analysis has grown substantially in its ability to study translational mechanisms in applied situations. Early in the use of single-case designs in educational research (see Chapter 2), $N = 1$ designs were used primarily to demonstrate that a particular intervention could effectively change behavior. Hence, designs like multiple-baseline or A-B-A-B designs were adequate for the analytical task.

In the 1990s and continuing today, researchers began asking more refined questions. Instead of asking whether an independent variable could change behavior, researchers began asking *why* a particular intervention changed behavior (see Kennedy et al., 2001; Lattal, 2008; Mace, 1994). That is, researchers began exploring the *mechanisms* responsible for the observed behavior change. Such questions, as noted by Baer et al. (1987), often require more complex experimental designs. Therefore, combined designs have been used more frequently to meet the analytical needs of *researchers seeking to explore causes, not just the effects, of behavior change.*

TACTICS IN COMBINED DESIGN

Table 15.1 shows possible combinations of single-case designs. The table shows possible combinations of two or more single-case designs in various configurations. As with many aspects of experimental design, the primary limitations on how different single-case designs are combined are parsimony and tractability. Combining too many designs may result in an intractable or impossible-to-implement experimental analysis, which, despite its elegance on paper or in verbal description, is essentially useless. Parsimony becomes an issue because, as a researcher,

TABLE 15.1 ■ Illustrative Tactics Used in Combined Designs	
Combination Tactics	**Possible Combinations**
Combining Two Single-Case Designs	A-B-A-B and Multielement Design
	A-B-A-B and Multiple-Baseline Design
	A-B-A-B and Repeated-Acquisition Design
	Multielement and Multiple-Baseline Design
	Multielement and Repeated-Acquisition Design
	Multiple-Baseline and Repeated-Acquisition Design
Combining Three or More Single-Case Designs	A-B-A-B, Multielement, and Multiple-Baseline Design
	Et cetera

you want to demonstrate functional relations as simply as the phenomenon allows. Using an unnecessarily complex experimental design is wasteful and merely an exercise in fitting the experimental question to the experimental design, rather than vice versa (see Chapter 3).

Figure 15.1 shows an example of a design that combines multiple-baseline and A-B-A-B design elements. This study by Lee et al. (2002) analyzed how schedules of reinforcement can alter the variability of behavior (see also Neuringer, 2002). Participants were three people of various ages with autism. The dependent variable was the number of varied and appropriate verbalizations made in response to questions. The baseline consisted of a differential reinforcement of appropriate (DRA) behaviors schedule in which rewards were delivered contingent on appropriate utterances. The independent variable was a combined DRA plus a lagged reinforcement schedule in which the response needed to differ from a previous utterance and be appropriate (Lag 1/DRA). The results shown in Figure 15.1 for David, Charles, and Larry show that the DRA baseline produced little variability in verbal behavior. However, when the Lag 1/DRA schedule was introduced, response variability increased within the conversational context. Not only was the effect of the independent variable analyzed sequentially across participants, but for David and Charles an A-B-A-B design was added to the multiple-baseline design. Thus, the experimental analysis showed the independent variable entering into a functional relation with behavior, and that effect could be reversed by returning to baseline reinforcement contingencies.

A somewhat more complex combination of multiple-baseline and A-B-A-B designs is shown in Figure 15.2. In this experiment by Kelley et al. (2002), the challenging behavior and alternative communicative responses of three children with developmental disabilities were analyzed. The experimental question focused on how competing reinforcement contingencies influence the acquisition of novel forms of communication serving the same operant function as problem behavior (see Carr & Durand, 1985; Tiger et al., 2008). The dependent measures were the occurrence per minute of problem behavior or alternative communication. Baseline consisted of a variable-ratio reinforcement schedule for challenging behavior and no programmed contingencies for communication responses. Two independent variables were studied. First, a functional communication training (FCT) procedure without extinction was analyzed. In this contingency arrangement, communication was reinforced as was problem behavior. In the second independent variable arrangement, the same FCT procedure was used for communication, but challenging behavior was placed on extinction. Initially, the FCT without extinction procedure was sequentially introduced in a multiple-baseline across-participants arrangement. This was followed by a change to the FCT with extinction procedure for two participants (Gary and Jennifer). For Gary, the procedures were then reversed to baseline and back to the FCT with extinction procedure. For Jennifer, an additional procedure (FCT, extinction, and response blocking) was introduced, withdrawn (i.e., returned to baseline), and then reintroduced. It is important to note that this experimental arrangement could not have been planned a priori but, instead, was a response to how each child responded to the initial intervention. Hence, Kelley et al. used a combined design, tailored to each child's behavior, to explore the behavioral processes that influenced their challenging behavior and possible interventions to reduce it.

Figure 15.3 shows a combined A-B-A-B and multielement design used by Ringdahl et al. (2002) to analyze the effects of various stimuli on behavior. The dependent variables were the frequency of aggression (Tony) or switch activation (Roland). The multielement component of the design was

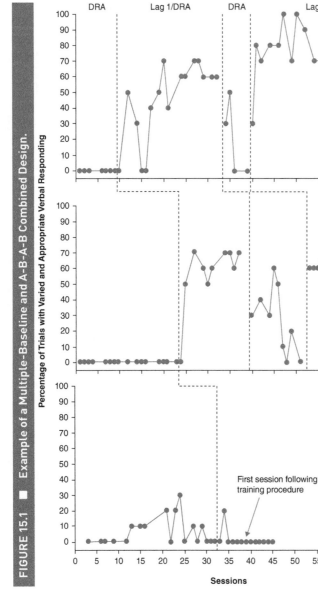

FIGURE 15.1 ■ Example of a Multiple-Baseline and A-B-A-B Combined Design.

Note: The study analyzed how schedules of reinforcement can alter the variability of behavior. Participants were three people of various ages with autism. The dependent variable was the number of varied and appropriate verbalizations made in response to questions. The baseline consisted of a differential reinforcement of appropriate (DRA) behaviors schedule in which rewards were delivered contingent on appropriate utterances. The independent variable was a combined DRA plus a lagged reinforcement schedule in which the response needed to differ from a previous utterance and be appropriate (Lag 1/DRA). (Figure 1, p. 396, from: Lee, R., McComas, J. J., & Jawor, J. (2002). The effects of differential and lag reinforcement schedules on varied verbal responding by individuals with autism. *Journal of Applied Behavior Analysis, 35*, 391–402. Copyright 2002 by the Society for the Experimental Analysis of Behavior. Reprinted by permission.)

FIGURE 15.2 ■ Variation of the Multiple-Baseline and A-B-A-B Combined Design.

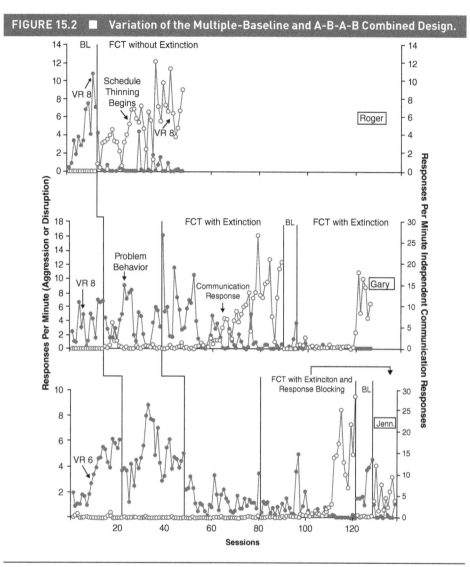

Note: This design was individualized according to each child's pattern of behavior. The experimental question focused on how competing reinforcement contingencies influence the acquisition of novel forms of communication that serve the same operant function as problem behavior (see Carr & Durand, 1985). The dependent measures were the occurrence per minute of challenging behavior or alternative communication. Baseline consisted of a variable-ratio (VR) reinforcement schedule for problem behavior and no programmed contingencies for communication responses. Two independent variables were studied. First, a functional communication training (FCT) procedure without extinction was analyzed. In this contingency arrangement, communication was reinforced as was challenging behavior. In the second independent variable arrangement, the same FCT procedure was used for communication, but problem behavior was placed on extinction. (Figure 2, p. 62, from: Kelley, M. E., Lerman, D. C., & Van Camp, C. M. (2002). The effects of competing reinforcement schedules on the acquisition of functional communication. *Journal of Applied Behavior Analysis, 35,* 59-63. Copyright 2002 by the Society for the Experimental Analysis of Behavior. Reprinted by permission.)

FIGURE 15.3 ■ Example of a Combined A-B-A-B and Multielement Design used to Analyze the Effects of Various Stimuli on Behavior.

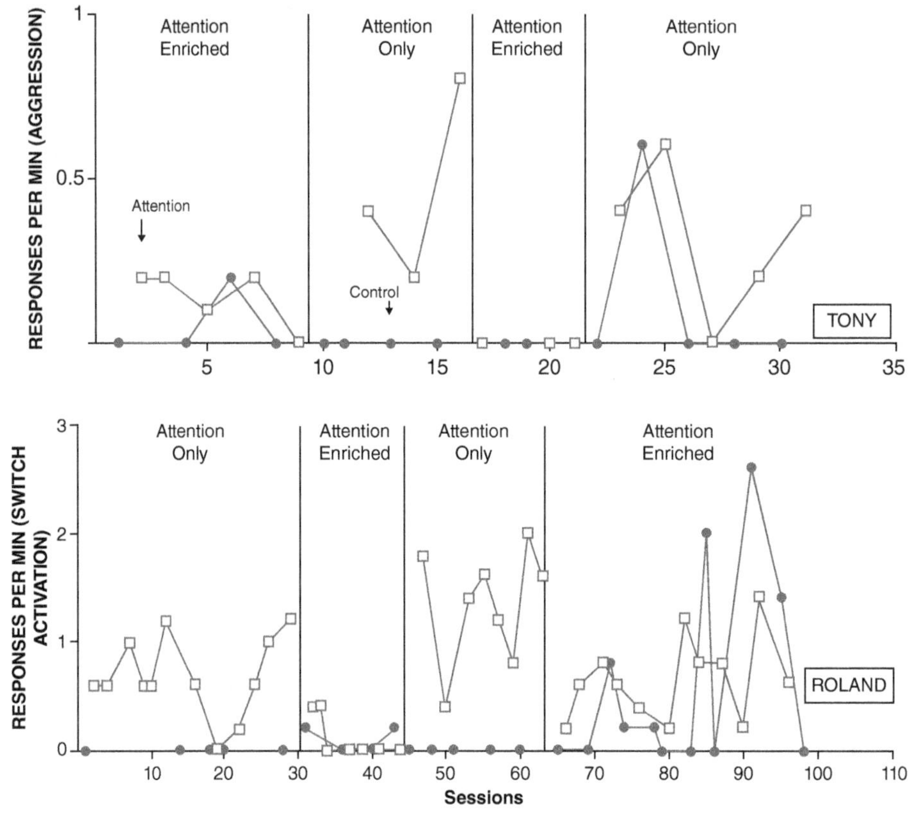

Note: The dependent variables were the frequency of aggression (Tony) or switch activation (Roland). The multielement component of the design was used to compare enriched stimulation (i.e., control) (closed circle) versus contingent attention (open square) for the behaviors of interest. The A-B-A-B component of the design compared enriched attention and attention only, with the former involving the addition of extra contingent stimuli along with attention. (Figure 1, p. 409, from: Ringdahl, J. E., Winborn, L. C., Andelman, M. S., & Kitsukawa, K. (2002). The effects of noncontingently available alternative stimuli on functional analysis outcomes. *Journal of Applied Behavior Analysis, 35*, 407–410. Copyright 2002 by the Society for the Experimental Analysis of Behavior. Reprinted by permission.)

used to compare enriched stimulation (i.e., control) (closed circle) versus contingent attention (open square) for the behaviors of interest. The A-B-A-B component of the design compared enriched attention and attention only, with the former involving the addition of extra contingent stimuli along with attention. The results of the Ringdahl et al. study showed that adding an additional form of stimulation enhanced the positively reinforcing effects of the attention intervention.

In a more elaborate design, Richman et al. (2001) analyzed the interaction between response effort and *concurrent operants* (see Box 15.1) on the aggression of a child with a disability (Mike). Mike's aggression (responses per minute) occurred to access positive reinforcement in the form of adult attention (see Figure 15.4). The experiment contained two phases. In the first phase,

FIGURE 15.4 ■ Example of a Design Combining A-B-A-B and Concurrent-Operants Procedures.

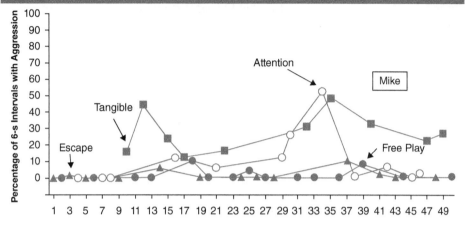

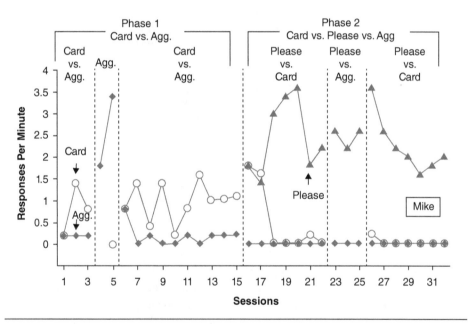

Note: The experiment contained two phases. In the first phase, an A-B-A comparison was conducted in which Mike could either aggress (closed circles) or use a response card (open circles) to access attention. When the card was available, he tended to use it at a rate of once per minute. In the second phase, a less effortful response (saying "Please") (closed triangles) was introduced and compared against each of the previous response options. (Figure 1, p. 75, from: Richman, D. M., Wacker, D. P., & Winborn, L. (2001). Response efficiency during functional communication training: Effects of effort on response allocation. *Journal of Applied Behavior Analysis, 34,* 73–76. Copyright 2001 by the Society for the Experimental Analysis of Behavior. Reprinted by permission.)

an A-B-A comparison was conducted in which Mike could either aggress (closed circles) or use a response card (open circles) to access attention. When the card was available, he tended to use it at a rate of once per minute. In the second phase, a less effortful response (saying "Please") (closed triangles) was introduced and compared against each of the previous response options. The results showed that Mike emitted the please response at a much higher rate than either the card or aggression, suggesting that the least effortful response was his preferred means of accessing attention. This design, then, combined A-B-A-B and concurrent-operants procedures to establish experimental control.

BOX 15.1: CONCURRENT OPERANTS AS AN ELEMENT IN COMBINED DESIGNS

Applied researchers began adopting procedures to demonstrate basic mechanisms originally developed in the experimental analysis of behavior (see Chapter 2). One of the most prominent findings from the basic research literature is the study of choice using concurrent schedules of reinforcement (see Herrnstein, 1970; McDowell, 2013). Using concurrent schedules, two separate reinforcement contingencies are simultaneously available, and the allocation of behavior to each option is assessed. This schedule of reinforcement establishes concurrent operants and is a model system for analyzing choice. By varying some parameter of the reinforcement schedule (e.g., reinforcer frequency or reinforcer magnitude), the influence of each variable on choice responding can be analyzed. This procedure has been widely adopted in applied behavior analysis, particularly in the analyses of why people choose to engage in challenging behaviors versus other more socially desirable alternatives (Fisher & Mazur, 1997; Poling et al., 2011). However, a concurrent-operants procedure is not a "stand-alone" single-case design. Instead, the use of a concurrent-operants procedure requires some other type of single-case design to establish a functional relation.

Another use of the concurrent-operants design is to combine it with a multiple-baseline design. Such a design is shown in Figure 15.5 from a study by Kennedy et al. (2000) that examined the stereotypical behaviors of students with autism. The dependent measures were the percentage of intervals with stereotypical behavior (closed circles) and frequency of signing (open circles) for a student named James. Baselines were conditions that established different reinforcement contingences (i.e., attention, demand, and no attention) for the same stereotypical response. When baselines were established, a FCT intervention was introduced that targeted a specific type of operant function. The design permitted an analysis of the degree to which a single behavior was maintained by multiple functions.

A similar design was used by Tang et al. (2003), but this combined design also incorporated an A-B-A-B element in the first tier of the multiple-baseline plus concurrent-operants arrangement (Figure 15.6). The independent and dependent variables were the same as in the Kennedy et al. (2000) study except that signing was also recorded using an interval-based estimation procedure. In this instance, the design was arranged to test whether a stereotypical response served multiple functions or only a single operant function. When it became clear that responding was only under control in the first tier of the multiple-baseline design, an A-B-A-B design was

FIGURE 15.5 ■ Example of a Concurrent-Operants Design Combined with a Multiple-Baseline Design.

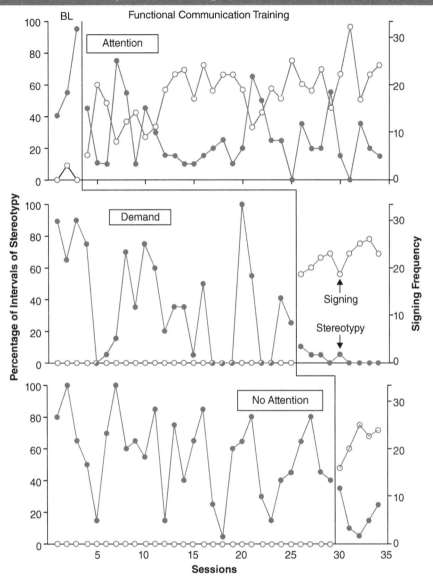

Note: This study analyzed the stereotypical behaviors of students with autism. The dependent measures were the percentage of intervals with stereotypical behavior (closed circles) and frequency of signing (open circles) for a student named James. Baselines were conditions that established different reinforcement contingences (i.e., attention, demand, and no attention) for the same stereotypical response. When baselines were established, an FCT intervention was introduced that targeted a specific type of operant function and associated sign. (Figure 2, p. 565, from: Kennedy, C. H., Meyer, K. A., Knowles, T., & Shukla, S. (2000). Analyzing the multiple functions of stereotypical behavior for students with autism: Implications for assessment and treatment. *Journal of Applied Behavior Analysis, 33,* 559–571. Copyright 2000 by the Society for the Experimental Analysis of Behavior. Reprinted by permission.)

FIGURE 15.6 ■ Example of a Combined Multiple-Baseline Across-Operants Functions, Concurrent-Operants, and A-B-A-B Design.

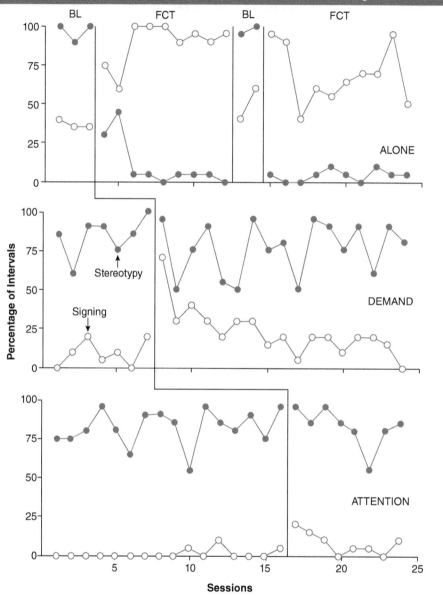

Note: The independent and dependent variables were the same as in Figure 15.5 except that signing was also recorded using an interval-based estimation procedure. In this instance the design was arranged to test whether a stereotypical response served multiple functions or only a single operant function. (Figure 6, p. 446, from: Tang, J.-C., Patterson, T. G., & Kennedy, C. H. (2003). Identifying specific sensory modalities maintaining the stereotypy of students with multiple profound disabilities. *Research in Developmental Disabilities, 24,* 433–451. Copyright 2003 by Elsevier Ltd. Reprinted by permission.)

added to demonstrate a functional relation. No experimental effect was shown for the second or third tiers of the multiple-baseline design, indicating that those reinforcement processes did not influence the student's stereotypy. Hence, in this example, a combined design was necessary to show some degree of experimental control over the behavior of interest.

A final example of a combined design is shown in Figure 15.7. The figure shows the results of a study by Martens et al. (2002) that analyzed the effects of a probabilistic reward contingency on the academic performance of three students in an elementary school mathematics class. The dependent variable was the number of correct problems solved. Baseline was comprised of the typical classroom procedures the general educator used. The independent variable was the introduction of a lottery system that provided students with rewards for completing different ratios of easy to hard problems. The design constituted a combined multielement design because it alternated between baseline (i.e., no lottery; closed ellipses) and lottery conditions (i.e., open rectangles) and a parametric A-B-A-B analysis of different easy-to-hard ratios. The results of the Martens et al. analysis showed that (a) in the absence of the lottery contingency few problems were completed correctly and (b) as the ratio emphasized harder questions, the lottery was less effective.

STRENGTHS AND LIMITATIONS

As noted in the beginning of this chapter, combined designs have emerged in recent years as an exciting means of exploring more complex behavioral processes than has previously been accomplished in educational settings (Epstein & Dallery, 2022; Smith, 2012). Combined designs allow for a more in-depth analysis of the variables maintaining responding and have the flexibility to be changed as an experiment progresses. An excellent example of this flexibility was provided by the Kelley et al. (2002) data shown in Figure 15.2. By using a combined design, Kelley et al. were able to extend a design noted for its inflexibility (i.e., the multiple-baseline across-students design) and individually tailor the analysis to the variables influencing each child's behavior. For this reason, when researchers are interested in understanding the basic mechanisms influencing variables of educational interest, combined designs are often the analytical tool of choice.

Additional strengths of combined designs are the ability to demonstrate experimental control in multiple ways and the opportunity to show a functional relation even if one aspect of the design does not show control over responding. The primary limitations of combined designs are twofold. First, one can "overdesign" an experiment and build in too much experimental control at the cost of parsimony. *Simplicity has its virtues and benefits.* A second concern is that these designs require a fairly sophisticated understanding of single-case methodology. One of the chief benefits noted in favor of the multiple-baseline across-participants design was its simplicity and tractability. It was hoped that such designs could be used by a range of practitioners to test the effectiveness of their own educational innovations. Combined designs, by necessity, are complex and require knowledge not only of single-case designs but also of basic mechanisms. However, as noted previously, this limitation is also the greatest strength of the combined design.

FIGURE 15.7 ■ Effects of a Probabilistic Reward Contingency on the Academic Performance.

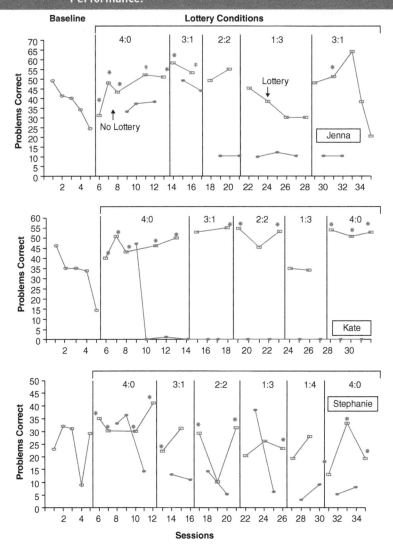

Note: Data are from three students in an elementary school mathematics class. The dependent variable was the number of correct problems solved individually on worksheets. Baseline was comprised of the typical classroom procedures. The independent variable was the introduction of a lottery system that provided students with rewards for completing different ratios of easy to hard problems. The design constitutes a combined multielement design because it alternated between baseline (i.e., no lottery; closed ellipses) and lottery conditions (i.e., open rectangles) and a parametric A-B-A-B analysis of different easy-to-hard ratios. (Figure 1, p. 405, from: Martens, B. K., Ardoin, S. P., Hilt, A. M., Lannie, A. L., Panahon, C. J., & Wolfe, L. A. (2002). Sensitivity of children's behavior to probabilistic reward: Effects of a decreasing-ratio lottery system on math performance. *Journal of Applied Behavior Analysis, 35*, 403–406. Copyright 2002 by the Society for the Experimental Analysis of Behavior. Reprinted by permission.)

In many respects this final chapter on single-case design tactics is not an ending but a starting point. By its nature, a book such as this presents experimental designs in a manner similar to how a cookbook presents recipes. Each one focuses on a single product with a fixed sequence of steps necessary to successfully complete the task. However, like good recipes, single-case designs are often the most interesting when you synthesize different approaches and tailor the processes to producing unique outcomes. For this reason, this final chapter on combined designs is really an invitation to learn more about single-case designs. There is no single, correct way to analyze behavior using single-case designs. It's a mode of thinking and problem solving that needs to be adapted to the task at hand, rather than approached in a rote and inflexible manner. This perspective on experimental designs is what led Baer et al. (1987) to write: "A good design is one that answers the question convincingly, and as such needs to be constructed in reaction to the question" (p. 319).

REFLECTION QUESTIONS

1. Describe the logic when using combined single-case designs. Does it differ from the analytical approaches used with individual single-case designs?

2. Can you describe a combined design that contains three distinct single-case designs?

3. What are the benefits of using a combined design approach?

4. Explain why a concurrent-operants analysis is, or is not, a stand-alone single-case research design.

5. What did Baer et al. (1987, p. 319) mean when they wrote, "A good design is one that answers the question convincingly, and as such needs to be constructed in reaction to the question"?

ANALYZING DATA

16 VISUAL ANALYSIS

LEARNING OBJECTIVES

After reading this chapter, you will be able to

16.1 Explain the various elements that make up a graph of quantitative data.

16.2 Define the dimensions of data available in a visual inspection of a graph.

16.3 Demonstrate the ways in which a data set may be analyzed using a graph.

16.4 Explain a protocol for teaching researchers how to consistently interpret visual data in graph form.

In single-case research, as data are collected, the information is graphed and analyzed on a continuous basis until the experiment is completed. The information from each session is plotted in a graphic display, and patterns in the data are studied to decide what the next step in the experiment will be. An example will help illustrate this process. After selecting the initial procedures for an experiment and deciding on a design tactic (e.g., an A-B-A-B design), data collection begins. After the first observational session, the data are scored, summarized, and charted in graphic form. The research team then visually inspects the data. After the first day, there are no trends or patterns in the data apart from the specific level obtained for each variable. However, as this process is repeated, visualizing the data begins to yield more complex patterns. For instance, the occurrence of challenging behavior and on-task behavior may occur at consistent levels day after day. If this pattern is replicated within a participant, decisions need to be made about the introduction of an independent variable. If the pattern in the data makes this a logical decision, then the intervention can be introduced. Or, if the pattern in the data has downward or upward trends or is highly variable, the research team may choose to continue baseline until a stable pattern is obtained. As the study unfolds, decisions are made on a daily basis whether to continue, change, or end a particular set of procedures. These decisions are ongoing during a study and always made in reference to the graphed data. This process is summarized in the expression often heard among single-case researchers, "Follow your data."

This is a dynamic process and roughly analogous to a chess match. The first observation is made (you move a chess piece), data are collected (your opponent makes their move), the results are analyzed (your next step is planned), the next move is executed, the data are collected, and so on. In chess, when errors are made or unexpected moves from an opponent occur, the tactical plan is changed accordingly and as often as needed to be successful. In single-case research, plans are changed as patterns in the data unfold, with the goal of revealing some type of behavioral process in the form of a functional relation. The use of graphic displays to visualize quantitative information is central to this process. The data, in graphic format, can be considered a road map for how a study is conducted that cannot be predicted in an a priori manner (Coopmans et al., 2014).

This process can be contrasted with group-comparison designs in which an experimental design (e.g., a pretest–posttest control group design; cf. Cook et al., 2002) is selected before the start of the study, data are then collected prior to and after intervention, the data are summarized, and the appropriate inferential statistic is used to test for an experimental effect. In such a case, the analysis occurs post hoc after the data are collected, and no change in the experimental design can be made without limiting internal validity. Unlike group-comparison designs, single-case designs are highly dynamic, and often the most exciting analyses unfold over time as patterns in the data emerge and the experimental tactic is adjusted in reaction to the data.

The process of inspecting graphic data is a very powerful way of revealing functional relations (Hacking, 1983; Smith et al., 2002). In single-case designs, the use of graphs to analyze data is as old as the method itself. In B. F. Skinner's seminal work that led to the development of behavior analysis, *The Behavior of Organisms* (1938), visual displays of data were prominently featured throughout the book as the primary means of data analysis. Figure 16.1 shows the first graph from Skinner (1938). In this figure, the cumulative number of responses by a rodent is shown during the initial shaping of a lever press. The data show that three lever presses occurred during the first 120 minutes of the session with large temporal gaps between responses. However, approximately 130 minutes into the conditioning session, the fourth response was emitted, and lever pressing began to occur at a rapid and regular rate for the remainder of the session. At this point, lever pressing had been brought under the control of a positive reinforcer. Figure 16.1 reveals this process in a manner that is easily accessed by other researchers. It is the most revealing way of analyzing the data and provides the most information to the viewer.

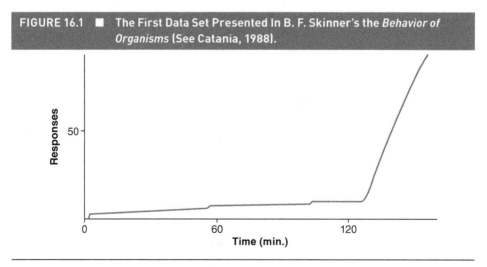

FIGURE 16.1 ■ The First Data Set Presented In B. F. Skinner's the *Behavior of Organisms* (See Catania, 1988).

Note. The *y*-axis displays the occurrence of individual responses as a cumulative function. The *x*-axis represents the passage of time. (Figure 2, p. 67, from: B. F. Skinner (1938). *The behavior of organisms: An experimental analysis.* Copley. Copyright 1991 by D. Appleton-Century Company, Inc. Reprinted by permission.)

The use of graphic analysis by Skinner (1938) was no accident. He was using the tools of experimental biology to analyze psychological phenomena (see Chapter 2). Graphic displays, because of their flexibility, ease of use, and ability to help researchers visualize functional relations, quickly became a mainstay in the experimental analysis of behavior. Not surprisingly, when researchers began to apply the behavioral mechanisms discovered in the laboratory to natural settings, such as public schools, the use of graphs was continued along with many other scientific practices. In fact, one of the most powerful interventions discovered for educators to be more effective in teaching others is to graph a student's performance and visually analyze the data on a regular basis, adjusting teaching procedures as indicated by the data (Binder & Watkins, 2013).

In this chapter, we will discuss how to use graphs in single-case research. Initially, we will review the elements comprising a graph. Then, we will discuss how to visually inspect data so that a conclusion about patterns in the data, and whether experimental control was demonstrated, can be reached. This will be followed by examples of how to use graphs to explore and analyze different facets of the data collected in an experiment. Finally, we will talk about how to teach people to visually inspect data so that there is a high level of consistency among those inspecting data.

ELEMENTS OF A GRAPH

Although there are a multitude of graphic formats that can be used to visually display data, there are some elements that most graphs share in common (see Parsonson & Baer [2015] for an extensive treatment of this topic). Figure 16.2 shows an example of a graph from a study

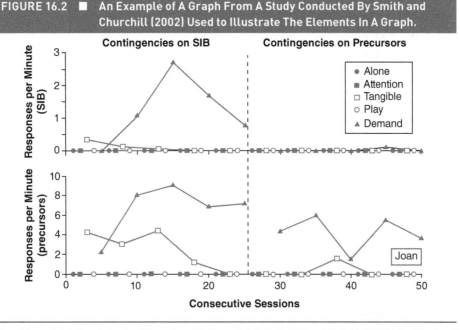

FIGURE 16.2 ■ An Example of A Graph From A Study Conducted By Smith and Churchill (2002) Used to Illustrate The Elements In A Graph.

Note. SIB = self-injurious behavior. (Figure 1, p. 130, from: Smith, R. G., & Churchill, R. M. (2002). Identification of environmental determinants of behavior disorders through functional analysis of precursor behaviors. *Journal of Applied Behavior Analysis, 35*, 125–136. Copyright 2002 by the Society for the Experimental Analysis of Behavior. Reprinted by permission.)

conducted by Smith and Churchill (2002). We will review the graph not for its content but for its structure and composition. This particular figure presents four panels in a two-by-two matrix configuration. The elements of the matrix are composed of two different independent variable manipulations labeled at the top of the graph and two different dependent variables labeled on the left-hand side of the graph.

The first place to start is with the y-*axis*, also referred to as the *vertical axis* or *ordinate*. The vertical line on the left-hand side of the graph demarks the y-axis of the graph and is marked according to some metric, in this case an equal-interval metric that is labeled 0 to 3 in units of 1 along the top panel and 0 to 10 in units of 2 along the bottom panel. Placement of the zero point of a graph varies among researchers, with some preferring to have the zero point raised above the x-axis while others prefer the zero point to rest on the x-axis. These metrics are then labeled with individual descriptors that provide information regarding the measurement unit and topography of behaviors. In this instance, the upper panel is labeled "Responses per Minute (SIB)," and the lower panel is labeled "Responses per Minute (precursors)." The information arrayed along the vertical axis of this graph informs the reader of what types of behaviors were measured, what measurement system was used to quantify responding, and what metric is being used to display the data.

The bottom of the graph is referred to as the x-*axis, horizontal axis*, or *abscissa*. The horizontal line running along the lower end of Figure 16.2 displays an equal-interval metric that ranges from 0 to 50 in units of 10. The metric label is presented below the numeric demarcations along the x-axis and identifies this part of the graph as "Consecutive Sessions." This part of the figure informs the reader, in this instance, that data are plotted on a session-by-session basis.

In this particular study, Smith and Churchill (2002) used a combined multielement and A-B design. The A-B components of the design are labeled with descriptors at the top of the graph, in this instance "Contingencies on SIB" (left side) and "Contingencies on Precursors" (right side). The phase change line—that is, the point in the experiment when conditions were changed from A to B—is designated as a solid line running vertically through the graph at midpoint. Some researchers prefer to use solid lines, and others prefer to use broken lines to denote phase changes.

Within Figure 16.2 are the data. In this example, five different experimental conditions were analyzed: Alone, Attention, Tangible, Play, and Demand. The experimental conditions are labeled in a legend contained within the graph and presented adjacent to the specific symbol (closed circle, closed square, open square, open circle, and closed triangle, respectively) that represents each condition. The quantitative outcomes from individual sessions are presented as individual data points connected by lines. Note that the data points are not connected across phase changes. Finally, the pseudonym or other identifier for the individual whose behavior is being analyzed in the study is placed in a box within the graph (in this case, "Joan"). Some researchers use boxes for the names and legends in a graph to clearly set them apart from the data, but others do not.

One last component of a graph is the *figure caption* that will be placed below or next to the figure if the study is published. The figure caption provides a written description of the information contained in the actual figure. Ideally, the reader should be able to look at the graph and read the figure caption and understand what the data represent without having to refer to the Method section or other text in the published paper. This information can include a general description of what the graph represents, a description of the y- and x-axes, and the phases and experimental conditions used in the study.

The components just reviewed comprise the basic elements of a graphic display. However, what specific form a graph takes depends on the nature of the data and the aspect of the experiment the investigators are trying to visualize (Holzinger, 2014; McInerny, 2013; Tufte, 1997). One stylistic issue to be considered when constructing graphs is Tufte's (1983) concept of *data ink* and *nondata ink*. Data ink refers to those elements in a graph that are drawn to display information that is critical for the visual analysis of the data. Nondata ink refers to those parts of the graph that could be erased without removing any information critical to the visual analysis. In general, data ink should be maximized within a graphic display, and nondata ink should be eliminated whenever possible. An example of this concept is displayed in Figure 16.3. In this figure, a histogram that might appear in a journal article is shown in the left-hand panel containing both data and nondata ink. In the center panel is only the nondata ink. In the right-hand

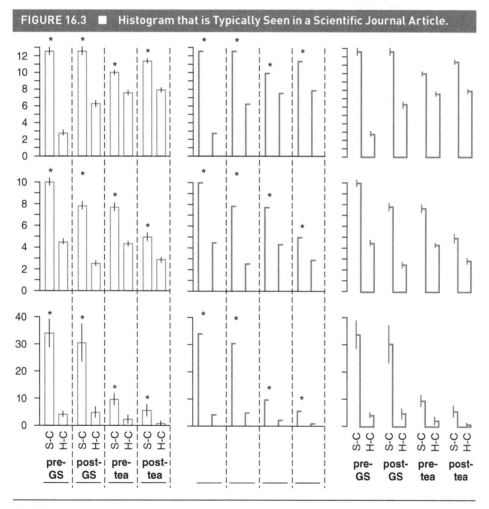

FIGURE 16.3 ■ Histogram that is Typically Seen in a Scientific Journal Article.

Note. The histogram is shown in the left-hand panel, containing both data and nondata ink. In the center panel is only the nondata ink. And in the right-hand panel is the remaining drawing that presents only the essential data ink that is necessary for analyzing the figure. (Copyright 1983 by Graphics Press, *The Visual Display of Quantitative Information.* Edward R. Tufte, 102, 1983. Reprinted by permission.)

panel is the remaining drawing that presents only the data ink necessary for analyzing the figure. Although the right-hand panel may be considered an extreme case of minimizing nondata ink, it nicely illustrates the point that graphs should be kept as simple and uncluttered as possible so the eye is drawn to the data.

VISUAL INSPECTION OF GRAPHS

The evaluation of quantitative information via visual inspection is accomplished by analyzing specific types of patterns in the data display. It may not seem obvious at first, but when a researcher looks at a graph, they look for a series of patterns that allow them to draw conclusions regarding what the data represent. These dimensions are familiar to someone who has been trained in their use, but for someone who is unfamiliar with them, their use is nonintuitive. In this section, we will review various dimensions of data that are visualized in graphs and used for analysis.

Within-Phase Patterns

The first dimension used in visual analysis is the *level* of the data. Level refers to the average of the data within a condition, typically calculated as the mean or median. The left-hand panel in Figure 16.4 shows a baseline data set with the level drawn over the data. There are six data points in the panel, with a mean of 4.7. Attending to the level of data within a phase allows for the estimation of the central tendency of the data during a particular part of an experiment. It also allows for comparison of patterns between phases (see discussion as follows). Although the absolute level within a phase is important, it should be noted, particularly in applied research, that the last few data points contain the most essential information regarding the level of behavior before a phase change. The pattern of data shown in the right-hand panel of Figure 16.4 illustrates this point. Although the mean level of the data is 6.7, the last three data points deviate from this level enough to warrant special emphasis.

A second dimension used to visually inspect graphs is the *trend* of the data. Trend refers to the best-fit straight line that could be placed over the data within a phase. Trend has two distinct elements that must be simultaneously evaluated: *slope* and *magnitude*. Slope is the

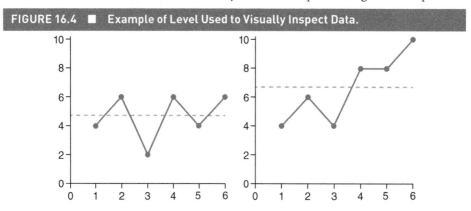

FIGURE 16.4 ■ Example of Level Used to Visually Inspect Data.

Note. The left-hand panel in the figure shows a baseline data set with the level drawn over the data. There are six data points in the panel, with a mean of 4.7. The right-hand panel in the figure shows a data set in which the most essential information is within the last three data points, rather than the overall average.

upward or downward slant or inclination of the data within a phase. Slopes are generally *positive (upward), flat,* or *negative (downward)*. A positive slope is one in which the data points are increasing in value within a phase (see upper left-hand panel of Figure 16.5). A negative slope is just the opposite, a downward pattern in the data within a phase (see lower left-hand panel of Figure 16.5). The second element of a trend is magnitude, which is the size or extent of the slope. The magnitude of a trend is qualitatively estimated as *high, medium,* or *low* (much the same as a correlation or effect size statistic). A high-magnitude slope is a rapidly increasing or decreasing pattern in the data (see upper right-hand panel of Figure 16.5). A low-magnitude slope is a gradually increasing or decreasing pattern in the data (see lower right-hand panel of Figure 16.5). It is important to note that the greater the slope, the less meaningful level is as a general estimate of the data pattern (see right-hand panel of Figure 16.4).

In judging the trend of a data set within a phase, a person simultaneously estimates the slope and magnitude of the data. For example, using Figure 16.5, the upper left-hand panel has a moderate positive trend, and the lower left-hand panel has a moderate negative trend. There are at least two ways of quantitatively estimating the trend of data. The first, *least-squares regression,* fits a straight line to the slope of the data set by minimizing the sum of squared deviations of the observed data from the line. Figure 16.6 shows a diagram of how to calculate a least-squares regression line (from Parsonson & Baer, 2015, p. 21).

FIGURE 16.5 ■ Examples of Slope and Magnitude Used to Estimate Trend.

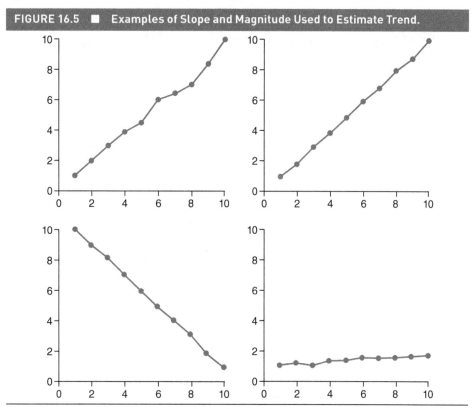

Note. Slope is the upward or downward slant or inclination of the data within a phase. Slopes are generally positive, flat, or negative. The magnitude of a trend is qualitatively estimated as high, medium, or low.

FIGURE 16.6 ■ Diagram Outlining the Process for Calculating a Least-Squares Regression Coefficient.

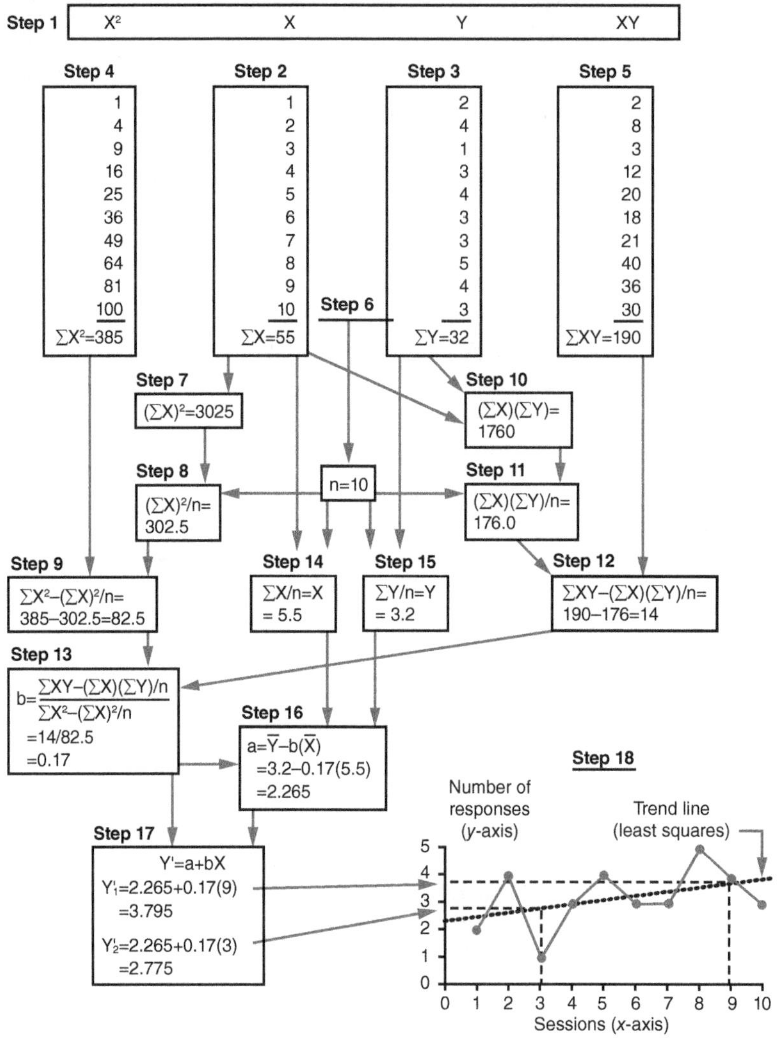

Note. See also Table 16.1 for a textual description of the process. (Figure 2.21, p. 21, from: Parsonson, B. S., & Baer, D. M. (2015). The visual analysis of data, and current research into the stimuli controlling it. In T. R. Kratochwill & J. R. Levin (Eds.), *Single-case research design and analysis: New directions for psychology and educa-tion* (pp. 15–40). Taylor & Francis. Copyright 1978 by Routledge, an imprint of Taylor & Francis Ltd. Permission conveyed through the Copyright Clearance Center Inc.)

Table 16.1 describes how to calculate the same data shown in Figure 16.6. The second method for quantitatively estimating trend is the *split-middle technique* (Lane & Gast, 2014; White, 1971). Using the split-middle technique requires seven or more data points within a phase and splits the data set in half, establishes a median for each half, and then plots a line that intersects the two medians (see Figure 16.7 from Kazdin, 1982, p. 313). A procedure for calcu-lating the trend of a data set using the split-middle technique is presented in Table 16.2.

TABLE 16.1 ■ *How to Calculate a Least-Squares Regression Line for the Data Shown in* Figure 16.6[a]	
Step-by-Step Outline of Procedure for Fitting a Straight-Line Trend by the Method of Least Squares	Examples of Computation Using Data From Figure 16.6
1. Head four columns as follows: X^2, X, Y, XY.	
2. Fill out the X column with the number of days, sessions, or trails—in ascending numerical order—in the phase being analyzed, and their sum $(\sum X)$.	$\sum X = 55$
3. In the Y column, enter the scores obtained on each successive day, session, etc., and their sum $(\sum Y)$.	$\sum Y = 32$
4. Fill out the X^2 column with the *square* of each of the corresponding X entries, and their sum $(\sum X^2)$.	$\sum X^2 = 385$
5. The XY column is composed of the cross products obtained by multiplying each Y column entry by its paired X column entry, and their sum $(\sum XY)$.	$\sum XY = 190$
6. The number of *pairs* of X and Y entries, n, is obtained by counting the number of entries in either the X or Y columns.	$n = 10$
7. Square $\sum X$ to obtain $(\sum X)^2$.	$(\sum X)^2 = 3025$
8. Divide $(\sum X)^2$ by n.	$\frac{(\sum X)^2}{n} = 302.5$
9. Subtract $\frac{(\sum X)^2}{n}$ from $\sum X^2$.	$\sum X^2 - \frac{(\sum X)^2}{n} = 385 - 302.5 = 82.5$
10. Multiply $\sum X$ and $\sum Y$ to obtain $(\sum X)(\sum Y)$.	$(\sum X)(\sum Y) = 1760$
11. Divide $(\sum X)(\sum Y)$ by n.	$(\sum X)\frac{(\sum Y)}{n} = 176.0$
12. Subtract $(\sum X)\frac{(\sum Y)}{n}$ from $\sum XY$.	$\sum XY - (\sum X)\frac{(\sum Y)}{n} = 190 - 176 = 14$
13. Divide $\sum XY - (\sum X)\frac{(\sum Y)}{n}$ by $\sum X^2 - \frac{(\sum X)^2}{n}$ (Step 9) to obtain b.	$b = \frac{14}{82.5} = 0.17$
14. Divide $\sum X$ by n to obtain mean of X, $\bar{X}$.	$\bar{X} = 5.5$
15. Divide $\sum Y$ by n to obtain mean of Y, $\bar{Y}$.	$\bar{Y} = 3.2$
16. To obtain a, multiply $\bar{X}$ by b and subtract $b(\bar{X})$ from $\bar{Y}$.	$a = \bar{Y} - b(\bar{X}) = 3.2 - 0.17(5.5) = 2.265$

(Continued)

TABLE 16.1 ■ *How to Calculate a Least-Squares Regression Line for the Data Shown in* Figure 16.6[a] *(Continued)*	
Step-by-Step Outline of Procedure for Fitting a Straight-Line Trend by the Method of Least Squares	**Examples of Computation Using Data From Figure 16.6**
17. The regression equation $Y' = a + bX$ is solved by substituting the values of a and b, and values of X from the X column. Two solutions, for different values of X give two values of Y'.	$Y_1' = 2.265 + 0.17(X)$ Let $X = 9$ (ninth X entry); $Y_1' = 2.265 + 0.17(9) = 3.795$ Let $X = 3$ (third X entry): $Y_2' = 2.265 + 0.17(3) = 2.775$
18. Locate Y_1' on the Y axis of the graph and the selected value of X on the X axis of the graph and mark the point at which they intersect. Similarly, locate Y_2' on the Y axis, and mark their point of intersection. A straight line drawn through the two points is the line of best fit and describes the trend in the data.	

[a] From: Parsonson, B. S., & Baer, D. M. (2015). The visual analysis of data, and current research into the stimuli controlling it. In T. R. Kratochwill & J. R. Levin (Eds.), *Single-case research design and analysis: New directions for psychology and education* (pp. 15–40). Taylor & Francis. Copyright 1978 by Routledge, an imprint of Taylor & Francis Ltd. Permission conveyed through the Copyright Clearance Center Inc.

A third dimension used to judge within-phase data patterns is *variability*. Variability can be defined as the degree to which individual data points deviate from the overall trend. Or, stated another way, variability is the degree to which the data points are dispersed relative to the best-fit straight line. Like the magnitude of a trend line, the terminology used to refer to variability is largely qualitative. Variability is typically referred to as being *high, medium*, or *low*. Figure 16.8 shows two examples of variability. The left-hand panel shows a graph with low variability. That is, the data points are very close to the best-fit straight line. This can be contrasted with the right-hand panel of Figure 16.8, which shows a data set with high variability. In this instance, the data points are scattered widely around the best-fit straight line. As a rule of thumb, the greater the variability in your data, the more data points required to document a consistent pattern.

In general, level, trend, and variability are used to describe the patterns that occur within each phase of a study. How these three dimensions change across phases is the primary means by which data are analyzed through visual inspection. For example, in baseline there might be a level of 50% along the *y*-axis with low variability and a moderate upward trend, but following intervention there might be a level of 5% with moderate variability and a slight downward trend. Another pattern of data that can occur within a phase deserves to be mentioned. In some cases, *within-phase changes* in data patterns can emerge. That is, there can be *curvilinear* or *cyclical* changes in the data. Figure 16.9 shows three examples of curvilinear data patterns. The top panel of the figure shows a curvilinear data pattern (also referred to as a *U* pattern). The center panel of Figure 16.9 shows an *inverse curvilinear* data pattern (also referred to as an *inverted* U) in which the data trend increases and then decreases during a particular phase. At the bottom of the figure is a cyclical data pattern where data increase and decrease in a phasic manner.

FIGURE 16.7 ■ Series of Graphs Illustrating How to Calculate Trend using the Split-middle Technique Described in Table 16.2.

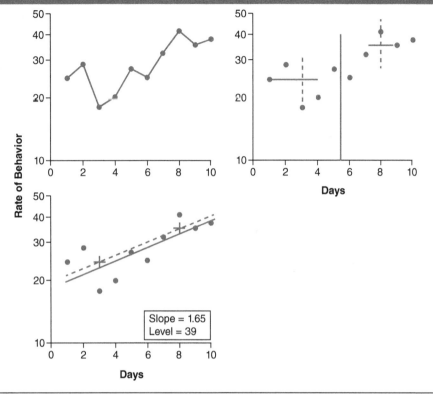

Note. Figure A-10, p. 313, from: Kazdin, A. E. (1982). *Single-case research designs.* Oxford University Press. Copyright 1982 by Oxford University Press. Reprinted by permission.

TABLE 16.2 ■ How to Calculate a Split-Middle Trend Estimation Line for the Data Shown in Figure 16.7

Step	Instruction
1	Count the number of data points in the phase that is being used for trend estimation.
2	Draw a line on the graph at the median data point to divide the graph into two halves.
3	Divide each of the halves in half using the technique described in Step 2.
4	Identify the median level of the data in each half of the split graph.
5	Mark the point at which the median number of sessions (x-axis) and median data level (y-axis) intersect for each half of the split graph.
6	Plot a straight line that intersects the two marks made in Step 5.
7	Adjust the straight line plotted in Step 6 so that 50% of the data points are above and 50% are below the line, making sure not to alter the slope of the line.

FIGURE 16.8 ■ Examples of two Different Degrees of Variability in Data.

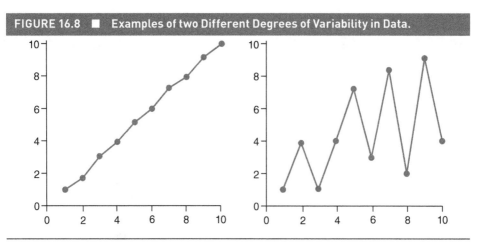

Note. The left-hand panel shows a graph with low variability. This can be contrasted with the right-hand panel, which shows a data set with high variability.

FIGURE 16.9 ■ Three Examples of Curvilinear and Cyclical Data Patterns.

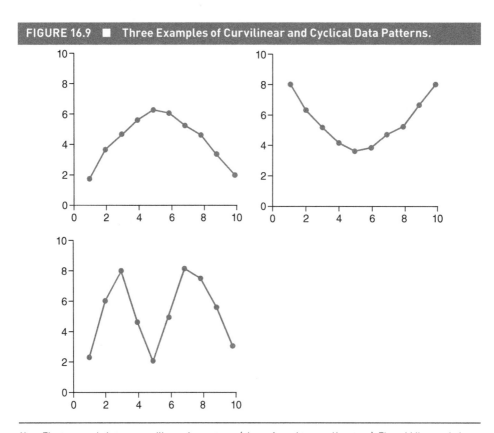

Note. The top panel shows a curvilinear data pattern (also referred to as a *U* pattern). The middle panel shows an *inverse curvilinear* data pattern (also referred to as an *inverted* U) in which the data trend increases and then decreases during a particular phase. At the bottom of the figure is a cyclical data pattern where data increase and decrease in phasic manner.

Between-Phase Patterns

Along with level, trend, variability, and curvilinear or cyclical patterns within a phase, there also are patterns occurring between phases that are used to visually inspect data. The first such pattern is referred to as *immediacy of effect* (or *rapidity of change*). This dimension of data displays can be defined as how quickly a change in the data pattern is produced after the phase change. This is typically expressed as changes in the level and trend of the data, although variability and curvilinear or cyclical relations can also contribute to the change. Like slope and variability, qualitative descriptors such as *rapid* or *slow* are used to describe this aspect of data. Figure 16.10 shows two examples of immediacy of effect. The top panel shows baseline (left side) and intervention phases (right side). The intervention had a rapid immediacy of effect because it quickly altered the pattern of data. This alteration in the data pattern across phases can be contrasted with the data in the lower panel of Figure 16.10. In this data set, there is no initial change in the pattern of behavior following introduction of the intervention, with the data then gradually decreasing over time. Such a pattern would be referred to as having a slow immediacy of effect.

FIGURE 16.10 ■ Two Examples of Immediacy of Effect.

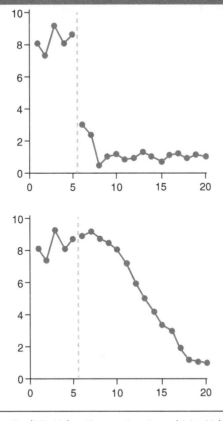

Note. The top panel shows baseline (left side) and intervention phases (right side). The intervention had a rapid immediacy of effect because it clearly altered the pattern of data represented in the graph. In the bottom panel there is no initial change in the pattern of behavior following introduction of the intervention with the data then gradually decreasing over time.

In general, the greater the immediacy of effect, the briefer a phase can be, and the more convincing the functional relation.

A second between-phase pattern is referred to as *overlap*. Overlap can be defined as the percentage or degree to which data in adjacent phases share similar quantitative values. Figure 16.11 shows three distinct patterns of overlap between baseline (left side) and intervention phases (right side). In the top panel of the figure, there is no overlap (i.e., 0%) between baseline

FIGURE 16.11 ■ Three Examples of Overlap in Data Between Phases.

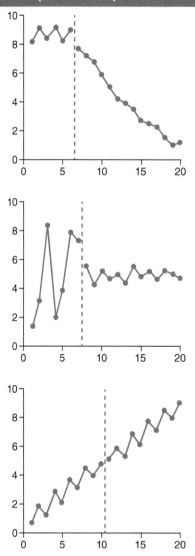

Note. In the top panel there is no overlap (i.e., 0%) between baseline and intervention phases. The center panel shows an example of complete (i.e., 100%) overlap between baseline and intervention phases. The final data set (bottom panel) presents a common data pattern that often leads to misinterpretation.

and intervention phases. This is because there are no overlapping data values between the two phases. The center panel of Figure 16.11 shows an example of complete (i.e., 100%) overlap between baseline and intervention phases. In this case, the intervention data completely overlap with the baseline data (although the converse is not true, so specifying the directionality of overlap is important). The final data set in Figure 16.11 (bottom panel) presents a common data pattern that leads to misinterpretation. Although there is no overlap between the data in adjacent phases, there is a trend that is continuous across phases. In such cases, trend overrides the importance of overlap in evaluating whether a functional relation has been established.

An Example

An illustration of how to use visual inspection to characterize a data set and arrive at a judgment regarding whether a functional relation has been established can be done using Figure 16.12. In this study by Cushing and Kennedy (1997) the percentage of time a student without disabilities (Cindy) was academically engaged served as the dependent variable. The baseline condition was Cindy working by herself in a general education classroom. During the initial baseline there was a high degree of variability with a mean of 42% (range, 0% to 76%) and a moderate downward trend. The intervention was comprised of Cindy serving as a peer support for a student with severe disabilities (Cathy). Following intervention, there was an immediate increase in the level of the dependent variable (M = 91%), with a small upward trend, little variability,

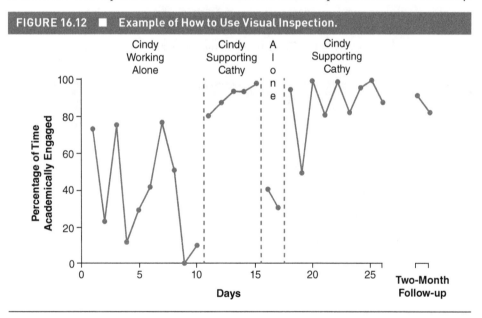

FIGURE 16.12 ■ Example of How to Use Visual Inspection.

Note. The percentage of time a student without disabilities (Cindy) was academically engaged served as the dependent variable. The baseline condition was Cindy working by herself in a general education classroom (i.e., home economics). The intervention was comprised of Cindy serving as a peer support for a student with severe disabilities (Cathy). (Figure 1, p. 145, from: Cushing, L. S., & Kennedy, C. H. (1997). Academic effects of providing peer support in general education classrooms on students without disabilities. *Journal of Applied Behavior Analysis, 30*, 139–151. Copyright 1997 by the Society for the Experimental Analysis of Behavior. Reproduced by permission.)

and no overlap with the previous baseline. The withdrawal of the intervention coincided with a reversal to baseline levels of performance ($M = 38\%$). Reintroducing the intervention resulted in an increase in academic engagement ($M = 85\%$) that after several sessions returned to levels similar to the previous intervention phase. Using the A-B-A-B withdrawal design, Cushing and Kennedy were able to demonstrate that Cindy was more academically engaged when she assisted Cathy than when she worked alone.

USING GRAPHS TO ANALYZE DATA

Now that we have reviewed the elements of line graphs and basic issues in visual analysis, we will focus on how to use graphs to explore various aspects of a data set. Data sets are often multifaceted and lend themselves to a variety of analyses. Depending on the approach taken, different aspects of the nature of the data will be revealed. Therefore, visual analysis of data is much more than simply putting data into a graphic template and describing the information. Instead, visual analysis is a process of using graphs to explore and visualize different aspects of the data so that researchers can arrive at a better understanding of the nature of their findings.

An example of how graphs can be used to focus on various aspects of a data set in educational research is provided by Haring and Kennedy (1988). These authors analyzed a *task analysis* data set using various graphic strategies. Task analysis is a process of breaking complex sequences of behavior into component parts that has proven effective at teaching people complex skills (Gold, 1976; McConomy et al., 2022). In this instance, a leisure activity was taught to a young man with severe disabilities. Table 16.3 lists the components of the leisure activity and

TABLE 16.3 ■ Task Analysis of a Leisure Skill	
Step	Instruction
1.	Gets radio and magazine[a]
2	Sits down in leisure area[a]
3	Turns radio on[a]
4	Selects radio station[a]
5	Puts headphones on appropriately
6	Looks at magazine[a]
7	Stops activity when signaled that break is finished[a]
8	Takes headphones off[a]
9	Turns radio off[a]
10	Puts magazine and radio away

[a]Critical steps.

notes the steps that were critical for independently completing the skill versus steps that were based on social convention.

Figure 16.13 shows five different approaches for visualizing the task analysis data, each showing different properties of the original data. Graph A is a standard line graph that presents the percentage of correct steps for each baseline and training session. This graphic approach

FIGURE 16.13 ■ Example of How Graphs can be used to Focus on Various Aspects of a Data Set in Educational Research.

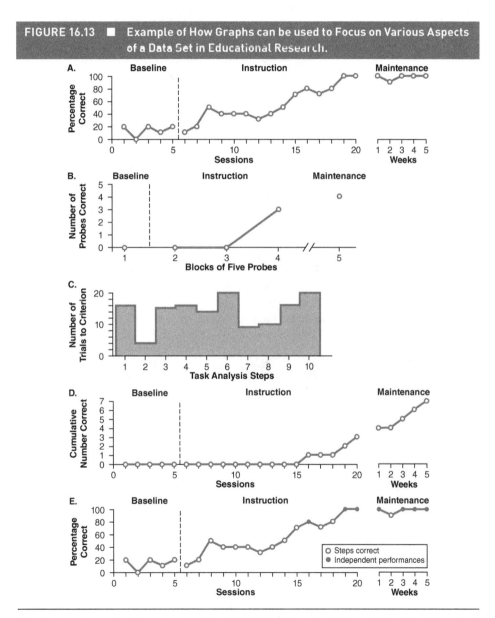

Note. Each graph reveals a different aspect of the original data. (Figure 1, p. 209, from: Haring, T. G., & Kennedy, C. H. (1988). Units of analysis in task-analytic research. *Journal of Applied Behavior Analysis, 21*, 207–216. Copyright 1988 by the Society for the Experimental Analysis of Behavior. Reproduced by permission.)

shows day-to-day variation in the data set, but does not provide information regarding when the skill was independently performed (i.e., all critical steps) and does not show the types of errors that occurred. Graph B shows the number of sessions (in blocks of five) that were independently completed. This second approach to visualizing the data allows for an analysis of independent performances, but does not show day-to-day variability or the types of errors that were made. Graph C displays the data as the number of sessions to criterion for each step in the task analysis (i.e., correctly performed three days in a row for a single step). This graphic approach shows the errors that were made in a summative fashion, but does not display day-to-day variation or when competent performances occurred. A fourth approach to visually displaying the data is shown in Graph D. This graph shows the cumulative number of times that the skill was performed independently. Using this approach, you can analyze if a session was independently performed and on what day (preserving day-to-day variation at a certain level), but no information is available regarding what types of errors were made. Graph E combines elements of Graphs A and D to display the percentage of steps correct (open circles) and the occurrence of independent performances (closed circles). By doing this, the graph shows all of the characteristics of the data previously described, with the exception of an error pattern analysis. A final graph was constructed by Haring and Kennedy (1988) that met each of the criteria previously discussed (see Figure 16.14). This final graph allows for a comprehensive visual analysis of the original data.

The previous examples illustrate how using various approaches to graphically displaying data can allow for the visualization of different aspects of a data set. The variety of means for visualizing data is enormous, and researchers need to select those graphic approaches that best represent salient aspects of their data. An issue that needs to be addressed when graphing data is the level at which the information will be summarized. In some instances, it may be more desirable to summarize data as averages (e.g., percentage of intervals), while at other times it may be best to graph

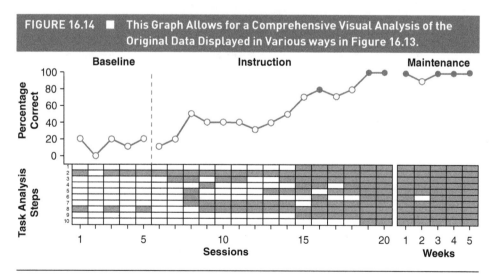

FIGURE 16.14 ■ This Graph Allows for a Comprehensive Visual Analysis of the Original Data Displayed in Various ways in Figure 16.13.

Note. Figure 2, p. 213, from: Haring, T. G., & Kennedy, C. H. (1988). Units of analysis in task-analytic research. *Journal of Applied Behavior Analysis, 21,* 207–216. Copyright 1988 by the Society for the Experimental Analysis of Behavior. Reproduced by permission.

data at a more fine-grained level (e.g., cumulative occurrences in real time). This former approach is sometimes referred as a *molar* approach and the latter as a *molecular* approach.

Figure 16.15 illustrates how the same data set can be visualized at various levels (Iversen, 1988). The data are from a laboratory experiment that analyzed the number of times a response was emitted following the delivery of a response-independent positive reinforcer. The *y*-axis displays this as the number of responses that occurred within 30 seconds of each reinforcing event. In the center panel of the graph are the raw data. It shows that on 1 occurrence 12 responses were emitted, on 4 occurrences 11 responses were emitted, on 1 occurrence 10 responses were emitted, and so on. If the data were summarized at a molar level, such as the mean and standard deviation of the raw data, it would look like the graph in the right-hand panel of Figure 16.15. If the data were analyzed at a more molecular level, one approach would be to adopt the strategy shown in the left-hand panel. In this instance, the data were further analyzed in terms of the contiguity between reinforcer delivery and the last response prior to the reinforcer delivery. The data in the left-hand panel clearly show that the greater the contiguity (e.g., 0 to 0.5 seconds) between prior responses and reinforcer delivery, the greater the number of postreinforcement responses.

The data displays in Figure 16.15 show how information can be summarized at different levels of aggregation and disaggregation. The raw data show the general distribution of events, the statistical data show central tendency and dispersion at the coarsest level, and the disaggregated data show specific patterns in the data. The information shown in the left-hand panel also illustrates the power of graphic displays to more completely analyze data. With the addition of a second variable along the horizontal axis, the author was able to account for variability in the behavior unexplained in the other panels. In this sense, graphs can be used to explore, visualize, and explain variability in behavior.

Another approach to visualizing information that is becoming increasingly common is to conduct *within-session analyses*. The information shown in Figures 16.2 through 16.15 has all been data summarizing events occurring during an entire session. That is, they represent the average level of events within the experimental session. However, in some instances, information regarding

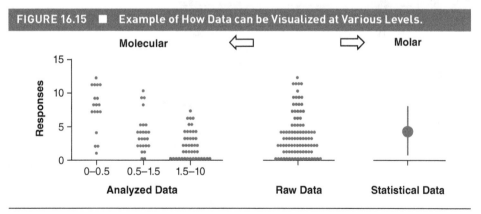

FIGURE 16.15 ■ Example of How Data can be Visualized at Various Levels.

Note. The data are from a laboratory experiment that analyzed the number of times a response was emitted following the delivery of a response-independent positive reinforcer. The vertical axis displays this as the number of responses that occurred within 30 seconds of each reinforcing event. Each of the panels aggregates the data at a different level of refinement. (Figure 6, p. 179, from: Iversen, I. H. (1988). Tactics of graphic design: A review of Tufte's *The visual display of quantitative information. Journal of the Experimental Analysis of Behavior, 49*, 171–189. Copyright 1988 by the Society for the Experimental Analysis of Behavior. Reproduced by permission.)

the pattern of events within a session can aid in the understanding of variables influencing behavior. One assumption that is implicit in summarizing whole-session data as individual data points is that the pattern of behavior observed in an experimental session was uniform throughout that session. For instances in which there are changes in responding during a session, within-session data analysis can reveal potentially important patterns that otherwise might not be discovered.

One of the first applied examples of within-session analysis was provided by Carr et al. (1980). Carr and colleagues were interested in understanding why aggression occurred in two boys with developmental disabilities. The analysis shown in Figure 16.16 indicated that the behavior was related to instructional demands: When demands were made, high levels of aggression occurred, while under no demand conditions, aggression rarely occurred. An important aspect of the experimental procedures was that the length of each session was fixed. Once the session was over, the demands stopped. Technically, if the children's

FIGURE 16.16 ■ Initial Analysis Conducted by Carr et al. (1980).

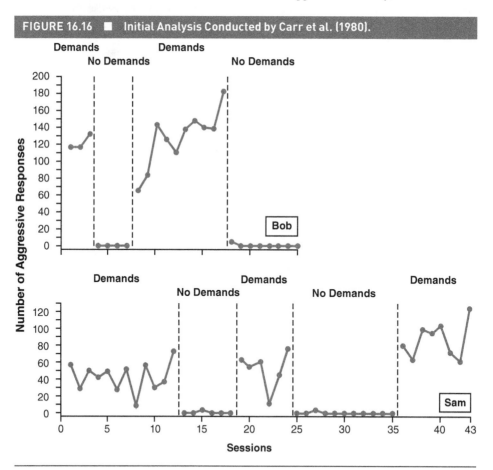

Note. The number of aggressive responses for Sam and Bob (two boys with developmental disabilities) served as the dependent variable. The independent variable was the presence or absence of instructional demands. (Figure 1, p. 105, from: Carr, E. G., Newsom, C. D., & Binkoff, J. A. (1980). Escape as a factor in the aggressive behavior of two retarded children. *Journal of Applied Behavior Analysis, 13*, 101–117. Copyright 1980 by the Society for the Experimental Analysis of Behavior. Reproduced by permission.)

behavior was reinforced by escape from instruction, termination of a session could constitute a fixed-interval (FI) schedule of negative reinforcement (see Catania, 2013a). An important characteristic of FI schedules is that they produce a scalloped pattern of behavior in which responding is less frequent early on but increases in probability as the end of the interval nears (i.e., reinforcement is more proximal). To see if the data they were obtaining fit this well-known pattern of behavior, Carr et al. conducted a within-session analysis that contrasted two conditions: the presence of a "safety signal" indicating no more demands would be made versus "no safety signal" in which demands were continued (see Figure 16.17). In the absence of the safety signal, aggression increased as the sessions continued,

FIGURE 16.17 ■ Within-Session Analysis Conducted by Carr et al. (1980) from the Between-Session Data Displayed in Figure 16.16.

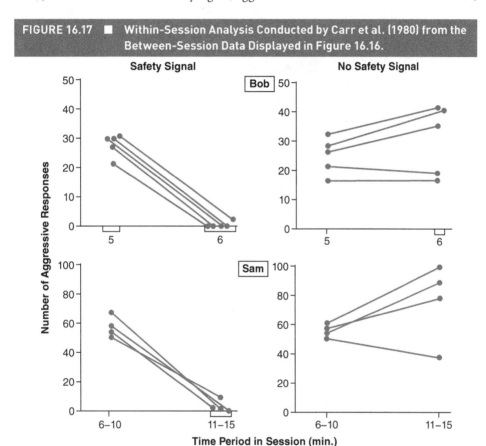

Note. As described in the Carr et al. paper, "Number of aggressive responses during the 5th and 6th min of each session in the second Demands condition for Bob (top half of figure) and during the 6th to 10th min and 11th to 15th min of each session in the third Demands condition for Sam (bottom half of figure). The left panels show data taken during Safety Signal sessions in which the experimenter signaled to each child that demands were no longer forthcoming. The signal was given to Bob at the start of the 6th min and to Sam at the start of the 11th min. The right panels show data taken during No Safety Signal sessions in which neither child received any cue that demands had ended. Some of the data points have been slightly displaced horizontally to enhance presentation clarity" (p. 106). (Figure 2, p. 106, from: Carr, E. G., Newsom, C. D., & Binkoff, J. A. (1980). Escape as a factor in the aggressive behavior of two retarded children. *Journal of Applied Behavior Analysis, 13,* 101–117. Copyright 1980 by the Society for the Experimental Analysis of Behavior. Reproduced by permission.)

but when the safety signal was presented, aggression decreased. This within-session analysis helped provide additional evidence that the aggression was negatively reinforced (see Beavers et al., 2013) and followed principles of behavior that were well established in basic research (see Catania, 2013b; Sidman, 1960).

Another example of within-session analysis is provided by Vollmer et al. (1997) in an analysis of adventitious positive reinforcement using noncontingent reinforcement (NCR) procedures to treat behavior problems. The top panel of Figure 16.18 shows an analysis of NCR to treat the behavior problem of an adolescent with developmental disabilities. During the second NCR phase (Sessions 14 through 20), problem behavior began to rapidly increase in frequency. Vollmer et al. conducted within-session analyses of these sessions, which are displayed in the

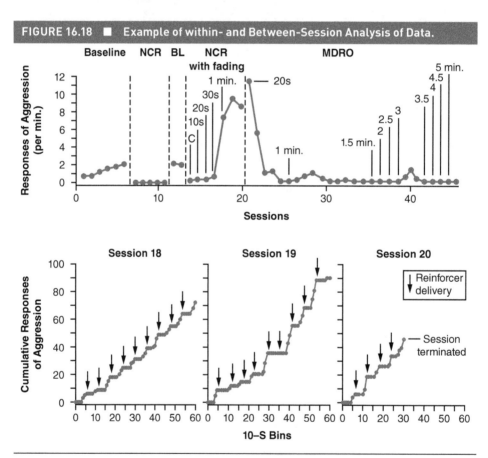

FIGURE 16.18 ■ Example of within- and Between-Session Analysis of Data.

Note. Vollmer et al. described this figure as "The upper panel shows aggression rates during baseline, continuous NCR, NCR with fading, and MDRO conditions (values for MDRO are shown in minutes). The fading steps are indicated by the lines and reinforcer delivery schedule values. The lower panel shows cumulative records of aggression during Sessions 18 through 20. Arrows indicate when reinforcers were presented" (p. 163). (Figure 1, p. 163, from: Vollmer, T. R., Ringdahl, J. E., Roane, H. S., & Marcus, B. A. (1997). Negative side effects of noncontingent reinforcement. *Journal of Applied Behavior Analysis, 30*, 161–164. Copyright 1997 by the Society for the Experimental Analysis of Behavior. Reproduced by permission.)

lower panels of the figure. Using the NCR procedure, a reinforcer was delivered on a response-independent fixed-time (FT) schedule. The pattern of responding and stimulus delivery on the NCR FT schedule showed a pattern of responding very similar to that previously discussed for FI schedules of reinforcement. That is, the authors had inadvertently (i.e., adventitiously) established a positive reinforcement contingency for the problem behavior, thus making it increase over time. Given the results of the within-session analysis, Vollmer et al. were able to arrange a momentary differential reinforcement of other (MDRO) schedule of reinforcement to counteract the adventitious positive reinforcement schedule established via the NCR procedure. In this example, the use of within-session analysis provided the ability to analyze the contiguity of events that were occurring on a moment-by-moment level that would not have otherwise been available for analysis.

In this section, I have attempted to highlight a few examples of *how graphs can be used to explore data*. This type of process is frequently done in experimental biology and the experimental analysis of behavior (see Chapter 2) but is far rarer in psychology or educational research (Smith et al., 2002). There are no prescribed limits to how data can be explored and visualized, nor are there templates for graphic analysis that are universally effective. Instead, researchers need to look carefully at their data, at multiple levels, and in conjunction with a range of events potentially serving as independent and dependent variables. The use of graphs can be extremely helpful in this process of exploring data and trying to more thoroughly understand what type(s) of functional relations may have been established in an experiment.

TRAINING PEOPLE TO VISUALLY ANALYZE DATA

One of the chief criticisms of the visual analysis of data by proponents of inferential statistics has been that judgments are inconsistent. That is, if two or three different researchers each inspect a graph, they may reach different conclusions. The basis for this concern was studies showing interrater variability when conducting visual analyses of data (e.g., DeProspero & Cohen, 1979; Furlong & Wampold, 1982; Jones et al., 1978). The findings showed that judges could differ under certain conditions when categorizing the size of experimental effects via visual analysis.

At the time these studies were conducted, they were interpreted by researchers not familiar with single-case methods as a damning critique of this research methodology (see Box 16.1). The criticism was that the data analysis methods of this new discipline were invalid, or at least inconsistent, rendering the methodology inadequate (Fisch, 2001; Shavelson & Towne, 2002). The logic was that if researchers varied in their visual interpretation of graphs, the data analysis methods used in behavior analysis were flawed. On the surface this criticism seems to have merit. However, the logic seems inconsistent with certain aspects of the scientific process. First, the judgment of raters differed primarily under conditions of small-level changes between conditions and high variability within phases. Few, if any, single-case researchers would attempt to claim functional relations under such circumstances. If they did, their claims would likely be challenged by other single-case researchers noting (a) any assertion regarding a functional relation needs to be highly qualified and (b) the finding would require direct replication with additional participants before it was publishable. Hence, the criticism that visual inspection may lead to increased Type I errors (i.e., claims of an effect when none exists) ignores the larger social context of how data are evaluated in science (see Smith et al., 2002). Rarely, in single-case research, do claims of an experimental effect rest on a single ambiguous A-B analysis. Such a claim would not survive the peer-review process that serves as the primary quality control system for introducing new findings into the research literature (see Chapter 1). Given that multiple individuals (i.e., researchers, reviewers, and editors) visually analyze each data set prior to publication, the odds of every person making a Type I error following this type of training is extremely small.

BOX 16.1: APPLIED PSYCHOLOGY'S DISFAVOR WITH VISUAL DATA ANALYSIS

Considerable attention was given to the emergence of applied behavior analysis when it emerged in the 1960s. Part of that attention was from applied psychologists who criticized the nascent field's primary approach to data analysis: graphic displays. This approach to data analysis contradicted the predominant approach in psychology, which was the use of inferential statistics. Applied psychologists have criticized researchers using single-case designs for not following proper scientific method (Shavelson & Towne, 2002). One of the underlying issues of this debate concerned two fundamentally different approaches to designing experiments and analyzing data. Using group-comparison methods, subjects are randomly assigned to prescribed conditions; after the data are collected, the results are analyzed to estimate the degree to which a particular finding is due to chance; and, if that probability is low enough, the results are accepted as due to experimental effects and not extraneous variables. In behavior analysis, experiments are designed to reveal how behavioral processes operate, and data analysis is focused on demonstrating functional relations via repeated experimental manipulations. The designs are inductive and changed as the data require. They exist as distinct approaches to conducting experiments. Criticizing one approach by using the experimental criteria of the other is logically unsatisfactory.

There is a long-standing truism among researchers that the appropriate analytical technique is tied not to a specific research methodology, but to the success of researchers in answering their experimental questions. Whether single-case designs are an adequate approach to answering experimental questions should be judged not by a particular person's aesthetic sense of what a research method should be, but by how useful that method adequately answers the experimental questions being posed. Given that research in the single-case research tradition has thrived for almost a century, from laboratory to applied settings, and is only showing signs of increasing in prevalence across a range of academic disciplines, this approach to experimental design must be producing useful results.

Otherwise, it would have ceased to be used as a tool for understanding human nature a long time ago.

Perhaps what is fundamentally at issue with applied psychology's disfavor of various methods used in single-case research is not the inadequacy of those methods, but critics' lack of familiarity with single-case methods and their underlying assumptions. To dismiss a functional relation derived from a single-case design as not adequate because inferential statistics were not used is no more substantive than behavior analysts complaining that group-comparison designs hide variability or are inefficient because they require too many participants to demonstrate experimental control. Ultimately, the adequacy of any particular experimental method will rest on researchers' ability to produce findings and solve problems by using that particular method.

A second flaw in criticisms leveled against visual inspection is that they ignore the self-corrective nature of the research process. If a researcher were to claim a functional relation from a limited data set with small effects, those findings would still need to be independently replicated. If the researcher did make a Type I error by overinterpreting the data, the researcher and others would be unable to replicate the original findings. The result would be the original finding being viewed as an anomaly and disregarded as a valid claim. It's important to remember that at the heart of the scientific method is a "quality control system" called replication (see Chapter 4).

A final limitation of critiques of visual analysis is that this approach to data analysis is demonstrably effective as a scientific technique. Ignoring for the moment the findings of experimental biology and medicine over the last two centuries (which often rely on visual analysis of data; see Latour & Woolgar, 2013), the single-case literature in educational research has repeatedly produced important findings over the last half century. Those findings, as noted in Chapter 2, have been repeatedly replicated, extended, and refined over time and have led to important insights into behavioral processes and innovative new teaching techniques. If the basis for data analysis in single-case research were fundamentally flawed, it is unclear how a continuous stream of important discoveries could be made (and repeatedly replicated).

A more adequate solution to concerns about interrater variability using visual analysis is one very familiar to educators and behavior analysts: teach people how to analyze graphed data. Such a process is done informally (or, at least, without an explicit curriculum) in every research team using visual analysis methods and is a standard component of university courses in behavior analysis. Recent data have shown that untrained observers can interpret graphed data (as indexed by a consensus of experts) with approximately 55% accuracy. However, following training, those same raters improve their performances to approximately 95% (Diller et al., 2016; Fisher et al., 2003; Kahng et al., 2010).

Fisher et al.'s (2003) validated approach to training visual analysis skills will be used as an example. (a) First, a set of A-B graphs is developed to show a range of effects relating to trend, level, variability, immediacy of effect, and overlap. (b) The graphs are then categorized into varying degrees of change between conditions as an index against which trainees' judgments can be indexed. (c) Trainees are then exposed to the concepts of visual inspection (reviewed in the previous sections of this chapter). (d) The A-B graphs are then presented individually to the trainees, who are asked to record whether an effect is present or not, and they are then provided with feedback regarding the accuracy of their performances. This relatively simple method can be used to train consistent visual inspectors in less than an hour according to multiple studies (DeRosa et al., 2021).

This type of formal training scenario, combined with regular reading and discussion of published research, seems to be the best approach to teaching people how to visually analyze data. Combine these approaches to the daily and weekly decisions that are required when engaging in either research or practice, and a rigorous training regimen is established. Many years after the debate over whether visual data analysis is an acceptable method, the focus has changed from whether the approach works to *how to effectively teach people to use this demonstrably effective data analysis technique*. In other words, with the vantage gained by hindsight, the issues regarding the use of visual data analysis are not if, but how.

CONCLUSION

The visual inspection of graphed data has proven to be one of the most powerful analytical techniques in science. By visualizing different aspects of a data set, the results of a study can be explored and described in a variety of ways. Such a process allows researchers to delve into various aspects and patterns of their data to gain a deeper understanding of the nature of their findings. The use of visual analysis techniques matches the inductive nature of single-case designs by facilitating data exploration and the provision of readily developed and updated data analysis formats. That is, as an experiment unfolds, the data can be tracked on a daily basis for decision-making purposes and the experimental procedures adjusted accordingly.

Because of these properties, graphed data have been the central means of data analysis for single-case researchers for almost 100 years. As basic laboratory findings were extended to socially relevant issues, the data analysis techniques of basic researchers were adopted by applied investigators. Although the use of graphs instead of inferential statistics as a primary means of data analysis is contrary to traditional approaches to psychology, it has proven itself in the biological and medical sciences as a useful technique. This chapter has attempted to provide an introduction to the visual analysis of data and provided a few examples of how graphic displays can be used to better understand the nature of functional relations that result from single-case research. However, like all aspects of research methodology, there is no single "correct way" of visualizing data. Instead, each researcher needs to adapt the techniques that are available to them to the analytical task at hand and use, or develop, the most appropriate means to reveal what patterns exist in their data.

1. Does the use of visual analysis in single-case designs produce a more sensitive, or less sensitive, ability to explore data and render a decision regarding experimental control?

2. Identify the elements in a graphic display and explain how each is necessary to identify experimental control.

3. When visually inspecting data, what are three within-phase dimensions of data and two between-phase data dimensions that are assessed?

4. How can an individual data set be analyzed along various criteria using graphic displays?

5. What does Tufte (1983) mean when he recommends that visual displays of data minimize nondata ink?

17 QUANTITATIVE ANALYSIS

It is clear at this point in the book that decisions regarding the internal validity of $N = 1$ experiments are arrived at through the analysis of visualized information. Single-case design experiments are conducted in an inductive manner where conditions are structured to allow comparisons between conditions, and the juxtaposition of those conditions constitutes the experimental design. Whether the experimental procedures follow a multiple-baseline design, an A-B-A-B withdrawal design, or some combination of designs, the investigator follows the data. The data patterns that emerge within and between conditions guide the researcher in deciding the length of an individual phase, whether to repeat a previous condition, or whether to alter the design of the planned experiment in an ad hoc manner. When Murray Sidman (1960, p. 214) wrote "there are no rules to experimental design," this process was what he was referring to. In many respects, if there is any "luck" in the outcome of $N = 1$ experiments, it is because of the design decisions of the researcher.

Researchers whose backgrounds are in other approaches to experimental design such as experimental and quasi-experimental group designs often view the single-case design process with skepticism (Barlow & Nok, 2009). The reality is that single-case designs are distinctly different from those of other experimental approaches. The inductive logic and focus on internal validity of $N = 1$ designs coupled with a lack of clear external validity are at odds with most of traditional psychology and its areas of application (Birnbrauer, 1983; Molenaar, 2004). Single-case designs are primarily focused on experimental control and consider the population generality of the findings a secondary issue. For experimental and quasi-experimental group designs, population generality is of primary interest, and internal validity is a threshold to be reached so the results can be extrapolated to representative groups of people. As was discussed in Chapters 2 and 5, both of these views are important; they just emphasize different experimental questions and goals. *There is, however, a more fundamental difference.*

A distinction between emphases on internal versus external validity in single-case versus group-comparison designs is not the core difference between these experimental methods. The core distinction is that each approach draws upon an orthogonal set of underlying assumptions about measurement. Group-comparison designs draw from a history based on psychometric measures from normal distributions that use statistical inference to differentiate among groups (Lord & Novick, 1968). The focus is on how groups are constituted with the person as an element in the larger group. This focus means that individual data points (i.e., a person) are independent of each other, each person contributes a single distinct data point, and measurement is designed to assess these interindividual differences. Classical test theory and its attendant statistical procedures were developed to describe groups of people and differentiate among groups based on statistical averages (Campbell, 1988). Assumptions such as the *independence* of data points, *random* samples representing a larger population, and *variance* among individual data points within a normal distribution are defining features of this measurement theory.

In contrast, the measurement assumptions implicit in $N = 1$ designs are entirely intraindividual in their focus. The focus is to measure (a) an individual's behavior (b) repeatedly over time (c) with the person serving as their own internal reference point. This intraindividual emphasis on experimental control was created independent of classic test theory and does not share many of its fundamental assumptions (Molenaar, 2008). First, data points sampled from a single participant over time are not independent of each other and tend to be highly autocorrelated (see Busk & Marascuilo, 1988; Shadish & Sullivan, 2011). Second, there is no expectation that individuals are representative of a larger group and that there is therefore homogeneity in data sets allowing generalizations about populations. Finally, the distribution of variance among intraindividual data points is not typically viewed as approximating normality (i.e., a normal distribution) and can fall along any type of distribution (in fact, distributions may change within an individual participant under different experimental conditions). In its essence, $N = 1$ designs do not follow the assumptions regarding data characteristics that are fundamental to group-comparison designs. However, single-case designs can demonstrate exceptionally high levels of internal validity, which is the purpose for which they were created.

These differences between interindividual and intraindividual experimental designs and their underlying measurement theories are often referred to as *nomothetic* versus *idiographic* or *vaganotic* versus *idemnotic* (see Johnston et al., 2020). The fundamental differences between these approaches, as just described, have existed in parallel for over 100 years as separate domains of psychological research. Neither approach is correct nor incorrect; they simply have different assumptions and goals. However, when a researcher from one tradition (e.g., interindividual measurement) encounters the other tradition (e.g., intraindividual measurement), the other approach is often indexed against the investigator's own research experiences. And, since each approach has fundamental assumptions that are orthogonal to the other, the result has often been an underappreciation of the other approach.

Although there are fundamental differences between these two approaches to experimentation in psychology and related social sciences, over the past several years there have been concerted efforts by both groups to identify opportunities for integration (e.g., Keren, 2014; Kratochwill & Levin, 2014). This rapprochement has several motivations. First, it proves the potential to generate new experimental tools that add quantitative precision and replicability to *describing patterns of data*. Second, it has produced several control techniques borrowed from group-comparison designs that may be used as *inferential statistical techniques*. Finally, this rapprochement has enabled the use of meta-analyses for single-case design findings that allow the integration of experimental findings across $N = 1$ designs.

Much of this work has been driven by the desire to incorporate single-case design findings into the larger educational research database (Shadish et al., 2008; Smith, 2012). The use of quantitative methods in $N = 1$ designs is a rapidly developing area of experimental research and offers great potential for single-case design researchers. In what follows, we will discuss three specific areas in which quantitative methods are used in single-case design research: *descriptive techniques, interferential techniques*, and *integrative techniques*. Each domain has its areas of innovation as well as interesting questions that are raised when integrating statistical techniques into an intraindividual design approach.

DESCRIPTIVE TECHNIQUES

The best starting place for quantifying single-case design data is with descriptive measures. And, since all data analysis in $N = 1$ designs begins with the visual analysis of graphed information, data displays are the natural starting point for numerically describing data. In this section we will review techniques for quantifying the primary data patterns in visual analysis: level, trend, variability, immediacy of effect, and overlap (see Chapter 16).

The level of data within a phase (or condition) is a general estimate of the central tendency of the pattern along the y-axis metric. Optimally, the level falls at the midpoint in the scale being used so that data can increase and/or decrease by an equal number of quantitative units. However, because we are discussing the application of single-case designs to applied educational problems, the level of data may begin or end at the end point of the measure being used (e.g., zero for skills to be learned or 100% for skills that are mastered). In general, there are two measures of central tendency that are used in single-case designs: the *mean* and *median*. Estimating level using the mean is the generally preferred technique because it is the more conservative description of data levels. However, researchers will use the median in cases where there are outliers present (i.e., skewed distributions) in which an extreme value shifts the mean away from its intended representative role (Nesselroade & Grimm, 2018).

A within-phase parameter that is essential to visually assessing patterns of data is the *trend*. Trends can be computed with as few as two data points, but the larger the N, the more compelling the estimate of slope becomes. The classic estimate of slope is to use a least-squares regression coefficient to calculate the trend (i.e., magnitude and direction of slope; see Figure 16.6). However, a simpler method that closely approximates the least-squares regression coefficient is the "split-middle trend estimate" introduced in Chapter 16. This metric, introduced by Owen R. White (1971; see also Gast & Spriggs, 2010; White & Haring, 1980), has become the preferred method in single-case design research for calculating trend because of its ease of computation and close approximation to the value arrived at using least-squares regression analyses.

The third aspect of within-phase data patterns is *variability*. This parameter of data is often calculated using range estimates. Two types of range estimates are used in describing variability: absolute range and relative range. The most commonly used estimate of variability is absolute range, which simply notes the lowest and highest values within a collection of data. The less frequently used variability estimate is relative range, which summarizes data dispersion by subtracting the smaller number from the larger value. The preference for one measure over the other is probably a combination of history and convention, rather than a clear scientific rationale.

An important quantitative parameter of within-phase data patterns that was only briefly mentioned in Chapter 16 is the *stability* of data from session to session. When $N = 1$ research methods emerged in the 1950s in the context of model systems experimentation, changes in the independent variable status were only introduced once "steady state" patterns of data were established (Sidman, 1960). A consistent pattern of data that changed little in level and had a well-established degree of variability is the optimal context for introducing a change in experimental conditions because of its sensitivity to changes in data patterns. However, in applied research extended baseline and intervention conditions are not always tractable or practical. Nonetheless, it may be pedagogically useful to discuss at least one technique developed to describe within-phase data stability.

Perhaps the most thorough treatment of data stability was presented by Killeen (1978) in which he presented the conclusion that a nomothetic-based measure provided a reasonable estimate of data stability. The nomothetic measure was based on changes in session-by-session values of difference decreasing over time until a magnitude of the difference fell within a specified criterion. A more contemporary measure that parallels Killeen's approach is the "stability envelope" (Lane & Gast, 2014; see also Barton et al., 2018). Figure 17.1 (top panel) shows a hypothetical data set from Lane and Gast (2014). For purposes of exposition, we will treat the A and B phases as distinct within-phase patterns to illustrate two examples of using the stability envelope. The calculation uses a measure of central tendency for data within a phase (mean or median) to represent an average value of data collected. Then, an estimate of variability is calculated for the same data points. A standard deviation derived from the data points (or a more conservative variability estimate) can be used to bound the level estimate, or, as Lane and Gast suggest, a percentage of the level can be used (e.g., ±25% of the mean). Figure 17.1 (bottom panel) shows the resulting numerical values and level/variability lines. This descriptive measure allows a researcher to estimate the percentage of data points within the range to illustrate the stability of the data. It would also be possible to use a trend estimate like the split middle to conduct a similar procedure for data that have clear upward or downward trends. Using a stability envelope allows single-case design researchers to quantify the pattern of variability within a phase that can provide additional evidence beyond visual inspection of the consistency in a data pattern.

Immediacy of effect is an important characteristic of the impact an independent variable has on the measure(s) of interest. Although there are no currently specified quantitative techniques for estimating immediacy of effect, there are some indexes worthy of attention. First is the degree to which the data following a phase change deviate from the mean and overall

FIGURE 17.1   ■   Example of Using A "Stability Envelope" to Assess Within-Phase Patterns of Behavior.

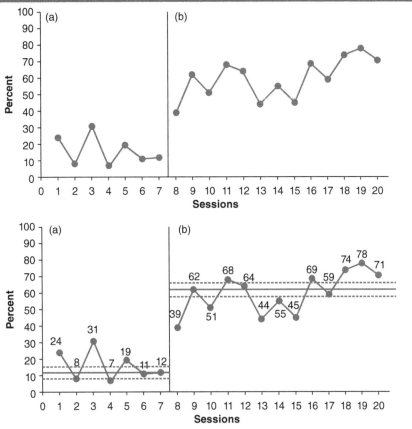

Note. A hypothetical data set for A-B phase data (top panel). The bottom panel shows the same data, but with individual data points quantified and ±25% variation metric (broken lines) surrounding the phase mean (solid line). (Figure 3, p. 450 (top), and Figure 4, p. 451 (bottom), from: Lane, J. D., & Gast, D. L. (2014). Visual analysis in single case experimental design studies: Brief review and guidelines. *Neuropsychological Rehabilitation, 24*(3–4), 445–463 (https://doi.org/10.1080/09602011.2013.815636). Copyright 2014 by Taylor & Francis Ltd. (http://www.tandfonline.com). Reproduced by permission.)

pattern of the previous phase. For example, an increase of 50% on the first day of intervention is more compelling than a 0% change. However, a corollary of initial change is the delay to a clear change in data pattern. Some interventions may be expected to have a delayed change following a phase transition (e.g., acquisition of sight words). Together the initial degree of effect and the degree the effect develops over time are the best quantitative parameters of immediacy of effect. Researchers have also suggested more qualitative parameters such as a hypothesis-driven prediction that a delay will occur (or an empirically derived prediction), and the consistency of the delay across participants and/or phases should also be considered (Lieberman et al., 2010).

The final parameter for quantifying behavior change in $N = 1$ research has received substantial attention in recent years. The degree of *overlap* in data between phases will be discussed in this section as a descriptive statistic and then later in the chapter as part of efforts to integrate data across studies using meta-analysis. The concept of overlap refers to the degree to which data from one phase are similar or deviate from the data in another phase based on the dependent variable(s) being used (see Chapter 16). In general, the less overlap between adjacent phases, the clearer the effect of the independent variable on the measures of interest.

Overlap metrics were first introduced in the late 1980s by Scruggs and colleagues (1987). The original conceptualization of this metric was referred to as the percentage of nonoverlapping data (PND). Figure 17.2 shows a figure used to illustrate the statistics from the original

FIGURE 17.2 ■ Hypothetical Data Showing Baseline and Treatment Conditions Across Sessions.

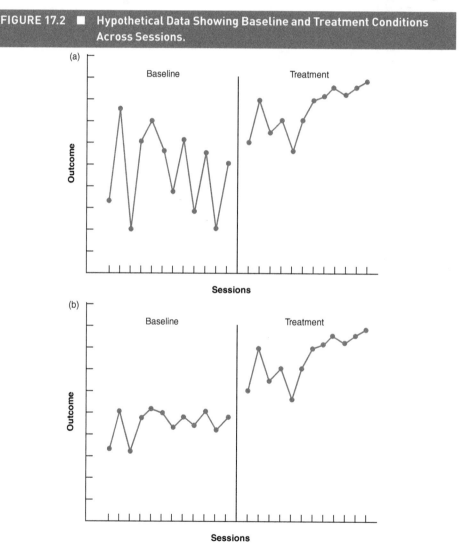

Note. Figure 1, p. 27, from: Scruggs, T. E., Mastropieri, M. A., & Casto, G. (1987). The quantitative synthesis of single-subject research: Methodology and validation. *Remedial and Special Education, 8*(2), 24–33. Copyright 1987 by Sage Publications. Reproduced by permission.

Scruggs et al. publication. The top panel of the figure shows an A-B phase with overlap between baseline and treatment, whereas the bottom panel of Figure 17.2 shows an analogous A-B data set without overlap. To compute PND, the investigator uses the total number of data points in the phase of interest (e.g., baseline) as the denominator and the number of data points that do not overlap with the adjacent phase (in this case treatment) as the numerator and multiplies the outcome by 100%. Figure 17.3 shows two examples of the PND calculation for the data illustrated in Figure 17.2. For the top panel of Figure 17.3, 6 data points overlapped between

FIGURE 17.3 ■ The Same Figure As Figure 17.2 But With The Percentage of Nonoverlapping Data (PND) Calculated.

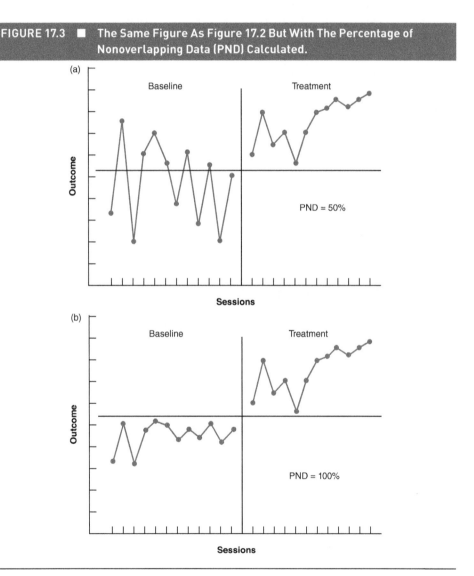

Note. Figure 1, p. 27, from: Scruggs, T. E., Mastropieri, M. A., & Casto, G. (1987). The quantitative synthesis of single-subject research: Methodology and validation. *Remedial and Special Education, 8*(2), 24–33. Copyright 1987 by Sage Publications. Reproduced by permission.

phases (6 did not overlap), and the number of baseline data points was 12; thus the calculation was 6/12, or 50% of the data points were nonoverlapping. The bottom panel of the figure has no overlapping data points, so the calculation would be 12/12, equaling 100%. Thus, the statistic provides a quantitative index of the degree of nonoverlap for data between phases on an experiment.

PND has become a frequently used statistic to estimate the degree of change from one phase to another in single-case design research. However, there are several limitations associated with this approach that should be noted. First, the statistic does not account for trends in the data across phases (White, 1987). Figure 17.4 shows data from Chapter 16 (Figure 16.11) illustrating a continuous upward trend in the data from baseline through treatment. As is noted in the figure, the calculation of PND results in 100% nonoverlapping data even though there is clearly no experimental effect. Second, the statistic does not take into account the magnitude of the experimental effect (Wolery et al., 2010). Figure 17.5 shows two different A-B graphs, with the top figure showing a small-magnitude change across phases (~15%) and the bottom figure showing a large-magnitude change across phases (~65%). However, when the PND is calculated, both figures produce a 100% outcome for nonoverlapping data. Thus, magnitude or degree of change in $N = 1$ experiments is not quantified by the statistic. Third, expected delays in intervention effects (e.g., for skill acquisition) are not accommodated by the statistic. Instead, the lag in the independent variable effect is counted as overlap between phases and reduces the reported size of the intervention effect (Wolery et al., 2010). Finally, the estimated PND outcome can be directly manipulated by increasing the number of either baseline or treatment data points collected to inflate the statistic (Pustejovsky, 2019). Given these limitations, although

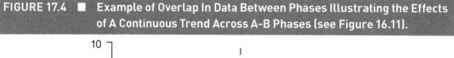

FIGURE 17.4 ■ Example of Overlap In Data Between Phases Illustrating the Effects of A Continuous Trend Across A-B Phases (see Figure 16.11).

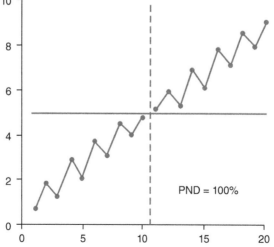

PND = 100%

Note. A PND calculation for these data yields a result of 100% nonoverlapping data despite the clear trend of the data across phases.

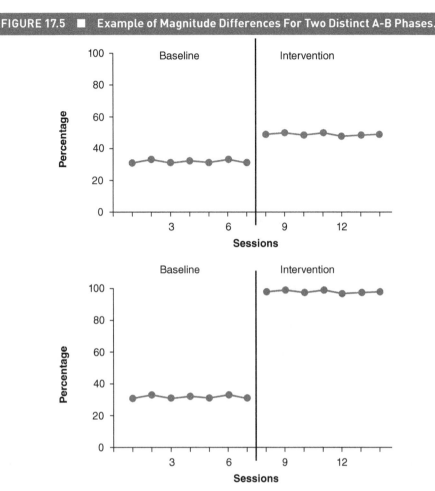

FIGURE 17.5 ■ Example of Magnitude Differences For Two Distinct A-B Phases.

Note. For both the top and bottom panels a PND calculation for these data yields a result of 100% nonoverlapping data despite the clear differences in level for the two different panels. (Figure 3, p. 25, from: Wolery, M., Busick, M., Reichow, B., & Barton, E. E. (2010). Comparison of overlap methods for quantitatively synthesizing single-subject data. *The Journal of Special Education, 44*(1), 18–28. Copyright 2010 by the Hammill Institute on Disabilities. Reproduced by permission.)

the PND statistic has become commonly used in single-case design studies, the use of the statistic is not warranted because of the limitations just reviewed (Becraft et al., 2020; Dowdy et al., 2021; Moeyaert et al., 2018; Pustejovsky, 2015; Tarlow, 2017; Salzburg et al., 1987; White, 1987; Wolery et al., 2010).

In light of these concerns, a number of variations in the PND statistic have been introduced. Some of these include the "percentage of data points exceeding the median" (PEM; Ma, 2006), "percentage of all nonoverlapping data" (PAND; Parker et al., 2007), "percentage of nonoverlapping corrected data" (PNCD; Manolov & Solanas, 2009), and "Tau-U" (Parker et al., 2011). The introduction of these more refined techniques has focused on minimizing a subset of the limitations mentioned previously for the PND, but they do not control for the entire range of concerns researchers have noted about the statistic. Thus, the most prudent observation would be that unless the authors of a study can clearly show that none of the concerns listed in the previous paragraph exist, the PND statistic and its variants should not be used. However, if these concerns can be addressed, then the PND or related techniques will be warranted.

INFERENTIAL TECHNIQUES

Researchers began working on integrating nomothetic inferential statistical techniques with $N = 1$ experiments in the 1960s (e.g., Revusky, 1967). These efforts have focused on providing single-case design researchers with the same basis to claim experimental effects as social scientists using experimental and quasi-experimental group-comparison designs. The logical basis of the approach is to be able to parse random variation in outcomes from those produced by the independent variable.

A number of approaches were proposed in the 1970s that met with various degrees of interest, but none became a commonly used test in either applied behavior analysis or the experimental analysis of behavior. For example, *time-series analysis*, a technique that was emerging for repeated-measures analyses in general psychology (Glass et al., 1975; Gottman et al., 1978), was proposed for use in single-case design studies. Time-series analyses used the repeated collection of data for a single entity and compared level and trend differences between two phases. However, there were practical limitations to the use of this technique that argued against its adoption in $N = 1$ designs. These limitations included the need to collect a large number of sessions per phase (estimates varied from 18 to ≥ 50 sessions per phase), the confound of serial dependency or autocorrelation (discussed previously in this chapter), and the need to fit relatively complex statistical models adapted to the particular conditions of an individual experiment.

However, interest in using inferential statistics with $N = 1$ designs has endured, with increased interest emerging over the last 20 years (e.g., Kratochwill & Levin, 2014). The primary focus of these recent efforts has been on *randomization techniques*. However, before we discuss these statistical tests, it is important to parse between two contemporary uses of randomization in single-case design research. The first approach to randomization was discussed in Chapter 11 and related to the assignment of experimental conditions to a random order within single-case designs. As was noted in Box 11.2, this type of randomization is *not a valid control technique* in idiographic research for the sequential assignment of individual experimental conditions.

A second approach, which focuses on the randomization of independent variable changes and/or participant assignment, has emerged as an option for interfacing inferential statistics with single-case designs (Kratochwill et al., 2023; Levin et al., 2018). Originally introduced by Revusky (1967), *randomization tests* were proposed based on randomizing conditions within a multiple-baseline design. This statistical approach was elaborated on and extended by Edgington (1969, 1980). The logic of this technique requires two or more independent conditions be randomly assigned to phase change time points and/or participants (or their "case" equivalent). According to Kratochwill et al. (2023), "randomization is used in one or more aspects of the study to increase the internal validity of the design" (p. 198) (see Box 17.1 for an alternative perspective). Randomization techniques have been proposed for A-B-A-B, multi-element, and multiple-baseline designs but may not be tractable for repeated-acquisition designs or brief experimental analyses.

BOX 17.1: RANDOMIZATION AND THREATS TO INTERNAL VALIDITY

Statistical procedures that access variation in data bounding some metric of central tendency and compare samples of data to assess whether the two data sets differ based on probability theory are the foundation of quantitative methods used in the social sciences. Within this process the use of randomization is placed on hallowed ground. In a statistical context, when parsing variation from independent variable effects and "noise in the signal," randomization of a variable allows for that construct to be "removed" from the signal-to-noise ratio. This is because randomizing a variable quantitatively distributes its presence evenly within large data sets. In this sense, randomization is a control technique. A question raised by the use of randomization in $N = 1$ designs is how this notion of "control" engages with the idiographic notion of directly controlling variables via experimental design. For example, does randomly assigning the start of an intervention phase, when indexed against a baseline, control for something? If so, what? If a baseline is increasing in trend and/or variability, randomly changing phases disrupts the design logic of single-case designs in which the data guide decision making. Is a threat to internal validity such as the unknown onset of psychotropic medication use or the initiation of at-home tutoring (i.e., history effects) controlled for by arbitrarily changing phases in a multiple-baseline design? It seems unlikely that the randomizing of phase changes, as an example, controls for threats such as history effects in single-case designs. One might view this as an example of imposing nomothetic measurement logic on an idiographic system that produces the appearance of "control" when there is little or none being produced by the randomization effort. Perhaps the one thing clearly controlled for by the use of randomization in $N = 1$ designs is the decision by the experimenter to change phases (or assign participants to tiers in a multiple baseline) that might introduce *experimenter bias*. If this is the case, and it seems reasonable to assume it is a possibility, then other decision-making logics would also suffice as alternatives to randomization. For example, when assigning participants to tiers of a multiple-baseline design, using students' ascending or descending shoe size to make assignments would serve the same function as randomization in minimizing experimenter bias (as would assignment by alphabetizing based on first names). Similarly, changing phases only on Mondays could serve as a proxy when deciding on phase transitions. The point is that randomization is not a "silver bullet" in single-case design research the way it can be used in experimental or quasi-experimental group-comparison designs. As with many aspects of $N = 1$ design research, it is up to the investigator to weigh the strengths and limitations of various procedural manipulations, such as randomization, and decide whether they act as controls for threats to internal validity or not.

An example of using randomization in a single-case multiple-baseline design across participants is provided by Gettinger et al. (2021). The authors studied the Academic and Behavior Combined Support (ABC Support) intervention to assess whether reading performance and academic engagement would improve for students whose behaviors required intervention. Six student–teacher dyads were each randomly assigned to a fixed intervention time point that was staggered across students, thus producing a multiple-baseline design. Figure 17.6 shows the

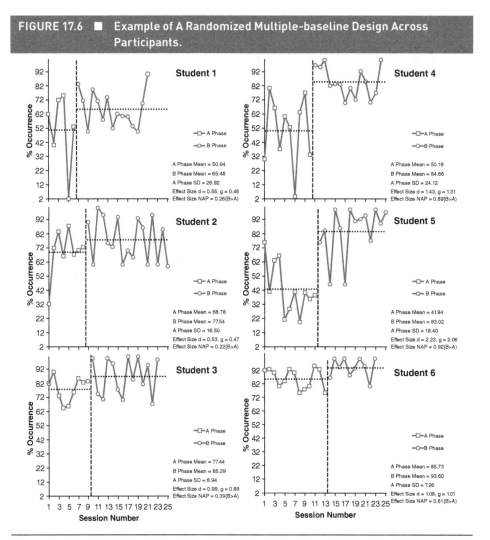

FIGURE 17.6 ■ Example of A Randomized Multiple-baseline Design Across Participants.

Note. The percent occurrence of academically engaged behavior is arrayed on the *y*-axis, and instructional sessions are arranged along the *x*-axis. The independent variable was the Academic and Behavior Combined Support (ABC Support) approach for improving social and academic functioning. The authors concluded that there were clear results via visual and statistical analysis (p = .001). (Figure 6, p. 13, from: Gettinger, M., Kratochwill, T. R., Eubanks, A., Foy, A., & Levin, J. R. (2021). Academic and behavior combined support: Evaluation of an integrated supplemental intervention for early elementary students. *Journal of School Psychology, 89*, 1–19. Copyright 2021 by the Society for the Study of School Psychology. Reproduced by permission.)

randomly staggered intervention assignment and effects on academically engaged behavior for the six participants. The figure shows the repeated-measures data typical of a single-case design along with phase mean and standard deviations for each condition (in addition, effect size estimates were included). The authors conducted randomization tests based on Wampold and Worsham (1986) and Ferron and Levin (2014) to arrive at a probability or p-value estimate. The outcomes for Figure 17.6, which are similar to the other data presented in the study, indicated a statistically significant outcome at the $p = .001$ level with the authors concluding through visual and statistical analysis that a clear effect was evident.

The reader, upon visually inspecting the data in Figure 17.6, may or may not draw the same conclusion about experimental control as the authors did. The level, trend, and overlap present for Students 1, 2, 3, and 6 would not generally meet the criteria via visual inspection for a clear experimental effect. The fact that a very clear statistical effect was achieved cannot be argued. This disparity in outcomes illustrates the still nascent status of randomization tests for single-case designs and why they have not received widespread adoption by researchers. Perhaps the most important issue raised by Figure 17.6 and similar experimental and analytic outcomes is how to interpret the results of an experiment when visual and statistical analyses show incompatible outcomes.

Nonetheless, a strength of randomization in single-case research is that it can control for intentional or unintentional bias in $N = 1$ designs. By randomly assigning a particular participant to a specific tier in a multiple-baseline design, a researcher avoids skewing results by assigning individuals who may be more likely (or less likely) to be responsive to the intervention. This logic can also be applied to the onset of interventions (and offset in the case of A-B-A-B designs); however, see Box 17.2 for a discussion of concerns that can be produced by randomly assigning phase changes. Overall, randomization techniques are emerging as potentially viable statistical methods for single-case experimental designs, although a great deal of work remains to be done to assess when visual analysis and statistical analysis results converge or diverge and how to interpret such instances. In addition, as noted in Boxes 17.1 and 17.2, reasonable questions remain regarding the degree to which the nomothetic logic of randomization techniques merges effectively with the idiographic logic of $N = 1$ design types.[1]

BOX 17.2: INADVERTENT EFFECTS OF RANDOMIZATION

Randomization techniques have been suggested for incorporation into $N = 1$ designs since the 1970s (e.g., Kratochwill, 1978) but have received mixed responses from single-case design researchers. Use of such techniques has an intuitive appeal since they are used effectively in group-comparison research on a regular basis. However, as noted in this chapter and several previous chapters in this book, mixing nomothetic and idiographic theories of measurement is akin to mixing oil and water and expecting a complete molecular integration of the substances: It is not possible, but some interesting by-products of the effort could result. One concerning by-product of using randomization techniques with $N = 1$

designs may occur when the time points for intervention onset and/or offset are determined by randomization methods rather than through visual inspection of the data. The concern is that an arbitrary change in phases (e.g., from baseline to intervention) may be contraindicated by patterns in the data (e.g., an upward trend that interferes with making intervention effects discernable). When a phase change is made at a time point when the data pattern does not warrant a phase change, the internal validity of the experiment can be compromised. *This is not an abstract concern, but a very real possibility.* For example, when a phase change is made at a point in an experiment that is not warranted by the data, the result may be a tier—or tiers—in a multiple-baseline design that does not show an experimental effect; following data trends by visual inspection, however, may have resulted in a clear experimental result. Thus, randomization techniques have the potential of compromising or abrogating the degree of experimental control in a study. When this occurs, it can result in a conclusion that underestimates the effectiveness of an intervention and may lead to the conclusion that the intervention is not effective. A cumulative result of such confounds in experimental design can be the underestimating of an intervention as evidence based. When an investigator is considering the use of randomization techniques in a single-case design experiment, it would be prudent to consider the possible plusses and minuses of randomization techniques when designing the study.

INTEGRATIVE TECHNIQUES

An accelerating trend in the social sciences over the past 40 years has been the development of quantitative methodologies allowing the integration of findings across experiments employing a similar intervention. As educational treatments have increased in number and effectiveness, researchers and policymakers have sought to understand how large and consistent the effects of a particular intervention might be. The obvious outcome of such an endeavor is an objective index of the usefulness of a particular treatment. A second outcome is that the use of such an index is to assist in the assessment of whether a particular intervention should be considered an evidence-based practice (Maggin & Odom, 2014; Slocum et al., 2014).

The quantitative synthesis of experimental results across multiple studies has come to rely on statistical techniques referred to as *meta-analysis*. The use of meta-analyses in group-comparison research has become the standard against which interventions—emerging or well established—are indexed. This is also becoming true in single-case design research, although there has been a time lag when compared with group-comparison analyses. Figure 17.7 shows the cumulative number of publications in which the keywords *meta-analysis* and *single-case designs* were used to describe the content of the paper (Becraft et al., 2020). As can be seen from the graph, there has been a clear and rapid increase in interest among single-case design researchers in meta-analysis. In the final section of this chapter, we will discuss what meta-analysis is, explore the statistical techniques used, and provide an example from the existing literature on how to use the techniques.

Meta-analytic techniques are based on *effect-size estimates*. The formulation of an effect size was originally introduced by Glass (1976) and Cohen (1977) and subsequently elaborated upon by Hedges (1982). This basic concept provides the foundation for meta-analytic methods, so we will begin with a brief primer on what an effect-size estimate is. The general idea behind this

FIGURE 17.7 ■ An Estimate of Interest by Single-case Design Researchers In the Use of Meta-analysis.

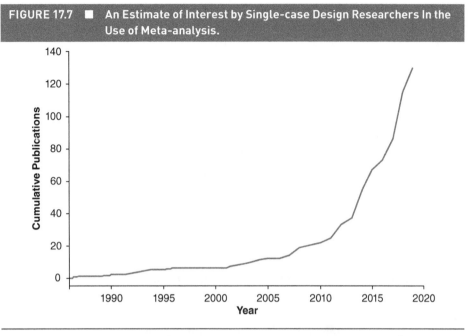

Note. The *y*-axis represents the cumulative number of published manuscripts using the indexes "meta-analysis" *and* "single-case design." (Figure 1, p. 1800, from: Becraft, J. L., Borrero, J. C., Sun, S., & McKenzie, A. A. (2020). A primer for using multilevel models to meta-analyze single case design data with AB phases. *Journal of Applied Behavior Analysis, 53*(3), 1799–1821. Copyright 2020 by the Society for the Experimental Analysis of Behavior. Reproduced by permission.)

statistical concept is that you compare two experimental conditions (e.g., baseline and intervention, or A-B) to assess their differential degree of effect on a dependent measure while factoring in the degree of variability present in the data set. An easily accessible formulation of this concept can be expressed using Cohen's *d* statistic, where effect size (ES) is the difference between the mean of two conditions (M_1, M_2) divided by the combined variance of the two conditions in standard deviation (SD) units:

$$\text{ES} = \frac{M_1 - M_2}{\text{SD}_{pooled}}$$

In essence, the statistic is conceptually assessing the difference between two conditions while taking into account the amount of variability in the data. (It should be noted that this particular formulation of an effect size statistic is not widely used in meta-analyses for technical reasons we will not delve into.) When applied to the results of individual experiments, effect-size estimates provide a quantitative metric of the magnitude of an experimental effect and offer a common index across different experiments.

When these effect-size outcomes are combined across studies of a particular intervention, researchers can estimate the average effect of the treatment (Lipsey & Wilson, 2000; Shadish et al., 2014). Meta-analyses use the existing effect sizes across studies to estimate an average treatment effect. These techniques can also be used to look at how moderator variables embedded in the analyses might influence intervention outcomes (e.g., intervention by gender and/or cultural status interactions). In general, there are three types of meta-analysis measures commonly used in the literature that we will briefly review: (a) *overlap*, (b) *regression*, and (c) *mean-based metrics*.

Overlap

Meta-analyses based on the amount of overlap in the data between two conditions (e.g., A-B) have been commonly used by investigators, particularly early in the development of meta-analytic methods for single-case design research. Overlap methodologies rely on the statistics we reviewed in the descriptive statistics section of this chapter and include PND, PAND, and so on (e.g., Parker et al., 2007; Scruggs et al., 1987). These statistics, as previously noted, have several limitations. First, the statistics do not account for data trends across conditions. Second, overlap metrics do not estimate the magnitude of the effect across conditions. Finally, and particularly relevant for meta-analyses, overlap techniques do not typically account for autocorrelation in the data. Although overlap metrics were frequently used in the early 2000s, quantitative methodologists now avoid recommending these approaches because of the confounds just mentioned (Becraft et al., 2020; Dowdy et al., 2021; Moeyaert et al., 2018; Pustejovsky, 2015).

Regression

Regression-based methods use regression analysis to identify combined-intervention outcomes while also allowing for moderator analyses (Moeyaert et al., 2020). These techniques use multilevel models (also referred to as hierarchical linear models), statistical techniques with a long history in educational psychology (Shadish & Rindskopf, 2007). These models can account for autocorrelation in data and model trends, making them a particularly useful approach. A three-level hierarchical model is typically employed that analyzes (a) within-participant, (b) within-experiment, and (c) between-experiment effects (Moeyaert et al., 2020). Multilevel modeling techniques are increasing in use among investigators and may be particularly well suited to single-case designs experiments. For a primer on how to use these techniques with $N = 1$ designs, readers are referred to Becraft et al. (2020). We will also return to these techniques when we discuss an example of meta-analytic methods.

Mean-Based Metrics

Like regression metrics, mean-based techniques are increasing in usage and provide an additional method for meta-analyses. A strength of mean-based metrics includes the ability to estimate the magnitude of effect within participants and between participants or experiments (Pustejovsky & Ferron, 2017). The majority of these analytic techniques are based on log response ratios, but there is also emerging interest in standardized mean differences (Hedges et al., 2012, 2013). A particular strength of mean-based metrics is that they incorporate estimates of magnitude and readily integrate percent-based direct observation measures commonly used in single-case designs (e.g., percentages derived from partial-, whole-, or momentary-interval sampling techniques; see Chapter 8). Again, like regression metrics, single-case design researchers may find mean-based metrics intuitively accessible. A related primer on the use of log response ratios is provided by Common et al. (2017) and Pustejovsky (2018).

An Example Using Regression

Richman et al. (2015) conducted meta-analysis of noncontingent reinforcement using hierarchical linear modeling, a form of regression analysis. Their goal was to answer these questions: What is the effect of noncontingent reinforcement on behavior, and is there a difference between functional reinforcers and nonfunctional reinforcers? The authors reviewed 55 experiments with a total of 91 individual participants across studies. They adopted a "top-down" approach that focused on an overall (omnibus) estimation of effect size across experiments followed by moderator analyses of potentially relevant variables (see Parker & Vannest, 2012).

Richman and colleagues (2015) chose two levels of analysis: (a) data points collected for individual participants, or "Level 1," and (b) possible interactive variables (e.g., functional vs. nonfunctional reinforcers) across participants, or "Level 2." For purposes of this discussion, we will focus only on the Level 1 results. The general effect-size estimate for NCR relative to baseline conditions was $d = -1.58$ (see Raudenbush et al., 2005). Interpretations of effect-size estimates can be qualitative (like correlation coefficients) and/or quantitative (e.g., amount of data variance accounted for). For comparison, when this type of effect size is calculated for group-comparison studies, d-value outcomes of ±0.5 to ±0.8 would qualitatively be considered "moderate" and "large," respectively. Thus, the Richman et al. outcome of $d = -1.58$ demonstrates that noncontingent reinforcement had an exceptionally large decelerative effect on behavior across the 55 studies analyzed. In quantitative terms, that difference was expressed as the intervention accounting for 60% of variance in all behavioral variability (an equally impressive estimate to the d value). As a result of this analysis, Richman et al. were able to conclude that noncontingent reinforcement "is an effective and empirically supported treatment for decreasing problem behavior" (p. 145).

Summary

Meta-analysis has emerged over the past two decades as a viable and welcomed analytical tool in single-case design research. The use of meta-analyses to summarize independent variable effects across experiments allows for the quantitative comparison of interventions primarily developed using $N = 1$ designs to be compared to the results of experimental and quasi-experimental group designs in a direct and rigorous manner. While meta-analysis metrics based on overlap estimates are decreasing in use because of methodological limitations, metrics based on regression and mean-based measures continue to increase in frequency.

CONCLUSION

The quantitative analysis of single-case design data has progressed rapidly over the past two decades. More and more, researchers employing $N = 1$ experimental designs are adopting descriptive, inferential, and integrative techniques to analyze experimental outcomes. Perhaps in no other area of single-case design research has progress been so furtive. As a result, researchers now have a cadre of descriptive and integrative techniques that are well developed and validated for use in $N = 1$ research. Other areas, such as inferential randomization tests, await further refinement and adoption by a broad set of investigators. Nonetheless, there are many linkages between emerging quantitative methods and the designs discussed in this book.

REFLECTION QUESTIONS

1. Describe how idiographic versus nomothetic measurement theories deal with intraindividual phenomena.

2. Explain various approaches to quantifying steady states of behavior and what are their strengths and limitations.

3. Can randomization in single-case designs be used to control for threats to internal validity?

4. What are the similarities and differences among descriptive, inferential, and integrative quantitative methods?

5. What are current approaches to meta-analysis, and what are their strengths and limitations?

ENDNOTE

1. It should be noted that multielement designs may be unique among $N = 1$ designs in their capacity to be integrated with randomization techniques because of their rapid alternation of conditions in which randomization does not disrupt the basic design logic of the single-case design needed for statistical analysis (see Shadish et al., 2013; Weaver & Lloyd, 2019).

18 SOCIAL VALIDITY

LEARNING OBJECTIVES

After reading this chapter, you will be able to

18.1   Describe the rationale for conducting social validity assessments.

18.2   Delineate three general approaches to estimating social validity, and their respective strengths and weaknesses.

18.3   Explain proposed reasons for underutilization of social validity assessment in research.

In educational settings researchers are often working to ameliorate some type of problematic situation, whether it be increasing the acquisition of reading skills, improving a child's articulation, or intervening to reduce challenging behavior. In addition, because schools are community settings, other students, teachers, paraprofessionals, school administrators, and related services personnel are likely to be involved. Most directly affected are the student and their family. Such a research context, by definition, occurs within a social milieu in which multiple individuals may be affected by the behavior change intervention, even if that intervention is focused on a single student.

Because of the applied nature of educational research, additional analytical activities are necessary to evaluate the effects of interventions on a range of consumers. If a researcher wants to understand the impact of their intervention on a classroom, more may be needed than to graph a functional relation between the intervention and improvements in mathematics performance. Additional information may include: Did the teacher find the intervention easy or hard to implement? How did the students react to the new procedure? Did the teacher continue to use the intervention once the study was completed? Were there any positive or negative side effects associated with the intervention? Did the recipients of the intervention perform at levels typical of other students their age? Did the school-building principal view the results as worth replicating in other classrooms? Information like this helps an investigator understand the broader social context of their intervention. Such an understanding can help them interpret functional relations within the social contexts in which they occur and, potentially, improve the effectiveness, acceptability, and/or sustainability of educational interventions. In order to understand this broader social context within which single-case research is conducted, researchers have developed a concept referred to as *social validity*.

WHAT IS SOCIAL VALIDITY?

Social validity is the estimation of the social impact an intervention has on various people who experience it in various ways. If, after 18 chapters focusing on the scientific virtues of being precise, objective, and analytical, this seems somewhat subjective, that is because *it is subjective*. And that is the reason why social validity is so integral to understanding the effects produced in applied settings. Because educational research occurs in applied contexts, knowing how people in those settings react to an intervention is an important component in understanding the effects of an intervention.

The concept of social validity was introduced to the field of applied psychology by Kazdin (1977) and Wolf (1978). However, there were antecedents to this concept in other disciplines. In the 1930s, the business sector became interested in whether employees making products and consumers using those products were satisfied (e.g., Roethlisberger & Dickson, 1939). In psychotherapy, psychologists and psychiatrists were interested in the expectations their clients had toward what they would experience and whether they believed they benefited from therapy (e.g., Rogers, 1942). Finally, in medicine, researchers and clinicians became interested in measuring whether patients were satisfied with the medical treatments they received (e.g., Makeover, 1950). Each of these lines of inquiry focused on establishing what people expected, experienced, and/or perceived were the effects of a particular endeavor.

When Kazdin (1977) and Wolf (1978) developed the concept of social validity, it was during the initial, rapid growth of applied behavior analysis. As was noted in Chapter 2, applied behavior analysis had emerged from earlier laboratory research and by the early 1970s was a well-established discipline, but one that was controversial (Enright, 2018; Wolraich, 1997). Much of the controversy was due to public concern about researchers "controlling" the behavior of other people. These concerns, in part, were due to the effectiveness of behavioral interventions and their explicit, operationally defined procedures focusing on the consequences of responding (Goldiamond, 1976). Whatever the actual basis for concern, there was a great deal of public debate about whether "behavior modification" was ethical or desirable.

Unfortunately, when behavior analysts tried to address these public concerns, there were scant data from their own studies to buttress their arguments about the social acceptability of their work. Because behavior analysts tended to focus on carefully defined behaviors that are directly relevant to a particular experimental question, there were little available data about how people "felt" about a particular experiment. This left behavior analysts in the uncomfortable situation of having very little data upon which to argue in favor of their interventions, other than the changes in behavior they typically quantified. This historical context set the occasion for Kazdin (1977) and Wolf (1978) to suggest measuring the social impact of behavioral interventions using the construct of social validity.

In Wolf's (1978) original description of social validity, he focused on the use of subjective judgments regarding the adequacy and desirability of behavioral interventions (see Box 18.1).

He suggested that by understanding the subjective nature of interventions, applied behavior analysts could gain a better understanding of the social importance of their work. Specifically, he outlined three general domains for subjective analysis: (a) *goals*, (b) *procedures*, and (c) *outcomes*. Goals referred to the targets of an intervention, including individuals, settings, and specific behaviors. Procedures referred to the techniques used in a study to change behavior or, put another way, what the experimenter did to increase or decrease the probability of specific behaviors. Outcomes referred to the behavioral changes actually produced by an intervention, both direct and indirect.

BOX 18.1: SHOULD ALL APPLIED STUDIES ASSESS SOCIAL VALIDITY?

Given the value of understanding the social impact of an experiment, should all single-case research studies use social validity assessments? One could argue that any study seeking to change a person's behavior in an applied context should have the social validity of that endeavor assessed. However, the appropriateness of using social validity assessments depends on what you mean by "applied context." In many respects, the "applied" versus "basic" distinction is a false dichotomy. Rather than being a binary distinction, these concepts actually span a translational continuum from basic to applied research. That is, some researchers may use humans and even study a behavior of clear social importance (e.g., self-injurious behavior), but be focused on how basic behavioral processes produce these behaviors. In such instances, the use of social validity data may not meaningfully contribute to the interpretation of the experimental results. However, the rationale for such investigations is gaining a better understanding of behavioral processes impacting socially important situations so that more effective interventions can be developed (Lerman, 2024). If this is the case, and translational studies are successful at identifying new behavior–environment mechanisms, then such findings necessarily need to be translated into practical interventions. Because such a translation has a clear therapeutic intent, those studies would clearly need to assess the social validity of their goals, procedures, and/or outcomes. However, at this point in time, given the complex range of research occurring within educational settings, the use of social validity assessments should probably be reserved for studies in which some type of quality-of-life effects are being studied.

These three domains were a framework to begin the study of social validity in educational settings. Such a system allowed for the systematic study of subjective data. However, these suggestions ran contrary to decades of research in behavior analysis in which only objectively defined variables were permitted into experimental reports. The success of the empirical approach championed in behavior analysis was requiring these same researchers to incorporate subjective data into their studies in order to better understand the broader effects being produced. It was, and still is, somewhat of an ironic situation, but a necessary one for understanding the effects of interventions in educational settings (see Box 18.1).

This historical context led Wolf (1978) to write this concluding statement in his paper introducing social validity:

> Earlier in our history, Watson and Skinner argued forcefully against subjective measurement because they were concerned about the inappropriate causal roles that hypothetical internal variables, subjectively reported, were playing in social science. As a result, many of us concluded that all subjective measurement was inappropriate. A new consensus seems to be developing. It seems that if we aspire to social importance, then we must develop systems that allow our consumers to provide us feedback about how our applications relate to their values, to their reinforcers. This is not a rejection of our heritage. Our use of subjective measures does not relate to internal causal variables. Instead, it is an attempt to assess the dimensions of complex reinforcers in socially acceptable and practical ways. It is an evolutionary event that is occurring as a function of the contingencies of the applied research environment; contingences that our founders would probably say they appreciate, if we had the nerve to ask them for such subjective feedback on our behavior. (p. 213)

APPROACHES TO SOCIAL VALIDITY

Over the last 40 years, three approaches have been introduced to estimate social validity (see Box 18.2). Each approach focuses on a different aspect of the construct of "social importance." As one might deduce, each has its strengths and limitations, and no single approach to assessing social validity can be referred as "the gold standard." Therefore, in this section, we will review the different approaches to social validity estimation, explain the purpose of each approach, provide examples of their use, and critique the strategies.

BOX 18.2: ESTIMATING SOCIAL VALIDITY RATHER THAN BEING SOCIALLY VALID OR SOCIAL VALIDITY AS AN ADJECTIVE RATHER THAN A NOUN

Unlike most aspects of single-case research, which deal with objective events, social validity presents researchers with a different type of analytical situation. Single-case research tends to focus on physical events that can be operationalized and directly measured. This rigorous approach to experimental methodology has been one of the key aspects of the success of the research designs over the past century. With the introduction of social validity, however, this situation was altered in some respects. The essence of the argument for social validity, particularly in the use of subjective evaluation, is to allow verbal constructs such as "like," "acceptable," and "inappropriate" into experimental analyses. While this is entirely appropriate within the framework of studying the social validity, it has led to some confusion in the language used to describe social validity. Because social validity is a social construct—that is, it is based on social conventions and poorly defined concepts—it is not a *thing*. Therefore, its use as a noun, as in "We need to show that this intervention has *social validity,"* is inaccurate and misleading. Rather, social validity is an adjective that describes some characteristics of the goals, procedures, and/or outcomes of an experiment in light of some defined social context. Because of this aspect of language use, it is more accurate to refer to *estimating* or *assessing* social validity.

Subjective Evaluation

The original conceptualization of social validity focused on what Kazdin (1977) and Wolf (1978) referred to as *subjective evaluation*. This approach is used to gather information regarding people's personal perceptions of some dimension of the goals, procedures, and/or outcomes of an experiment. The purpose is to estimate how people view some dimension of the experimental situation. Which aspect of the experimental situation is assessed is largely a function of the experimental question and what the researcher wants to learn. For example, if the investigators are working on a novel applied problem, then they might gather social validity data on whether this topic is viewed as important and their goals for changing these behaviors are appropriate. However, if the investigators are focusing on the use of a novel intervention, then they might want to assess whether people view their new technique as acceptable. Or, the experimenters may want to demonstrate the desirable qualitative outcomes of their procedures, so they might have people subjectively evaluate the behavior of interest before and after intervention. Depending on what the experimenter wants to learn, any or all of these approaches to subjective evaluation could be used.

Selecting Foci

The first step in using subjective evaluation is to identify whether you are interested in receiving feedback about the goals, procedures, outcomes, or some combination thereof. Once this has been decided, the researchers need to identify who they will solicit information from. Schwartz and Baer (1991) identified four types of consumers: (a) *direct consumers*, (b) *indirect consumers*, (c) *members of the immediate community*, and (d) *members of the extended community*. Direct consumers are the immediate recipients of the intervention—for example, the student whose spelling is being improved or the teacher who is receiving professional development to improve their use of evidence-based practices. Indirect consumers are people involved in the situation that is being studied. These individuals can include the parents of a child who is receiving the spelling intervention or the building principal in charge of supervising the teacher who is learning to use new instructional techniques. Members of the immediate community are those who are indirectly impacted by the study, but who have some type of contact with the direct and indirect consumers. These individuals can include other children and their parents, other teachers in the school, or school board members. Members of the extended community are individuals who do not have direct contact with consumers, but who may be interested in the potential beneficial or detrimental effects of a study. Examples could include taxpayers, legislators, media reports, content experts, or anyone else who might be interested in the researcher's efforts (see Luiselli, 2021).

Consumer Group Selection

Again, which group(s) is the focus on the social validity assessment is a function of the question being posed. At one of end of the continuum, a researcher may want to understand how children and teachers react to a particular type of educational intervention. For example, researchers might compare lecture-based instruction with cooperative learning groups and ask the direct consumers which approach they preferred and why. At the other end of the continuum, researchers might be interested in polling a regionally representative group of homeowners (i.e., people who pay the property taxes that finance local school systems) about whether they view school violence as so important an issue that they would endorse cuts in other school programs (e.g., extramural sports) to increase services to reduce violence.

Assessment Strategies

Once the consumer group(s) are identified, researchers need to select the assessment strategy to be used. In general, there are four approaches to collecting subjective evaluation information: (a) *questionnaires*, (b) *forced-choice procedures*, (c) *structured interviews*, and (d) *open-ended interviews*. Questionnaires are the most frequently used method (Kennedy, 1992). Questionnaires typically present a series of questions to which a particular person responds in writing or some other medium. The questions focus on some aspect of the investigation that the experimenter wants to learn about. For example, the questionnaire might ask a series of questions regarding the acceptability of the intervention procedures given certain circumstances (see Kazdin, 1980). Forced-choice procedures require informants to make choices among possible goals, procedures, and/or outcomes. For example, individuals might be asked to sort a variety of interventions used to reduce behavior problems in order of acceptability. In some instances, these choices are abstractions sampling a person's opinion; in other instances, individuals may be asked to actually choose among possible goals or procedures that they will be the recipients of (see Luiselli, 2021; Schwartz & Baer, 1991).

Using structured interviews requires the development of a series of questions that are read to the respondent followed by an opportunity for that individual to answer. Typically, these questions have a fixed number of response options to choose from. For example, the interviewer may ask the informant a series of questions to which they respond "Yes," "No," or "Maybe." Open-ended interviews pose predetermined questions to a respondent that allow the individual to provide an extended and unstructured answer. For example, an experimenter may ask questions such as "What did you think of the cooperative learning intervention?" or "How did the students respond to whole-class instruction?" The answers are then recorded using some medium for later summarization and analysis.

Data Analysis

The final step in conducting a subjective evaluation assessment is data analysis. This step in the process is the least clearly defined in the research literature. If the data are based on discrete, quantifiable elements (e.g., Likert-type scales or Yes/No responses), then the use of descriptive statistics specifying the average and variation in responses would be appropriate. For example, in response to the question "This treatment is one that I would agree to use with my child," parental reports could be summarized as a mean of 4.3 (range, 2 to 5) on a 5-point Likert-type scale (with 1 being *strongly disagree* and 5 being *strongly agree*). Another option is summarizing the number of response options that were selected for each question. Table 18.1 shows the results of a treatment acceptability analysis of parent training using a telehealth intervention in the United States and other countries (Tsami et al., 2019).

If the data are qualitative in nature (i.e., verbal responses), most likely derived from structured or open-ended questions, then a qualitative analysis of the data may be required. A review of the research literature using social validity assessments suggests that *content analysis* is the most frequently published form of qualitative data analysis conducted on this type of

TABLE 18.1 ■ Results From an Intervention Acceptability Assessment		
Mean Ratings (With Ranges) on a 7-Point Scale for Each Item on the Social Validity Survey for 12 Parents in the Current Study (Left Column) and for a Comparison Sample of Parents Residing in the United States (Right Column).		
Items	**Participants**	**U.S.**
How acceptable do you find the functional analysis? (1 = *unacceptable*; 7 = *very acceptable*)	6.7 (4–7)	N/A
How acceptable do you find the treatment to be regarding your concerns about your child? (1 = *unacceptable*; 7 = *very acceptable*)	6.6 (6–7)	6.9 (6–7)
How likely is this treatment to make permanent improvements in your child's behavior? (1 = *unlikely*; 7 = *very likely*)	6.4 (5–7)	6.6 (5–7)
How costly will it be to carry out this treatment? (1 = *very costly*; 7 = *not at all costly*)	5.1 (1–7)	3.6 (1–7)
How willing are you to carry out this treatment? (1 = *not at all willing*; 7 = *very willing*)	6.4 (4–7)	6.9 (6–7)
How much time will be needed each day for you to carry out this treatment? (1 = *much time*; 7 = *little time*)	2.7 (2–6)	2.4 (1–7)
How confident are you that the treatment will be effective? (1 = *confident*; 7 = *very confident*)	6.3 (5–7)	6.7 (6–7)
How willing would you be to change your family routine to carry out this treatment? (1 = *not at all willing*; 7 = *very willing*)	6.3 (3–7)	6.7 (5–7)
How disruptive will it be for your family (in general) to carry out this treatment? (1 = *very disruptive*; 7 = *not at all disruptive*)	4.9 (1–4)	3.4 (1–7)
How effective is the treatment likely to be for your child? (1 = *not at all effective*; 7 = *very effective*)	6.4 (5–7)	6.7 (5–7)
How well will carrying out this treatment fit into your family routine? (1 = *not at all well*; 7 = *very well*)	5.7 (4–7)	6.6 (5–7)
How much do you like using your computer for assessment and treatment? (1 = *not at all*; 7 = *very much*)	6.5 (5–7)	N/A

Note. From: Tsami, L., Lerman, D., & Toper-Korkmaz, O. (2019). Effectiveness and acceptability of parent training via telehealth among families around the world. *Journal of Applied Behavior Analysis, 52*(4), 1113–1129. Copyright 2019 by the Society for the Experimental Analysis of Behavior. Reproduced by permission.

data (see Brantlinger, 2005; Leko et al., 2021). In content analysis, the responses to each question are copied onto response cards or some other medium. Members of the research team then individually read and thematically sort them, resorting into self-constructed categories. Once two or more members have done this, then the research team meets to discuss their categorization, and the group revises the categorization scheme as appropriate and then agrees on how to sort each response item to a particular question. A similar process is undertaken for each question asked of respondents. These data can be summarized in at least two ways. A study by Cox and Kennedy (2003) will be used to illustrate both types of data summarization. The data reflect parental responses to open-ended questions about the hospitalization and subsequent recovery of their child who had a multiple disability. Table 18.2 shows a

TABLE 18.2 ■ Parent Responses to Open-Ended Questions	
Responses to Questions	**%**
1. What Did Your Child's School Do That Was Helpful?	
● Nothing	14.3%
● Offered Support	85.7%
2. What Could the School Have Done to Be More Helpful?	
● More Communication and Coordination	35%
● Nothing	50%
● School Not Responsible	15%
3. What Did The Hospital Do That Was Helpful?	
● Nothing	20%
● Provided Health Services to Child	24%
● Provided Support Services to Parents	8%
● Supportive Staff	48%
4. What Could the Hospital Have Done to Be More Helpful?	
● Improve Support for Parents	13.3%
● Improve Care	26.7%
● Increase Continuity and Collaboration	13.3%
● More Staff Education	26.7%
● Nothing	20%
5. How Successful Was Home-School-Hospital Communication?	
● Communication Not an Issue	10.5%
● No Communication Among Entities	47.4%
● Parent Assumed Lead	26.3%
● Satisfactory	15.8%

TABLE 18.2 ■ Parent Responses to Open-Ended Questions *(Continued)*	
Responses to Questions	**%**
6. What Could Have Been Done to Improve Home-School-Hospital Communication?	
● Improved Communication	26%
● Not Sure What to Recommend	8.7%
● School and Hospital Separate Issues	65.3%
7. What Was the Effect of the Hospitalization on Your Child's Education?	
● Improved Performance	15.8%
● No or Little Effect	42.1%
● Small Negative Effect	21%
● Substantial Negative Effect	21.1%

From: Cox, J. A., & Kennedy, C. H. (2003). Transitions between school and hospital for students with multiple disabilities: A survey of causes, educational continuity, and parental perceptions. *Research and Practice for People With Severe Disabilities (formerly JASH), 28,* 1–6. Copyright 2003 by TASH. Reproduced by permission.

content analysis that specified general response categories to each question and summarized the percentage of answers from respondents included in each category. Another technique for presenting these same data would be to present subcategories of answers to questions and exemplars of the actual responses that were received.

Table 18.3 shows the data from Question 1 of Table 18.2 in this more detailed format. As with the visual analysis of data, what is most important in analyzing this type of data is that the process and presentation reveal the character of the data that are obtained in as clear and concise a manner as possible.

There are several strengths and limitations to using subjective evaluation as a technique for estimating social validity. An important strength, and one championed by Kazdin (1977) and Wolf (1978), is that subjective evaluation allows qualitative information to be added to data gathered through a quantitative single-case design process. A second strength of subjective evaluation is that its use broadens the range of dependent variables in a study. Both strengths are based on including people's perceptions and opinions in the interpretation of what was done and resulted from an experiment designed to have beneficial outcomes to particular individuals. An important limitation of subjective evaluation is that *the questions posed are often biased toward receiving a positive outcome.* That is, researchers often develop questions or present them in ways in which the situation predisposes respondents toward favorable answers. A second limitation of this technique is that people's perceptions of situations may not meaningfully reflect changes in a participant's behavior. A third limitation is that most instruments developed for subjective evaluation studies have unknown psychometric properties. That is, the reliability and validity of the instruments are typically unknown, and the degree to which they accurately and consistently measure what the author(s) intend to measure is highly questionable (see Finn & Sladeczek, 2001). Overall, the use of subjective evaluation can be an important tool, if a particular experimental question is developed in which this information would be useful.

TABLE 18.3 ■ Examples of Responses to Types of Support Provided in Question 1 of Table 18.2	
Type of Support	**Response**
Provided General Support	"PT [physical therapist] and teachers called and came to hospital."
	"Teacher called and brought homework."
Offered General Support	"Called once they heard child was in the hospital."
	"School offered homebound services but we declined."
Homebound Services	"Homebound teacher was already part of IEP [individualized education plan]. The teacher just came to the hospital."
	"Homebound teacher provided laptop at the hospital."

Note. From: Cox, J. A., & Kennedy, C. H. (2003). Transitions between school and hospital for students with multiple disabilities: A survey of causes, educational continuity, and parental perceptions. *Research and Practice for People With Severe Disabilities (formerly JASH), 28*, 1–6. Copyright 2003 by TASH. Reproduced by permission.

Normative Comparison

A second approach to estimating social validity was developed largely in response to concerns about the highly qualitative nature of the data derived from subjective evaluations. The approach, referred to as *normative comparison*, was outlined by Van Houten (1979) shortly after the Kazdin (1977) and Wolf (1978) papers were published. In normative comparison, a particular behavior(s) engaged in by a participant is compared to some reference sample of individuals. Typically, the reference group is chosen because it can serve as an exemplar of desirable levels or topographies of the behavior(s) of interest. The focus is to reference the behavior change goals and outcomes for the participants in a study against some normative group whose behavior is considered typical or desirable.

One of the first examples of the use of normative comparisons is provided by Walker and Hops (1976). These authors focused on improving the behavior of students considered to have conduct problems in general education classrooms. As a reference regarding the treatment goals and as an index of intervention outcomes, Walker and Hops sampled levels of appropriate and inappropriate behaviors among classroom peers identified by teachers as behaving appropriately. The children with conduct problems were then given an intervention in a separate setting until their behavior approximated those of their peers in the general education classrooms (see Figure 18.1). The children with conduct problems were then reintroduced into the general education classroom and maintained similar behavioral levels to those of their peers. Such a demonstration shows quantitatively that the appropriate behavior of the students who originally had conduct problems was similar to those of their peers without behavior problems following intervention.

Identifying Behaviors

To conduct normative comparisons, the researcher needs to begin by identifying the behaviors of interest in the group of students whose behaviors will receive intervention. Then, a decision

FIGURE 18.1   ■   One of the First Examples of the Use of Normative Comparison.

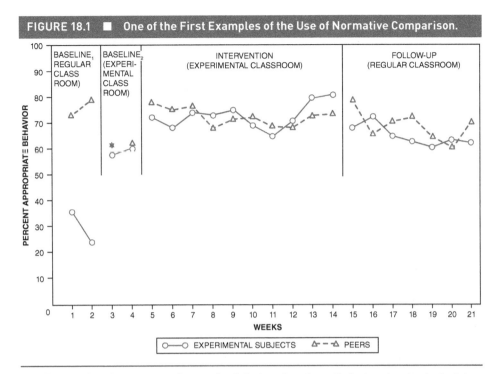

Note. The data show the percentage of appropriate behaviors along the vertical axis and weeks of school along the horizontal axis. Open circles designate the behavior of children with conduct problems. Open triangles designate the behavior of peers in the classroom deemed to behave appropriately by teachers. (Figure 1, p. 164, from: Walker, H. M., & Hops, H. (1976). Use of normative peer data as a standard for evaluating classroom treatment effects. *Journal of Applied Behavior Analysis, 9*, 159–168. Copyright 1976 by the Society for the Experimental Analysis of Behavior. Reproduced by permission.)

is made whether to base the goals, outcomes, or both aspects of intervention on a normative sample. If goals, alone, are chosen for comparison, then the researchers will have an intervention target to reach but no information on normative outcomes. If only outcomes are the focus of comparison, then the researchers will have a metric of the normative outcomes of their intervention effects but no quantitative goals to guide their efforts. For these reasons, it is probably best to use normative comparison to both identify the goals to be achieved and then further demonstrate that after those goals have been met they are still normative values.

Comparison Groups

Once these decisions are made, the researchers will need to identify an *appropriate reference group* to sample data from. Often the choice is made to sample from a group of individuals who already show desirable levels of the behavior of interest. Then, levels of those behaviors need to be measured in the environments in which they would naturally occur. These data, when summarized, provide the basis for comparing the goals and outcomes of the intervention that will then be experimentally analyzed.

Benefits of this approach to assessing social validity are primarily that there is a clear and defendable basis for setting the goals of an intervention. It is likely that in educational research when a child is identified as "deviant" in some aspect, the subsequent expectations for changes in their behavior are higher than for their peers who were not viewed as needing to receive some particular intervention (Foster & Mash, 1999). Collecting normative data may help with this concern. An additional strength of this approach is that it provides a reference after interventions have been implemented regarding whether the person's behavior is within the range of their peers whose behavior has been deemed acceptable. A final strength of this approach is the logical foundation for basing treatment gains that gives this strategy a high degree of face validity. That is, at face value most experts would say it is a reasonable and rationale approach to identifying intervention goals and evaluating outcomes.

Limitations of normative comparison include concerns regarding whether the group chosen as the normative sample is, indeed, itself normative. It is possible that the group sampled displays either too high a level or too low a level of behaviors to be considered a truly representative sample. In addition, as noted by Van Houten (1979), the goals chosen for a particular person in reference to the normative sample may be unobtainable. In some cases, an individual may not need to be "average" to be successful within some type of social or academic context, and the overreliance on normative values may interfere with the evaluation of what it takes for a particular person to be successful, even if that does not mean normative.

Sustainability

A more recent index of social validity is the degree to which the effects of a particular intervention are sustained over time (Kennedy, 2002). *Sustainability* is an index of whether the procedures and outcomes of an experiment continue once the research is completed and the researchers are no longer involved. If the consumers present in a particular context consider the procedures being used and the behavioral change that results from the intervention to be desirable, then they are likely to maintain the program. The use of sustainability as an index of social validity comes from this observation: "If an intervention is socially invalid, it can hardly be effective, even if it changes its target behaviors thoroughly and with an otherwise excellent cost-benefit ratio; social validity is not sufficient for effectiveness but is necessary to effectiveness" (Baer et al., 1987, p. 323). Therefore, if an intervention is sustained over time, it must have some qualities that are consistent with what we mean when we say something "has social validity."

An example of sustainability is provided by Reid et al. (2017). Reid et al. studied a collaborative team strategy used to increase the use of functional skills instruction for individuals with significant support needs. The intervention was originally demonstrated to be effective in 1985 in a series of studies using single-case designs. The procedure for increasing functional skill engagement was institutionalized into a set of procedures overseen by a supervisor, and performance feedback to staff was embedded into ongoing team meetings. The intent was to make these original research practices a routine part of the staff's work expectations. As shown in Figure 18.2, 30 years later the procedures were still being used with appropriate updates and refinements, and the intervention effects had improved over the decades of implementation. Such a result suggests that this intervention was useful and acceptable to those using it.

A focus on *maintenance* was first proposed by Rusch and Kazdin (1981) within the context of experimentally analyzing the factors involved in intervention success over time. These

FIGURE 18.2 ■ Example of Sustainability.

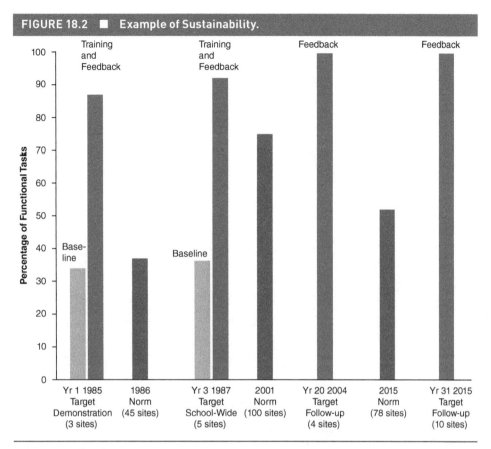

Note. Reid et al. (2017) studied a collaborative team strategy used to increase the use of functional skills instruction for individuals with significant support needs. The intervention was originally demonstrated to be effective in 1985 in a series of studies using single-case designs. The procedure for increasing functional skill engagement was institutionalized into a set of procedures overseen by a supervisor, and performance feedback to staff was embedded into ongoing team meetings. The intent was to make these original research practices a routine part of the staff's work expectations. Thirty years later, the procedures were still being used with appropriate updates and refinements, and the intervention effects had improved over the decades of implementation. (Figure 1, p. 15, from: Reid, D. H., Parsons, M. B., & Jensen, J. M. (2017). Maintaining staff performance following a training intervention: Suggestions from a 30-year case example. *Behavior Analysis in Practice, 10*(1), 12–21. Copyright 2015 by the Association for Behavior Analysis International. Reproduced with permission from Springer Nature Customer Service Center.)

authors suggested that withdrawal designs over extended time periods can be used to analyze the maintenance of interventions and their effects on behavior. Figure 18.3 shows several hypothetical examples of withdrawal designs proposed to experimentally study maintenance. If we put Rusch and Kazdin's suggestions within the framework put forward in Chapter 5 regarding experimental questions, such an analytical scheme sets the occasion for conducting component and parametric analyses (Kennedy, 2002). Component analyses allow investigators to remove one or more aspects of an independent variable, assess its effects on behavior, and then return to the previous conditions. Such analyses could be used to identify those components of an intervention that are necessary for it to be sustained by consumers. Conducting parametric analyses

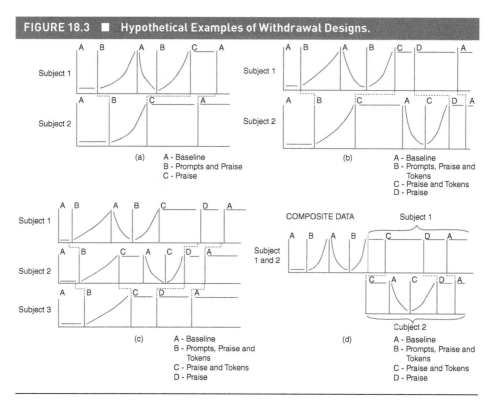

FIGURE 18.3 ■ Hypothetical Examples of Withdrawal Designs.

Note. A systematic withdrawal of a two-component treatment across two participants is represented in the upper-left graph (a). Withdrawal of a three-component treatment across two subjects is indicated in the upper-right graph (b). A systematic withdrawal of a three-component treatment across three subjects is shown in the lower-left portion of the figure (c). Finally, withdrawal of a three-component treatment across two subjects within an A-B-A-B reversal is depicted in the lower-right portion (d). (Figure 2, p. 137, from: Rusch, F. R., & Kazdin, A. E. (1981). Toward a methodology of withdrawal designs for the assessment of response maintenance. *Journal of Applied Behavior Analysis, 14,* 131–140. Copyright 1981 by the Society for the Experimental Analysis of Behavior. Reproduced by permission.)

would permit a cost-benefit analysis of differing levels of intervention, their effects on behavior, and whether consumers choose to sustain the intervention. Such experiments could produce important information, not only of how interventions are sustained over time but of why they are, or are not, sustained over time.

The primary strength of sustainability as an index of social validity is its face validity. If a group of consumers maintain an intervention over extended periods of time, there must be something about the intervention and its effects that are meaningful to those consumers. *This, perhaps, is an empirical test of what subjective evaluation seeks to assess.* However, there are several limits to the concept of sustainability. First, it requires an extended period of time to conduct analyses, something that might not be logistically feasible. Second, other variables not known to the experimenters may influence the adoption and maintenance of an intervention (e.g., federal policy or court rulings). Finally, sustainability is an indirect index of the degree to which the procedures and outcomes of an investigation have some degree of social validity.

TRENDS IN THE USE OF SOCIAL VALIDITY

Following the logic just outlined for the sustainability of interventions, if researchers find social validity assessments a useful analytical tool, then their use should be prevalent in the extant literature. If the data derived from such assessments are useful to investigators, they are likely to draw on such information when they conduct their studies. Conversely, if the social validity data are not useful or too cumbersome to make their collection experimentally helpful, we might see limited use of these procedures.

Such archival data are available and they are not encouraging. Kennedy (1992), Carr et al. (1999), and Ferguson et al. (2019) have documented the degree to which social validity assessments are incorporated into applied behavior-analytic research. The results of the Ferguson et al. analysis are presented in Figure 18.4. Arrayed along the vertical axis are the percentage of research articles and the total number of articles published in the *Journal of Applied Behavior Analysis* reporting data relating to social validity. The horizontal axis represents the year of publication. Approximately 15% of the studies analyzed used social validity assessments during the decade studied. This pattern largely replicates the previous Kennedy and Carr et al. findings. In addition, the Kennedy and Carr et al. reports noted that less than 5% of published studies used normative comparison methods.

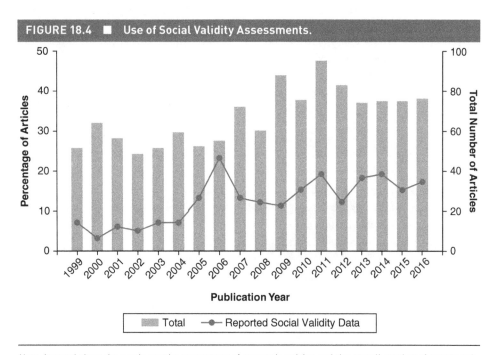

FIGURE 18.4 ■ Use of Social Validity Assessments.

Note. Arrayed along the *y*-axis are the percentage of research articles and the overall number of papers published in the *Journal of Applied Behavior Analysis* that reported data relating to social validity. The *x*-axis represents the year of publication. (Figure 1, p. 6, from: Ferguson, J. L., Cihon, J. H., Leaf, J. B., Van Meter, S. M., McEachin, J., & Leaf, R. (2019). Assessment of social validity trends in the *Journal of Applied Behavior Analysis*. *European Journal of Behavior Analysis, 20*(1), 146–157 (https://doi.org/10.1080/15021149.2018.1534771). Copyright 1991 by Taylor & Francis (http://www.tandfonline.com). Reproduced by permission.)

These data seem to suggest that researchers are only occasionally incorporating social validity assessments into their experimental methods. Two possible explanations have been put forward for this pattern. First, as noted in Box 18.1, not all studies in applied behavior analysis are directly focused on improving a person's quality of life via intervention. Many experiments, referred to as translational studies, focus on analyzing the underlying mechanisms of behavior change and fall between basic and applied research (Critchfield, 2011; Poling & Edwards, 2011). This could account for some percentage of applied studies not using social validity assessments. However, a perusal of the literature over the past several decades reveals that a number of studies that are explicitly focused on interventions to improve behavior do not incorporate social validity assessments into their data collection protocols.

A second possible explanation for the underutilization of social validity assessments is that the procedures may not be yielding data that researchers find useful in interpreting the outcomes of their research. It might be that the nature of the data collected in many social validity assessments is not as beneficial as is the cost of collecting the data. Part of this might relate to the rigor used in gathering social validity data. For example, Fawcett (1991) has suggested increasing the psychometric rigor of social validity assessments so that the reliability and validity of assessments are established prior to their being used in a research study. Schwartz and Kelly (2021) have argued that the incorporation of consumer input should be central to social validity analyses, rather than something that is conducted as a secondary experimental effort. Finally, Hawkins (1991) has suggested that social validity should not only be assessed but be subjected to experimental analyses that yield functional relations relating to the social importance of research findings, rather than descriptive data. Each of these suggestions, if incorporated into studies of social validity, would improve the quality of the information obtained and, potentially, increase researchers' efforts to incorporate this important construct into their applied studies.

CONCLUSION

An interest in studying social validity emerged during the 1970s in applied behavior analysis and was then extended to other areas of applied psychology and education. The impetus for this development was public concern that behavior-analytic methods might be effective, but they may not be socially acceptable. In order to better understand whether these concerns were warranted, Kazdin (1977) and Wolf (1978) introduced the construct of social validity to applied researchers. These methods have come to incorporate *subjective evaluation, normative comparison*, and *sustainability* as procedures for collecting social validity information.

If used as intended, social validity assessments allow the study of how behavioral interventions impact a range of individuals directly and indirectly involved in the investigation. Subjective evaluations allow the collection of data relating to personal perceptions of the appropriateness of the goals, procedures, and outcomes of a study. Normative comparisons provide a method for indexing the goals and outcomes of a study against some social standard or reference. Finally, sustainability permits an assessment of the extent to which the procedures and outcomes of an experiment are adopted and maintained by a group of individuals. Each approach to social validity assessment can provide important information about the effects of an intervention above and beyond what is typically reported in terms of dependent variables in applied research.

REFLECTION QUESTIONS

1. Describe the different foci of social validity assessments.

2. Why is it more accurate to describe social validity as an estimation technique as opposed to a confirmatory analysis?

3. What are the strengths and limitations of the three approaches to assessing social validity?

4. Do all applied studies need to use an estimate of social validity?

5. Can you describe an instance in which combining ethnographic (qualitative) methods with single-case designs could produce useful information regarding social validity?

REFERENCES

CHAPTER 1

Allum, N., Sturgis, P., Tabourazi, D., & Brunton-Smith, I. (2008). Science knowledge and attitudes across cultures: A meta-analysis. *Public Understanding of Science, 17*(1), 35–54.

Alsbury, T. L. (2008). *The future of school board governance: Relevancy and revelation*. Rowman and Littlefield Education.

American Psychological Association. (2020). *Publication manual of the American Psychological Association* (7th ed.). American Psychological Association.

Baldwin, J. D. (1987). *George Herbert Mead: A unifying theory for sociology*. Sage.

Bristow, W. (2010). *Enlightenment*. Stanford University Press.

Burgos, J. E. (2021). The real problem with hypothetical constructs. *Perspectives on Behavior Science, 44*, 683–704.

Cohen, M. R., & Nagel, E. (1962). *An introduction to logic*. Hackett.

Curry, J. H., Johnson, S., & Peacock, R. (2020). Robert Gagné and the systematic design of instruction. In J. K. McDonald & R. E. West (Eds.), *Design for learning: Principles, processes, and praxis*. EdTech Books.

Dewey, J. (1958). *Experience and nature*. Dover.

Fisher, W. W., Piazza, C. C., & Roane, H. S. (2002). Sleep and cyclical variables related to self-injurious and other destructive behaviors. In S. R. Schroeder, M. L. Oster-Granite, & T. Thompson (Eds.), *Self-injurious behavior: Gene-brain-behavior relationships* (pp. 205–222). American Psychological Association.

Goldenweiser, A. (1938). The concept of causality in the physical and social sciences. *American Sociological Review, 3*(5), 624–636.

Haack, S. (2011). *Defending science—within reason: Between scientism and cynicism*. Prometheus Books.

Halle, J. W., Marshall, A. M., & Spradlin, J. E. (1979). Time display: A technique to increase language use and facilitate generalization in retarded children. *Journal of Applied Behavior Analysis, 12*, 431–439.

Horn, A. L., Roitsch, J., & Murphy, K. A. (2023). Constant time delay to teach reading to students with intellectual disability and autism: A review. *International Journal of Developmental Disabilities, 69*(2), 123–133.

Horner, R. H., Day, H. M., & Day, J. R. (1997). Using neutralizing routines to reduce problem behaviors. *Journal of Applied Behavior Analysis, 30*, 601–614.

Kantor, J. R. (1963). *The scientific evolution of psychology* (Vol. 1). Principia Press.

Kennedy, C. H. (2021). How does health impact challenging behavior? *Research and Practice for Persons With Severe Disabilities, 46*(3), 208–215.

Kennedy, C. H., & Itkonen, T. (1993). Effects of setting events on the problem behavior of students with severe disabilities. *Journal of Applied Behavior Analysis, 26*, 321–328.

Kennedy, C. H., Meyer, K. A., Werts, M. G., & Cushing, L. S. (2000). Effects of sleep deprivation on free-operant avoidance. *Journal of the Experimental Analysis of Behavior, 73*, 333–345.

Kirby, M., & Kennedy, C. H. (2003). Effects of variable-interval length on behavioral tolerance to REM sleep deprivation. *Journal of the Experimental Analysis of Behavior, 80*(2), 253–260.

Kuhn, T. S. (1957). *The Copernican revolution: Planetary astronomy in the development of western thought*. Harvard University Press.

Land, D. (2002). Local school boards under review: Their role and effectiveness in relation to students' academic achievement. *Review of Educational Research, 72*(2), 229–278.

Lehrer, R., & Schauble, L. (2015). The development of scientific thinking. In L. S. Liben, U. Müller, & R. M. Lerner (Eds.), *Handbook of child psychology and developmental science: Cognitive processes* (pp. 671–714). John Wiley & Sons.

Linn, M. C. (1990). What constitutes scientific thinking. *Contemporary Psychology, 35*(1), 16–17.

MacCorquodale, K., & Meehl, P. E. (1948). On a distinction between hypothetical constructs and intervening variables. *Psychological Review, 55*, 95–107.

Mager, R. F. (1962). *Preparing instructional objectives*. Fearon.

Marr, M. J. (1986). Mathematics and verbal behavior. In T. Thompson & M. D. Zeiler (Eds.), *Analysis and integration of behavioral units* (pp. 161–183). Lawrence Erlbaum Associates.

Maxwell, S. E., Lau, M. Y., & Howard, G. S. (2015). Is psychology suffering from a replication crisis? What does "failure to replicate" really mean? *American Psychologist, 70*(6), 487.

Morey, L. C. (1991). *Classification of mental disorder as a collection of hypothetical constructs* (Vol. 100, No. 3).

American Psychological Association.

National Science Board. (2014). *Science and engineering indicators 2014. Chapter 7 Science and technology: Public attitudes and understanding*. National Science Foundation.

O'Reilly, M. F. (1995). Functional analysis and treatment of escape-maintained aggression correlated with sleep deprivation. *Journal of Applied Behavior Analysis, 28*, 225–226.

Pashler, H., & Wagenmakers, E. J. (2012). Editors' introduction to the special section on replicability in psychological science: A crisis of confidence? *Perspectives on Psychological Science, 7*(6), 528–530.

Pearl, J. (2009). *Causality*. Cambridge University Press.

Sidman, M. (1960). *Tactics of scientific research: Evaluating experimental data in psychology*. Basic Books.

Simmons, J. P., Nelson, L. D., & Simonsohn, U. (2011). False-positive psychology: Undisclosed flexibility in data collection and analysis allows presenting anything as significant. *Psychological Science, 22*(11), 1359–1366.

Simon, H. A. (1987). *Psychology of scientific discovery*. Carnegie Mellon University Press.

Simon, H. A. (2013). Understanding the processes of science: The psychology of scientific discovery. In *Progress in science and its social conditions: Nobel symposium 58 held at Lidingö, Sweden, 15–19 August 1983* (p. 159). Elsevier.

Skinner, B. F. (1948). "Superstition" in the pigeon. *Journal of Experimental Psychology, 38*(2), 62–64.

Skinner, B. F. (1950). Are theories of learning necessary? *Psychological Review, 57*, 193–216.

Skinner, B. F. (1954). The science of learning and the art of teaching. *Harvard Educational Review, 24*, 86–97.

Skinner, B. F. (1983). *A matter of consequences*. Alfred A. Knopf.

Street, D. J. (1990). Fisher's contributions to agricultural statistics. *Biometrics, 46*(4), 937–945.

Symons, F. J., Davis, M. L., & Thompson, T. (2000). Self-injurious behavior and sleep disturbance in adults with developmental disabilities. *Research in Developmental Disabilities, 21*, 115–123.

Taubes, G. (1993). *Bad science: The short life and weird times of cold fusion*. Random House.

Tomlinson, S. (1997). Edward Lee Thorndike and John Dewey on the science of education. *Oxford Review of Education, 23*(3), 365–383.

Touchette, P. E. (1971). Transfer of stimulus control: Measuring the moment of transfer. *Journal of the Experimental Analysis of Behavior, 15*, pp. 347–354. Underwood, B.J (1957) *Psychological research*. Prentice-Hall.

Vyse, S. (2022). Superstition and learning. In S. Hupp & R. Wiseman (Eds.), *Investigating pop psychology* (pp. 38–46). Routledge.

Watson, J. B. (1924). *Behaviorism*. W. W. Norton.

Whitehead, A. N., & Russell, B. (1925). *Principia mathematica* (2nd ed.). Cambridge University Press.

CHAPTER 2

Alper, T. G., & White, O. R. (1971). Precision teaching: A tool for the school psychologist and teacher. *Journal of School Psychology, 9*, 445–454.

Ayllon, T., & Michael, J. (1959). The psychiatric nurse as a behavioral engineer. *Journal of the Experimental Analysis of Behavior, 2*, 323–334.

Bacon, F. (2000). *The new organon* (L. Jardine & M. Silverthorne, Trans.). Cambridge University Press. (Original work published 1620)

Baer, D. M. (1962). Laboratory control of thumbsucking by withdrawal and re-presentation of reinforcement. *Journal of the Experimental Analysis of Behavior, 5*, 525–528.

Baer, D. M., & LeBlanc, J. M. (1977). *New developments in behavioral research: Theory, method, and application: In honor of Sidney W. Bijou.* Lawrence Erlbaum Associates.

Baer, D. M., Wolf, M. M., & Risley, T. R. (1968). Some current dimensions of applied behavior analysis. *Journal of Applied Behavior Analysis, 1*, 91–97.

Baum, W. M. (2002). The Harvard Pigeon Lab under Herrnstein. *Journal of the Experimental Analysis of Behavior, 77*, 347–355.

Bernard, C. (1927). *An introduction to the study of experimental medicine* (H. Copley &

A. M. Greene, Trans.). Macmillan. (Original work published 1865)

Bijou, S. W. (1963). Theory and research in mental (developmental) retardation. *Psychological Record, 13*, 95–110.

Bijou, S. W. (1995). *Behavior analysis of child development* (2nd ed.). Context Press.

Bjork, D. W. (1993). *B. F. Skinner: A life.* Basic Books.

Boakes, R. A. (1984). *From Darwin to behaviorism: Psychology and the minds of animals.* Cambridge University Press.

Boring, E. G. (1950). *A history of experimental psychology* (2nd ed.). Appleton-Century-Crofts.

Brittan, G. G., Jr. (2015). *Kant's theory of science.* Princeton University Press.

Catania, A. C. (2013). *Learning* (5th ed.). Sloan.

Chiesa, M. (1994). *Radical behaviorism: The philosophy and the science.* Authors Cooperative.

Collins, F. S., Green, E. D., Guttmacher, A. E., & Guyer, M. S. (2003). A vision for the future of genomics research: A blueprint for the genomic era. *Nature, 422*, 835–847.

Cooter, R., & Pickston, J. (2000). *Medicine in the twentieth century.* Harwood Academic Publishers.

Darwin, C. (1859). *On the origin of species by means of natural selection, or the preservation of favoured races in the struggle for life.* Murray.

Davison, M., & McCarthy, D. (1987). *The matching law: A*

research review. Lawrence Erlbaum Associates.

Dews, P. B. (1987). An outsider on the inside. *Journal of the Experimental Analysis of Behavior, 48*, 459–462.

Dinsmoor, J. A. (1990). Academic roots: Columbia University, 1943–1951. *Journal of the Experimental Analysis of Behavior, 54*, 129–150.

Ferster, C. B., & DeMyer, M. K. (1961). The development of performances in autistic children in an automatically controlled environment. *Journal of Chronic Diseases, 13*, 312–345.

Ferster, C. B., & Skinner, B. F. (1957). *Schedules of reinforcement.* Appleton-Century-Crofts.

Fuller, P. R. (1949). Operant conditioning of a vegetative human organism. *American Journal of Psychology, 62*, 587–590.

Goldiamond, I. (1965). Stuttering and fluency as manipulatable operant response classes. In L. Krasner & L. P. Ullmann (Eds.), *Research in behavior modification: New developments and implications* (pp. 231–259). Holt, Rinehart, & Winston.

Gould, S. J. (2002). *The structure of evolutionary theory.* Harvard University Press.

Guess, D., Sailor, W., Rutherford, G., & Baer, D. M. (1968). An experimental analysis of linguistic development: The productive use of the plural morpheme. *Journal of Applied Behavior Analysis, 1*, 297–306.

Hall, R. V., Lund, D., & Jackson, D. (1968). Effects of teacher attention on study behavior. *Journal of Applied Behavior Analysis, 1*, 1–12.

Haring, N. G. (2016). Republication of "Educational services for the severely and profoundly handicapped.". *Journal of Special Education, 50*(2), 69–74.

Haring, N. G., & Phillips, E. L. (1972). *Analysis and modification of classroom behavior.* Prentice-Hall.

Healy, A. F., Kosslyn, S. M., & Shiffrin, R. M. (1992a). *Essays in honor of William K. Estes: Vol. 1. From learning theory to connectionist theory.* Lawrence Erlbaum Associates.

Healy, A. F., Kosslyn, S. M., & Shiffrin, R. M. (1992b). *Essays in honor of William K. Estes: Vol. 2. From learning processes to cognitive processes.* Lawrence Erlbaum Associates.

Herrnstein, R. J. (1990). Rational choice theory: Necessary but not sufficient. *American Psychologist, 45*, 356–367.

Hodos, W., & Ator, N. A. (1994). A festschrift in honor of Joseph V. Brady in his 70th year. *Journal of the Experimental Analysis of Behavior, 61*, 131–134.

Johnston, J. M., Pennypacker, H. S., & Green, G. (2020). *Strategies and tactics of behavioral research and practice* (4th ed.). Routledge.

Joncich, G. (1968). *The sane positivist: A biography of Edward L. Thorndike.* Wesleyan University Press.

Journal of Applied Behavior Analysis. (1968–present). Society for the Experimental Analysis of Behavior.

Journal of the Experimental Analysis of Behavior . (1958–present). Society for the Experimental Analysis of Behavior.

Kazdin, A. E. (1978). *History of behavior modification.* University Park Press.

Keller, F. S. (1968). Good-bye, teacher.. . . *Journal of Applied Behavior Analysis, 1*, 79–89.

Keller, E. F. (2002). *Making sense of life: Explaining biological development with models, metaphors, and machines.* Harvard University Press.

Keller, F. S., & Schoenfeld, W. N. (1950). *Principles of psychology: A systematic text in the science of behavior.* Appleton-Century-Crofts.

Kennedy, C. H. (1995). A lesson learned (Thomas G. Haring, 1953–1993). *Journal of Behavioral Education, 5*, 119–121.

Kennedy, C. H., Caruso, M., & Thompson, T. (2001). Experimental analyses of gene-brain-behavior relations: Some notes on their application. *Journal of Applied Behavior Analysis, 34*, 539–549.

Kirschner, P. A., Sweller, J., & Clark, R. E. (2006). Why minimal guidance during instruction does not work: An analysis of the failure of constructivist, discovery, problem-based, experiential, and inquiry-based teaching. *Educational Psychologist, 41*(2), 75–86.

Lagemann, E. C. (2002). *An elusive science: The troubling history of education research.* University of Chicago Press.

Lamarck, J.-B. (2011). *Philosophical zoology: An exposition with regard to the natural history of animals.* Cambridge University Press. (Original work published 1809)

Lane, H. (1963). The autophonic scale of voice level for congenitally deaf subjects. *Journal of Experimental Psychology, 66*, 328–331.

Leicester, J., Sidman, M., Stoddard, L. T., & Mohr, J. P. (1971). The nature of aphasic responses. *Neuropsychologia, 9*, 141–155.

Leschner, A. I., Schultz, A. M., Terry, S. F., & Liverman, C. T. (2013). *The CTSA program at the NIH: Opportunities for advancing clinical and translational research.* National Academies Press.

Lindsley, O. R. (1956). Operant conditioning methods applied to research in chronic schizophrenia. *Psychiatric Research Reports, 5*, 118–139.

Lindsley, O. R. (1991). Precision teaching's unique legacy from B. F. Skinner. *Journal of Behavioral Education, 1*, 253–266.

Lovaas, O. I., Freitag, G., Gold, V. J., & Kassorla, I. C. (1965). Experimental studies in childhood schizophrenia: Analysis of self-destructive behavior. *Journal of Experimental Child Psychology, 2*, 67–84.

Lovaas, O. I., Schreibman, L., Koegel, R. L., & Rehm, R. (1971). Selective responding by autistic children to multiple sensory input. *Journal of Abnormal Psychology, 77*, 211–222.

Lovitt, T. C., & Curtiss, K. A. (1969). Academic response rate as a function of teacher- and self-imposed contingencies. *Journal of Applied Behavior Analysis*, *2*, 49–53.

MacCorquodale, K., & Meehl, P. E. (1948). On a distinction between hypothetical constructs and intervening variables. *Psychological Review*, *55*, 95–107.

McDowell, E. (1817). Three cases of extirpation of diseased ovaria. *Eclectic Repertory, and Analytical Review, Medical and Philosophical*, *7*, 242–244.

Meehl, P. E. (2016). Trait language and behaviorese. In M. D. Zeiler & T. Thompson (Eds.), *Analysis and integration of behavioral units* (pp. 343–362). Routledge.

Molenaar, P. C., & Campbell, C. G. (2009). The new person-specific paradigm in psychology. *Current Directions in Psychological Science*, *18*(2), 112–117.

Moore, J. (1984). On privacy, causes, and contingencies. *The Behavior Analyst*, *7*, 3–16.

Moore, J. (2008). *Conceptual foundations of radical behaviorism*. Sloane.

Nathan, D. G., & Varmus, H. E. (2000). The National Institutes of Health and clinical research: A progress report. *Nature Medicine*, *6*(11), 1201–1204.

Pavlov, I. P. (1960). *Conditioned reflexes: An investigation of the physiological activity of the cerebral cortex* (G. V. Anrep, Trans.). Dover. (Original work published 1897)

Scott, J. (2000). Rational choice theory. In G. Browning, A. Halcli, & F. Webster (Eds.),

Understanding contemporary society: Theories of the present (pp. 126–138). Sage.

Sechenov, I. M. (1965). *Reflexes of the brain: An attempt to establish the physiological basis of psychological processes* (S. Belsky, Trans.). MIT Press.

Shadish, W. R., Cook, T. D., & Campbell, D. T. (2002). *Experimental and quasi-experimental designs for generalized causal inference*. Houghton, Mifflin and Company.

Sherman, J. A. (1965). Use of reinforcement and imitation to reinstate verbal behavior in mute psychotics. *Journal of Abnormal Psychology*, *70*, 155–164.

Sherrington, C. E. (1975). Charles Scott Sherrington (1857–1952). *Notes and Records of the Royal Society of London*, *30*, 45–63.

Sherrington, C. S. (1989). The Integrative action of the nervous system. *Classics of Medicine*. (Original work published 1906)

Sidman, M. (1952). A note on functional relations obtained from group data. *Psychological Bulletin*, *49*, 263–269.

Sidman, M. (1960). *Tactics of scientific research*. Basic Books.

Sidman, M. (1989). *Coercion and its fallout*. Authors Cooperative.

Skinner, B. F. (1938). *The behavior of organisms: An experimental analysis*. Appleton-Century-Crofts.

Skinner, B. F. (1953). *Science and human behavior*. Free Press.

Skinner, B. F. (1961). Why we need teaching machines. *Harvard Educational Review*, *31*, 377–398.

Skinner, B. F. (1981). Charles B. Ferster: A personal memoir. *Journal of the Experimental Analysis of Behavior*, *35*, 259–261.

Skinner, B. F. (1983). *A matter of consequences: Part three of an autobiography*. Alfred A. Knopf.

Spradlin, J. E., Cotter, V. W., & Baxley, N. (1973). Establishing a conditional discrimination without direct training: A study of transfer with retarded adolescents. *American Journal of Mental Deficiency*, *77*, 556–566.

Staats, C. K., Staats, A. W., & Schutz, R. E. (1962). The effects of discrimination pretraining on textual behavior. *Journal of Educational Psychology*, *53*, 32–37.

Strain, P. S., Shores, R. E., & Kerr, M. M. (1976). An experimental analysis of spillover effects on the social interaction of behaviorally handicapped preschool children. *Journal of Applied Behavior Analysis*, *9*, 31–40.

Strain, P. S., & Timm, M. A. (1974). An experimental analysis of social interaction between a behaviorally disordered preschool child and her classroom peers. *Journal of Applied Behavior Analysis*, *7*, 583–590.

Sulzer, B., & Mayer, G. R. (1972). *Behavior modification procedures for school personnel*. Dryden.

Thaler, R. H. (2016). Behavioral economics: Past, present, and future. *American Economic Review, 106*(7), 1577–1600.

Thaler, R. H., & Ganser, L. J. (2015). *Misbehaving: The making of behavioral economics.* W. W. Norton.

Thompson, T. (1984). The examining magistrate for nature: A retrospective review of Claude Bernard's An introduction to the study of experimental medicine. *Journal of the Experimental Analysis of Behavior, 41*, 211–216.

Thorndike, E. L. (1898). Animal intelligence: An experimental study of the associative processes in animals. *Psychological Review Monograph Supplement, 73*, 16–43.

Thorndike, E. L. (2011). *Educational psychology* (Vol. 2). Teachers College, Columbia University Press.

Todd, J. T., & Morris, E. K. (1994). *Modern perspectives on John B. Watson and classical behaviorism.* Greenwood.

Todd, J. T., & Morris, E. K. (1995). *Modern perspectives on B. F. Skinner and contemporary behaviorism.* Greenwood.

Trent, J. W. (1994). *Inventing the feeble mind: A history of mental retardation in the United States.* University of California Press.

Underwood, B. J. (1957). *Psychological research.* Prentice-Hall.

van den Bergh, S. (1995). An astronomical life. *Comments on Astrophysics, 18*, 181–190.

von Neumann, J., & Morgenstern, O. (1947). *Theory of games and economic behavior* (2nd ed.). Princeton University Press.

Walker, H. M., & Buckley, N. K. (1968). The use of positive reinforcement in conditioning attending behavior. *Journal of Applied Behavior Analysis, 1*, 245–250.

Wallace, A. R. (1875). *Contributions to the theory of natural selection.* Macmillan.

Watson, J. B. (1924). *Behaviorism.* W. W. Norton.

Winzer, M. A. (2009). *From integration to inclusion: A history of special education in the 20th century.* Gallaudet University Press.

Wolery, M. (2005). Norris G. Haring: Biographical sketch. In G. M. Sugai & R. H. Horner (Eds.), *Encyclopedia of behavior modification and cognitive behavior therapy* (Vol. 3). Sage.

Wolf, M. M., Risley, T. R., & Mees, H. (1964). Application of operant conditioning procedures to the behavior problems of an autistic child. *Behaviour Research and Therapy, 1*, 305–312.

CHAPTER 3

Campbell, D. T., & Stanley, J. C. (2015). *Experimental and quasi-experimental designs for research.* Ravenio.

Carr, E. G., & Durand, V. M. (1985). Reducing behavior problems through functional communication training. *Journal of Applied Behavior Analysis, 18*, 111–126.

Cushing, L. S., & Kennedy, C. H. (1997). Academic effects of providing peer support in general education classrooms on students without disabilities.

Journal of Applied Behavior Analysis, 30, 139–151.

Dugan, E., Kamps, D., Leonard, B., Watkins, N., Rheinberger, A., & Stackhaus, J. (1995). Effects of cooperative learning groups during social studies for students with autism and fourth-grade peers. *Journal of Applied Behavior Analysis, 28*, 175–188.

Ghaemmaghami, M., Hanley, G. P., & Jessel, J. (2021). Functional communication training: From efficacy to effectiveness. *Journal of Applied Behavior Analysis, 54*(1), 122–143.

Johnston, J. M., Pennypacker, H. S., & Green, G. (2020). *Strategies and tactics of behavioral research and practice* (4th ed.). Routledge.

Kennedy, C. H. (2004). Facts, interpretations, and explanations: A review of Evelyn Fox Keller's *Making sense of life. Journal of Applied Behavior Analysis, 37*(4), 539–553.

Kennedy, C. H., & Meyer, K. A. (1996). Sleep deprivation, allergy symptoms, and negatively reinforced problem behavior. *Journal of Applied Behavior Analysis, 29*, 133–135.

Kennedy, C. H., Meyer, K. A., Knowles, T., & Shukla, S. (2000). Analyzing the multiple functions of stereotypical behavior for students with autism: Implications for assessment and treatment. *Journal of Applied Behavior Analysis, 33*, 559–571.

Kuntz, E. M., Santos, A. V., & Kennedy, C. H. (2020). Functional analysis and intervention of perseverative speech in students with high-functioning autism and related neurodevelopmental disabilities. *Journal of Applied Behavior Analysis, 53*(4), 2421–2428.

Merriam-Webster. (2024, June 20). *Relationship*. https://www.merriam-webster.com/dictionary/relationship

Rucker, D. D., McShane, B. B., & Preacher, K. J. (2015). A researcher's guide to regression, discretization, and median splits of continuous variables. *Journal of Consumer Psychology, 25*(4), 666–678.

Shadish, W. R., Cook, T. D., & Campbell, D. T. (2001). *Experimental and quasi-experimental designs for generalized causal inference* (2nd ed.). Cengage Learning.

Sidman, M. (1960). *Tactics of scientific research*. Basic Books.

Simmons, J. P., Nelson, L. D., & Simonsohn, U. (2011). False-positive psychology: Undisclosed flexibility in data collection and analysis allows presenting anything as significant. *Psychological Science, 22*(11), 1359–1366.

CHAPTER 4

Birnbrauer, J. S. (1981). External validity and experimental investigation of individual behavior. *Analysis and Intervention in Developmental Disabilities, 1*, 117–132.

Branch, M. N. (2019). The "reproducibility crisis:" Might the methods used frequently in behavior-analysis research help? *Perspectives on Behavior Science, 42*(1), 77–89.

Camerer, C. F., Dreber, A., Holzmeister, F., Ho, T. H., Huber, J., Johannesson, M., Kirchler, M., Nave, G., Nosek, B. A., Pfeiffer, T., Altmejd, A., Buttrick, N., Chan, T., Chen, Y., Forsell, E., Gampa, A., Heikensten, E., Hummer, L., Imai, T., Isaksson, S., Manfredi, D., . . . Wu, H. (2018). Evaluating the replicability of social science experiments in *Nature* and *Science* between 2010 and 2015. *Nature Human Behaviour, 2*(9), 637–644.

Campbell, D. T., & Stanley, J. C. (2015). *Experimental and quasi-experimental designs for research*. Ravenio.

Cook, T. D., Campbell, D. T., & Shadish, W. (2002). *Experimental and quasi-experimental designs for generalized causal inference*. Houghton Mifflin.

Critchfield, T. S., & Vargas, E. A. (1991). Self-recording, instructions, and public self-graphing: Effects on swimming in the absence of coach verbal interaction. *Behavior Modification, 15*, 95–112.

Deno, S. L., Fuchs, L. S., Marston, D., & Shin, J. (2001). Using curriculum-based measurement to establish growth standards for students with learning disabilities. *School Psychology Review, 30*, 507–524.

Freese, J., & Peterson, D. (2017). Replication in social science. *Annual Review of Sociology, 43*, 147–165.

Hains, A. H., & Baer, D. M. (1989). Interaction effects in multielement designs: Inevitable, desirable, and ignorable. *Journal of Applied Behavior, 22*, 57–69.

Johnston, J. M., Pennypacker, H. S., & Green, G. (2020). *Strategies and tactics of behavioral research and practice* (4th ed.). Routledge.

Kame'enui, E. J., Fuchs, L., Francis, D. J., Good, R., III, O'Connor., R, E., Simmons, D. C., Tindal, G., & Torgesen, J. K. (2006). The adequacy of tools for assessing reading competence: A framework and review. *Educational Researcher, 35*(4), 3–11.

Logan, K. R., Jacobs, H. A., Gast, D. L., Murray, A. S., Daino, K., & Skala, C. (1998). The impact of typical peers on the perceived happiness of students with profound multiple disabilities. *Journal of the Association for Persons With Severe Handicaps, 23*, 309–318.

Maxwell, S. E., Lau, M. Y., & Howard, G. S. (2015). Is psychology suffering from a replication crisis? What does "failure to replicate" really mean? *American Psychologist, 70*(6), 487.

McKenzie, T. L., & Rushall, B. S. (1974). Effects of self-recording on attendance and performance in a competitive swimming training environment. *Journal of Applied Behavior, 7*, 199–206.

Merriam-Webster. (2024, June 12). *Replication*. https://www.merriam-webster.com/dictionary/replication

Parsons, M. B., Reid, D. H., Green, C. W., & Browning, L. B. (1999). Reducing individualized job coach assistance provided to persons with multiple severe disabilities in work settings. *Journal of the Association for Persons With Severe Handicaps, 24*, 292–297.

Sidman, M. (1960). *Tactics of scientific research: Evaluating experimental data in psychology*. Basic Books.

Simmons, J. P., Nelson, L. D., & Simonsohn, U. (2011). False-positive psychology: Undisclosed flexibility in data collection and analysis allows presenting anything as significant. *Psychological Science, 22*, 1359–1366.

Stroebe, W., & Strack, F. (2014). The alleged crisis and the illusion of exact replication. *Perspectives on Psychological Science, 9*(1), 59–71.

Walker, S. G., & Carr, J. E. (2021). Generality of findings from single-case designs: It's not all about the *"N." Behavior Analysis in Practice, 14*(4), 991–995.

Ward, P., & Carnes, M. (2002). Effects of posting self-set goals on collegiate football players' skill execution during practice and games. *Journal of Applied Behavior Analysis, 35*,1–12.

CHAPTER 5

Baer, D. M., Wolf, M. M., & Risley, T. R. (1968). Some current dimensions of applied behavior analysis. *Journal of Applied Behavior Analysis, 1*, 91–97.

Barrish, H. H., Saunders, M., & Wolf, M. M. (1969). Good behavior game: Effects of individual contingencies for group consequences on disruptive behavior in a classroom. *Journal of Applied Behavior Analysis, 2*, 119–124.

Common, E. A., Bross, L. A., Oakes, W. P., Cantwell, E. D.,

Lane, K. L., & Germer, K. A. (2019). Systematic review of high probability requests in K–12 settings: Examining the evidence base. *Behavioral Disorders, 45*(1), 3–21.

Fisher, W. W., Piazza, C. C., & Roane, H. S (Eds.). (2021). *Handbook of applied behavior analysis*. Guilford Publications.

Garfinkle, A., & Kaiser, A. P. (2003). Communication. In C. H. Kennedy, & E. Horn (Eds.), *Including students with severe disabilities* (pp. 120–137). Allyn and Bacon.

Hayes, S. C., Rincover, A., & Solnick, J. V. (1980). The technical drift of applied behavior analysis. *Journal of Applied Behavior Analysis, 13*, 275–285.

Kim, J. Y., Fienup, D. M., Draus, C. J., & Wong, K. K. (2023). Differential mastery criteria impact sight word acquisition and maintenance: Application to individual operants and teaching trial doses. *Journal of Applied Behavior Analysis, 56*(2), 388–399.

Medland, M. B., & Stachnik, T. J. (1972). Good-behavior game: A replication and systematic analysis. *Journal of Applied Behavior Analysis, 5*, 45–51.

Murray, L. K., & Kollins, S. H. (2000). Effects of methylphenidate on sensitivity to reinforcement in children diagnosed with attention deficit hyperactivity disorder: An application of the matching law. *Journal of Applied Behavior Analysis, 33*, 573–592.

Spooner, F., Root, J. R., Saunders, A. F., & Browder, D. M. (2019). An updated evidence-based practice review on teaching mathematics to

students with moderate and severe developmental disabilities. *Remedial and Special Education, 40*(3), 150–165.

Thiemann, K. S., & Goldstein, H. (2001). Social stories, written text cues, and video feedback: Effects on social communication of children with autism. *Journal of Applied Behavior Analysis, 34*, 425–446.

Wacker, D. P., Steege, M. W., Northup, J., Sasso, G., Berg, W., Reimers, T., Cooper, L., Cigrand, K., & Donn, L. (1990). A component analysis of functional communication training across three topographies of severe behavior problems. *Journal of Applied Behavior Analysis, 23*, 417–430.

CHAPTER 6

American Psychological Association Presidential Task Force on Evidence-Based Practice. (2006). Evidence-based practice in psychology. *American Psychologist, 61*(4), 271–285.

Ayers, A. J. (1972). *Sensory integration and learning disorders*. Western Psychological Services.

Bauer, M. S., & Kirchner, J. (2020). Implementation science: What is it and why should I care? *Psychiatry Research, 283*, Article 112376.

Bodison, S. C., & Parham, L. D. (2018). Specific sensory techniques and sensory environmental modifications for children and youth with sensory integration difficulties: A systematic review. *American Journal of*

Occupational Therapy, 72(1), 7201190040p1–7201190040p11.

Byiers, B. J., Reichle, J., & Symons, F. J. (2012). Single-subject experimental design for evidence-based practice. *American Journal of Speech-Language Pathology, 21*(4), 397–414.

Camarata, S., Miller, L. J., & Wallace, M. T. (2020). Evaluating sensory integration/sensory processing treatment: Issues and analysis. *Frontiers in Integrative Neuroscience, 14*, 55.

Case-Smith, J., Weaver, L. L., & Fristad, M. A. (2015). A systematic review of sensory processing interventions for children with autism spectrum disorders. *Autism, 19*(2), 133–148.

Cook, B. G., & Odom, S. L. (2013). Evidence-based practices and implementation science in special education. *Exceptional Children, 79*(2), 135–144.

Deris, A. R., Hagelman, E. M., Schilling, K., & DiCarlo, C. F. (2006). *Using a weighted or pressure vest for a child with autistic spectrum disorder.* ERIC Clearinghouse.

Dunst, C. J., Trivette, C. M., & Cutspec, P. A. (2002). Toward an operational definition of evidence-based practices. *Centerscope, 1*(1), 1–10.

Fuchs, L. S., & Fuchs, D. (2007). A model for implementing responsiveness to intervention. *Teaching Exceptional Children, 39*(5), 14–20.

Gambrill, E. (2005). *Critical thinking in clinical practice: Improving the accuracy of judgements and decisions* (2nd ed.). Wiley.

Gersten, R., Fuchs, L. S., Compton, D., Coyne, M., Greenwood, C., & Innocenti, M. S. (2005). Quality indicators for group experimental and quasi-experimental research in special education. *Exceptional Children, 71*(2), 149–164.

Green, V. A., Pituch, K. A., Itchon, J., Choi, A., O'Reilly, M., & Sigafoos, J. (2006). Internet survey of treatments used by parents of children with autism. *Research in Developmental Disabilities, 27*(1), 70–84.

Griffiths, Y., & Stuart, M. (2013). Reviewing evidence-based practice for pupils with dyslexia and literacy difficulties. *Journal of Research in Reading, 36*(1), 96–116.

Greenhalgh, T., Howick, J., & Maskrey, N. (2014). Evidence based medicine: A movement in crisis? *British Medical Journal, 348*, 1–7.

Guyatt, G., Cairns, J., Churchill, D., Cook, D., Haynes, B., Hirsh, J., Irvine, J., Levine, Mark., Levine, Mitchell., Nishikawa, J., Sackett, D., Brill-Edwards, P., Gerstein, H., Gibson, J., Jaeschke, R., Kerigan, A., Neville, A., Panju, A., Detsky, A.Enkin, M. Frid, P., … Tugwell, P. (1992). Evidence-based medicine: A new approach to teaching the practice of medicine. *Journal of the American Medical Association, 268*(17), 2420–2425.

Halle, J. W., Baer, D. M., & Spradlin, J. E. (1981). Teachers' generalized use of delay as a stimulus control procedure to increase language use in handicapped children.

Journal of Applied Behavior Analysis, 14(4), 389–409.

Halle, J. W., Marshall, A. M., & Spradlin, J. E. (1979). Time delay: A technique to increase language use and facilitate generalization in retarded children. *Journal of Applied Behavior Analysis, 12*(3), 431–439.

Horner, R. H., Carr, E. G., Halle, J., McGee, G., Odom, S., & Wolery, M. (2005). The use of single-subject research to identify evidence-based practice in special education. *Exceptional Children, 71*(2), 165–179.

Howick, J., Phillips, B., Ball, C., Sackett, D., & Badenoch, D. (2009). *Oxford Centre for Evidence-Based Medicine levels of evidence.* University of Oxford, Centre for Evidence-based Medicine.

Hume, K., Steinbrenner, J. R., Odom, S. L., Morin, K. L., Nowell, S. W., Tomaszewski, B., Szendrey, S., McIntyre, N. S., Yücesoy-Öksan, S., & Savage, M. N. (2021). Evidence-based practices for children, youth, and young adults with autism: Third generation review. *Journal of Autism and Developmental Disorders, 51*, 4013–4032.

Johnston, J. M., Pennypacker, H. S., & Green, G. (2020). *Strategies and tactics of behavioral research and practice* (4th ed.). Routledge.

Kratochwill, T. R., Hitchcock, J. H., Horner, R. H., Levin, J. R., Odom, S. L., Rindskopf, D. M., & Shadish, W. R. (2013). Single-case intervention research design standards. *Remedial and Special Education, 34*(1), 26–38.

Ledford, J. R., Lambert, J. M., Pustejovsky, J. E., Zimmerman, K. N., Hollins, N., & Barton, E. E. (2023). Single-case-design research in special education: Next-generation guidelines and considerations. *Exceptional Children, 89*(4), 379–396.

Lloyd, J. W., & Therrien, W. J (Eds.). (2023, July). *Exceptional Children, 89*(4), 356–489. [Special issue.]

Lonigan, C. J., Elbert, J. C., & Johnson, S. B. (1998). Empirically supported psychosocial interventions for children: An overview. *Journal of Clinical Child Psychology, 27*(2), 138–145.

No Child Left Behind (NCLB) Act of 2001, Pub. L. No. 107-110, § 101, Stat. 1425 (2002).

Maggin, D. M., Barton, E., Reichow, B., Lane, K. L., & Shogren, K. A. (2022). Commentary on the What Works Clearinghouse *Standards and Procedures Handbook* (v. 4.1) for the review of single-case research. *Remedial and Special Education, 43*(6), 421–433.

Miller, L. J., Anzalone, M. E., Lane, S. J., Cermak, S. A., & Osten, E. T. (2007). Concept evolution in sensory integration: A proposed nosology for diagnosis. *American Journal of Occupational Therapy, 61*(2), 135–140.

Moeller, J. D., Dattilo, J., & Rusch, F. (2015). Applying quality indicators to single-case research designs used in special education: A systematic review. *Psychology in the Schools, 52*(2), 139–153.

Natesan Batley, P., McClure, E. B., Brewer, B., Contractor, A.

A., Batley, N. J., Hedges, L. V., & Chin, S. (2023). Evidence and reporting standards in N-of-1 medical studies: A systematic review. *Translational Psychiatry, 13*(1), Article 263.

Odom, S. L., Brantlinger, E., Gersten, R., Horner, R. H., Thompson, B., & Harris, K. R. (2005). Research in special education: Scientific methods and evidence-based practices. *Exceptional Children, 71*(2), 137–148.

Olson, L. J., & Moulton, H. J. (2004). Use of weighted vests in pediatric occupational therapy practice. *Physical and Occupational Therapy in Pediatrics, 24*(3), 45–60.

Riley-Tillman, T. C., Burns, M. K., & Kilgus, S. P. (2020). *Evaluating educational interventions: Single-case design for measuring response to intervention.* Guilford Publications.

Sackett, D. L., Rosenberg, W. M., Gray, J. M., Haynes, R. B., & Richardson, W. S. (1996). Evidence based medicine: What it is and what it isn't. *British Medical Journal, 312*, 71–72.

Shavelson, R. J., & Towne, L. (2002). *Scientific research in education.* National Academies Press.

Sidman, M. (1960). *Tactics of scientific research.* Basic Books.

Smith, B. J., Strain, P. S., Snyder, P., Sandall, S. R., McLean, M. E., Ramsey, A. B., & Sumi, W. C. (2002). DEC recommended practices: A review of 9 years of EllECSE research literature. *Journal of Early Intervention, 25*(2), 108–119.

Steinbrenner, J. R., Hume, K., Odom, S. L., Morin, K. L.,

Nowell, S. W., Tomaszewski, B., Szendrey, S., McIntyre, N. S., Yücesoy-Özkan, S., & Savage, M. N. (2020). *Evidence-based practices for children, youth, and young adults with autism.* The University of North Carolina at Chapel Hill, Fran Porter Graham Child Development Institute, National Clearinghouse on Autism Evidence and Practice Review Team

Stephenson, J., & Carter, M. (2009). The use of weighted vests with children with autism spectrum disorders and other disabilities. *Journal of Autism and Developmental Disorders, 39*, 105–114.

Tankersley, M., Cook, B. G., & Cook, L. (2008). A preliminary examination to identify the presence of quality indicators in single-subject research. *Education and Treatment of Children, 31*(4), 523–548.

Taylor, C. J., Spriggs, A. D., Ault, M. J., Flanagan, S., & Sartini, E. C. (2017). A systematic review of weighted vests with individuals with autism spectrum disorder. *Research in Autism Spectrum Disorders, 37*, 49–60.

Terrace, H. S. (1963a). Discrimination learning with and without "errors.". *Journal of the Experimental Analysis of Behavior, 6*(1), 1–27.

Terrace, H. S. (1963b). Errorless transfer of a discrimination across two continua. *Journal of the Experimental Analysis of Behavior, 6*(2), 223–232.

Tincani, M., & Travers, J. (2018). Publishing single-case research design studies that do not demonstrate experimental control. *Remedial* and Special Education, 39(2), 118–128.

Toste, J. R., Talbott, E., & Cumming, M. M. (2023). Special issue preview: Introducing the next generation of quality indicators for research in special education. Exceptional Children, 89(4), 357–358.

Touchette, P. E. (1971). Transfer of stimulus control: Measuring the moment of transfer. Journal of the Experimental Analysis of Behavior, 15(3), 347–354.

What Works Clearinghouse. (2020a). Procedures handbook (Version 4.1). National Center for Education Evaluation and Regional Assistance, Institute of Education Sciences, U.S. Department of Education. https://ies.ed.gov/ncee/WWC/Docs/referenceresources/WWC-Procedures-Handbook-v4-1-508.pdf

What Works Clearinghouse. (2020b). Standards handbook (Version 4.1). National Center for Education Evaluation and Regional Assistance, Institute of Education Sciences, U. S. Department of Education. https://ies.ed.gov/ncee/WWC/Docs/referenceresources/WWC-Standards-Handbook-v4-1-508.pdf

Whitehurst, G. J. (2003). The Institute of Education Sciences: New wine, new bottles. U.S. Department of Education.

Wolery, M. (2012). A commentary: Single-case design technical document of the What Works Clearinghouse. Remedial and Special Education, 34(1), 39–43.

Wolery, M., Ault, M. J., & Doyle, P. M. (1992). Teaching students with moderate to severe disabilities: Use of response prompting strategies. Longman.

Woolf, S. H. (1992). Practice guidelines, a new reality in medicine: II. Methods of developing guidelines. Archives of Internal Medicine, 152(5), 946–952.

CHAPTER 7

Anger, D. (1956). The dependence of interresponse times upon the relative reinforcement of different interresponse times. Journal of Experimental Psychology, 52, 145–161.

Baer, D. M. (1986). In application, frequency is not the only estimate of the probability of behavioral units. In T. Thompson & M. D. Zeiler (Eds.), Analysis and integration of behavioral units (pp. 117–136). Lawrence Erlbaum Associates.

Catania, A. C. (2013). Learning (5th ed.). Prentice-Hall.

Christle, C. A., & Schuster, J. W. (2003). The effects of using response cards on student participation, academic achievement, and on-task behavior during whole-class, math instruction. Journal of Behavioral Education, 12, 147–165.

Evans, A. L., Bulla, A. J., & Kieta, A. R. (2021). The precision teaching system: A synthesized definition, concept analysis, and process. Behavior Analysis in Practice, 14(3), 559–576.

Hagopian, L. P., Rush, K. S., Lewin, A. B., & Long, E. S. (2001). Evaluating the predictive validity of a single stimulus engagement preference assessment. Journal of Applied Behavior Analysis, 34, 475–485.

Johnston, J. M., & Hodge, C. (1989). Describing behavior with ratios of count and time. The Behavior Analyst, 12, 177–185.

Johnston, J. M., Pennypacker, H. S., & Green, G. (2020). Strategies and tactics of behavioral research and practice (4th ed.). Routledge.

Kostewicz, D. E., Kubina, R. M., & Cooper, J. O. (2000). Managing aggressive thoughts and feelings with daily counts of non-aggressive thoughts and feelings: A self-experiment. Journal of Behavior Therapy and Experimental Psychiatry, 31, 177–187.

Lindsley, O. R. (1991). Precision teaching's unique legacy from B. F. Skinner. Journal of Behavioral Education, 1, 253–266.

Lippman, L. G., & Tragesser, S. L. (2003). Contingent magnitude of reward in modified human-operant DRL-LH and CRF schedules. The Psychological Record, 53, 429–442.

Merriam-Webster. (2024, June 29). Metaphor. https://www.merriam-webster.com/dictionary/metaphor

Ross, D. F., Read, J. D., & Toglia, M. P. (2003). Adult eyewitness testimony: Current trends and developments. Cambridge University Press.

Schoenfeld, W. N. (1995). "Reinforcement" in behavior theory. The Behavior Analyst, 18, 173–185.

Skinner, B. F. (1945). The operational analysis of psychological terms. *Psychological Review, 52,* 270–277.

Skinner, B. F. (1950). Are theories of learning necessary? *Psychological Review, 57,* 193–216.

Skinner, B. F. (1985). Cognitive science and behaviorism. *British Journal of Psychology, 76,* 291–301.

Todd, J. T., & Morris, E. K. (1994). *Modern perspectives on John B. Watson and classical behaviorism.* Greenwood.

Todd, J. T., & Morris, E. K. (1995). *Modern perspectives on B. F. Skinner and contemporary behaviorism.* Greenwood.

Watson, J. B. (1924). *Behaviorism.* W. W. Norton.

Wehby, J. H., & Hollahan, M. S. (2000). Effects of high-probability requests on the latency to initiate academic tasks. *Journal of Applied Behavior Analysis, 33,* 259–262.

CHAPTER 8

Annett, J. (2004). Hierarchical task analysis. *The handbook of task analysis for human-computer interaction.* University of Chicago Press.

Bakeman, R., & Gottman, J. M. (1997). *Observing interaction: An introduction to sequential analysis* (2nd ed.). Cambridge University Press.

Bakeman, R., & Quera, V. (2012). *Behavioral observation.* American Psychological Association.

Bijou, S. W., Peterson, R. F., & Ault, M. H. (1968). A method to integrate descriptive and experimental field studies at the level of data and empirical concepts. *Journal of Applied Behavior Analysis, 1,* 175–191.

Catania, A. C. (2013). *Learning* (5th ed.). Prentice-Hall.

Cooper, J. O., Heron, T. E., & Heward, W. L. (2020). *Applied behavior analysis* (3rd ed.). Pearson.

Gresham, F. M., Gansle, K. A., & Noell, G. H. (1993). Treatment integrity in applied behavior analysis with children. *Journal of Applied Behavior Analysis, 26,* 257–263.

Harrop, A., & Daniels, M. (1986). Methods of time sampling: A reappraisal of momentary time sampling and partial interval recording. *Journal of Applied Behavior Analysis, 19,* 73–77.

Kahng, S., Ingvarsson, E. T., Quigg, A. M., Seckinger, K. E., Teichman, H. M., & Clay, C. J. (2021). Defining and measuring behavior. In W. W. Fisher, C. C. Piazza, & H. S. Roane (Eds.), *Handbook of applied behavior analysis* (pp. 135–154). Guilford Publications.

Kelly, M. B. (1977). A review of the observational data-collection and reliability procedures reported in the Journal of Applied Behavior Analysis. *Journal of Applied Behavior Analysis, 10,* 97–101.

Kennedy, C. H. (1994). Manipulating antecedent conditions to alter the stimulus control of problem behavior. *Journal of Applied Behavior Analysis, 27,* 161–170.

Kennedy, C. H. (2003). Peer-to-peer relationships as a foundation for inclusive education. In D. Fisher (Ed.), *Inclusive education in urban schools* (pp. 145–156). Paul H. Brookes.

Kieras, D. E., & Butler, K. A. (1997). Task analysis and the design of functionality. *The Computer Science and Engineering Handbook, 23,* 1401–1423.

Ledford, J. R., & Gast, D. L. (2014). Measuring procedural fidelity in behavioural research. *Neuropsychological Rehabilitation, 24*(3-4) 332–348.

Lerman, D. C. (2003). From the laboratory to community application: Translational research in behavior analysis. *Journal of Applied Behavior Analysis, 36,* 415–419.

Malouf, D. B., & Schiller, E. P. (1995). Practice and research in special education. *Exceptional Children, 61,* 414–424.

Mayer, G. R., Sulzer-Azaroff, B., & Wallace, M. (2012). *Behavior analysis for lasting change.* Sloan Publishing.

Miltenberger, R. G., Rapp, J. T., & Long, E. S. (1999). A low-tech method for conducting real-time recording. *Journal of Applied Behavior Analysis, 32,* 119--120.

Nunes, E. V., Carroll, K. M., & Bickel, W. K. (2002). Clinical and translational research: Introduction to the special issue. *Experimental and Clinical Psychopharmacology, 10,* 155–158.

Peterson, L., Homer, A. L., & Wonderlich, S. A. (1982). The integrity of independent variables in behavior analysis. *Journal of Applied Behavior Analysis, 15,* 477–492.

Powell, J., Martindale, A., & Kulp, S. (1975). An evaluation of time-sample measures of behavior. *Journal of Applied Behavior Analysis, 8*, 463–469.

Repp, A. C., Roberts, D. M., Slack, D. J., Repp, C. F., & Berkler, M. S. (1976). A comparison of frequency, interval, and time-sampling methods of data collection. *Journal of Applied Behavior Analysis, 9*, 501–508.

Schall, J. V. (2007). *The order of things*. Ignatius Press.

Springer, B., Brown, T., & Duncan, P. K. (1981). Current measurement in applied behavior analysis. *The Behavior Analyst, 4*, 19–32.

Tang, J.-C., Patterson, T. G., & Kennedy, C. H. (2003). Identifying specific sensory modalities maintaining the stereotypy of students with multiple profound disabilities. *Research in Developmental Disabilities, 24*, 433–451.

Thompson, T., Felce, D., & Symons, F. (1999). *Behavioral observation: Technology and applications in developmental disabilities*. Paul H. Brookes.

Trout, J. D. (1998). *Measuring the intentional world: Realism, naturalism, and quantitative methods in the behavioral sciences*. Oxford University Press.

Wacker, D. P. (2000). Building a bridge between research in experimental and applied behavior analysis. In J. C. Leslie & D. Blackman (Eds.), *Experimental and applied analysis of human behavior* (pp. 205–234). Context Press.

Walker, H. M., & Severson, H. H. (1992). *Systematic screening for behavior disorders (SSBD)*. Sopris West.

Whaley, D. L. (1973). *Psychological testing and the philosophy of measurement*. Behaviordelia.

CHAPTER 9

Araujo, J., & Born, D. G. (1985). Calculating percentage agreement correctly but writing its formula incorrectly. *The Behavior Analyst, 8*(2), 207–208.

Artman, K., Wolery, M., & Yoder, P. (2012). Embracing our visual inspection and analysis tradition: Graphing interobserver agreement data. *Remedial and Special Education, 33*(2), 71–77.

Baer, D. M., Wolf, M. M., & Risley, T. R. (1987). Some still-current dimensions of applied behavior analysis. *Journal of Applied Behavior Analysis, 20*(4), 313–327.

Barrish, H. H., Saunders, M., & Wolf, M. M. (1969). Good behavior game: Effects of individual contingencies for group consequences on disruptive behavior in a classroom. *Journal of Applied Behavior Analysis, 2*(2), 119–124.

Bijou, S. W., Peterson, R. F., & Ault, M. H. (1968). A method to integrate descriptive and experimental field studies at the level of data and empirical concepts. *Journal of Applied Behavior Analysis, 1*, 175°191.

Billingsley, F. F, White, O. R., & Munson, R. (1980). Procedural reliability: A rationale and an example. *Behavioral Assessment, 2*, 229–241.

Cohen, J. A. (1960). A coefficient of agreement for nominal scales. *Educational and Psychological Measurement, 20*, 37–46.

Deitz, S. M. (1988). Another's view of observer agreement and observer accuracy. *Journal of Applied Behavior Analysis, 21*, 113.

DiGennaro Reed, F. D., & Codding, R. S. (2014). Advancements in procedural fidelity assessment and intervention: Introduction to the special issue. *Journal of Behavioral Education, 23*(1), 1–18.

Essig, L., Rotta, K., & Poling, A. (2023). Interobserver agreement and procedural fidelity: An odd asymmetry. *Journal of Applied Behavior Analysis, 56*(1), 78–85.

Gresham, F. M., Gansle, K. A., & Noell, G. H. (1993). Treatment integrity in applied behavior analysis with children. *Journal of Applied Behavior Analysis, 26*(2), 257–263.

Hartmann, D. (1977). Considerations in the choice of interobserver reliability estimates. *Journal of Applied Behavior Analysis, 10*, 103–116.

Hausman, N. L., Javed, N., Bednar, M. K., Guell, M., Schaller, E., Nevill, R. E., & Kahng, S. (2022). Interobserver agreement: A preliminary investigation into how much is enough? *Journal of Applied Behavior Analysis, 55*(2), 357–368.

Hawkins, R. P., & Dotson, V. A. (1975). Reliability scores that delude: An Alice in Wonderland trip through misleading characteristics of interobserver agreement scores in interval recording. In E. Ramp & G. Semb (Eds.), *Behavior analysis: Areas of research and application* (pp. 359–376). Prentice-Hall.

Horner, R. H., Carr, E. G., Halle, J. W., McGee, G., Odom, S. L., & Wolery, M. (2005). The use of single-subject research to identify evidence-based practice in special education. *Exceptional Children, 71*(2), 165–179.

Johnson, S. M., & Bolstad, O. D. (1973). Methodological issues in naturalistic observation: Some problems and solutions for field research. In L. A. Hamerlynck, L. C. Handy, & E. J. Mash (Eds.), *Behavior change: Methodology, concepts, and practice* (pp. 7–67). Research Press.

Johnston, J. M., Pennypacker, H. S., & Green, G. (2020). *Strategies and tactics of behavioral research and practice* (4th ed.). Routledge.

Kazdin, A. E. (1977). Artifact, bias, and complexity of assessment: The ABCs of reliability. *Journal of Applied Behavior Analysis, 10*, 141–150.

Kelly, M. B. (1977). A review of the observational data-collection and reliability procedures reported in the Journal of Applied Behavior Analysis. *Journal of Applied Behavior Analysis, 10*, 97–101.

Ledford, J. R., & Wolery, M. (2013). Procedural fidelity: An analysis of measurement and reporting practices. *Journal of Early Intervention, 35*(2), 173–193.

Pennington, B., & McComas, J. J. (2017). Effects of the good behavior game across classroom contexts. *Journal*

of Applied Behavior Analysis, *50*(1), 176–180.

Peterson, L., Homer, A. L., & Wonderlich, S. A. (1982). The integrity of independent variables in behavior analysis. *Journal of Applied Behavior Analysis, 15*(4), 477–492.

Repp, A. C., Deitz, D. E. D., Boles, S. M., Deitz, S. M., & Repp, C. F. (1976). Differences among common methods for calculating interobserver agreement. *Journal of Applied Behavior Analysis, 9*, 109–113.

Shoukri, M. M. (2003). *Measures of interobserver agreement and reliability.* CRC Press.

Strain, P., Fox, L., & Barton, E. E. (2021). On expanding the definition and use of procedural fidelity. *Research and Practice for Persons With Severe Disabilities, 46*(3), 173–183.

Watkins, M. W., & Pacheco, M. (2000). Interobserver agreement in behavioral research: Importance and calculation. *Journal of Behavioral Education, 10*, 205–212.

Yeaton, W. H., & Sechrest, L. (1981). Critical dimensions in the choice and maintenance of successful treatments: Strength, integrity, and effectiveness. *Journal of Consulting and Clinical Psychology, 49*(2), 156–167.

CHAPTER 10

Angell, M. E., Nicholson, J. K., Watts, E. H., & Blum, C. (2011). Using a multicomponent adapted power card strategy to decrease latency during interactivity transitions for

three children with developmental disabilities. *Focus on Autism and Other Developmental Disabilities, 26*(4), 206–217.

Baer, D. M., Wolf, M. M., & Risley, T. R. (1968). Some current dimensions of applied behavior analysis. *Journal of Applied Behavior Analysis, 1*(1), 91–101.

Cooper, J. O., Heron, T. E., & Heward, W. L. (2020). *Applied behavior analysis.* Pearson UK.

De Prey, R. L., & Sugai, G. (2002). The effect of active supervision and pre-correction on minor behavioral incidents in a sixth-grade general education classroom. *Journal of Behavioral Education, 11*, 255–262.

Furlonger, B. E., Oey, A., Moore, D., Busacca, M., & Scott, D. (2017). Improving amateur indoor rock climbing performance using a changing criterion design within a self-management program. *The Sport Journal, 19*(1), 1–16.

Goldstein, H., Kaczmarek, L., Pennington, R., & Shafer, K. (1992). Peer-mediated intervention: Attending to, commenting on, and acknowledging the behavior of preschoolers with autism. *Journal of Applied Behavior Analysis, 25*(2), 289–305.

Hall, R. V. (1971). *Managing behavior: Behavior modification, the measurement of behavior.* H & H Enterprises.

Hall, R. V., Lund, D., & Jackson, D. (1968). Effects of teacher attention on study behavior. *Journal of Applied Behavior Analysis, 1*(1), 1–12.

Hartmann, D. P., & Hall, R. V. (1976). The changing criterion design. *Journal of*

Applied Behavior Analysis, 9(4), 527–532.

Journal of Applied Behavior Analysis. (1968–present). *Society for the Experimental Analysis.* https://onlinelibrary.wiley.com/journal/19383703

Kennedy, C. H., & Souza, G. (1995). Functional analysis and treatment of eye poking. *Journal of Applied Behavior Analysis, 28,* 27–37.

Klein, L. A., Houlihan, D., Vincent, J. L., & Panahon, C. J. (2017). Best practices in utilizing the changing criterion design. *Behavior Analysis in Practice, 10*(1), 52–61.

Leitenberg, H. (1973). The use of single-case methodology in psychotherapy research. *Journal of Abnormal Psychology, 82,* 87–101.

Maguire, R. W., & Allen, R. F. (2022). *Stimulus equivalence for students with developmental disabilities.* Routledge.

McDaniel, S. C., & Bruhn, A. L. (2016). Using a changing-criterion design to evaluate the effects of check-in/check-out with goal modification. *Journal of Positive Behavior Interventions, 18*(4), 197–208.

McDougall, D. (2005). The range-bound changing criterion design. *Behavioral Interventions: Theory and Practice in Residential and Community-Based Clinical Programs, 20*(2), 129–137.

McHugh, C. L., Dozier, C. L., Diaz de Villegas, S. C., & Kanaman, N. A. (2022). Using synchronous reinforcement to increase mask wearing in adults with intellectual and developmental disabilities.

Journal of Applied Behavior Analysis, 55(4), 1157–1171.

Pace, G. M., & Toyer, E. A. (2000). The effects of a vitamin supplement on the pica of a child with severe mental retardation. *Journal of Applied Behavior Analysis, 33,* 619–622.

Shadish, W. R., Cook, T. D., & Campbell, D. T. (2002). *Experimental and quasi-experimental designs for generalized causal inference.* Houghton Mifflin.

Sidman, M. (1960). *Tactics of scientific research.* Basic Books.

Sidman, M. (1994). *Equivalence relations and behavior: A research story.* Authors Cooperative.

Weis, L., & Hall, R. V. (1971). Modification of cigarette smoking through avoidance of punishment. In R. V. Hall (Ed.), *Managing behavior: Behavior modification applications in school and home* (pp. 77–102). H & H Enterprises.

CHAPTER 11

Agras, W. S., Leitenberg, H., Barlow, D. H., & Thomson, L. E. (1969). Instructions and reinforcement in the modification of neurotic behavior. *American Journal of Psychiatry, 125,* 1435–1439.

Barlow, D. H., & Hayes, S. C. (1979). Alternating treatments design: One strategy for comparing the effects of two treatments in a single subject. *Journal of Applied Behavior Analysis, 12,* 199–210.

Barlow, D. H., & Hersen, M. (1984). *Single case*

experimental designs: Strategies for studying behavior change (2nd ed.). Pergamon.

Berg, W. K., Peck, S., Wacker, D. P., Harding, J., McComas, J., Richman, D., & Brown, K. (2000). The effects of presession exposure to attention on the results of assessments of attention as a reinforcer. *Journal of Applied Behavior Analysis, 33,* 463–477.

Browning, R. M. (1967). A same-subject design for simultaneous comparison of three reinforcement contingencies. *Behavior Research and Therapy, 5,* 237–243.

Campbell, D. T., & Stanley, J. C. (1963). *Experimental and quasi-experimental designs for research.* Houghton Mifflin.

Catania, A. C., Matthews, T. J., Silverman, P. J., & Yohalem, R. (1977). Yoked variable-ratio and variable-interval responding in pigeons. *Journal of the Experimental Analysis of Behavior, 28,* 155–162.

Ferster, C. B., & Skinner, B. F. (1957). *Schedules of reinforcement.* Prentice-Hall.

Flood, W. A., Wilder, D. A., Flood, A. L., & Masuda, A. (2002). Peer-mediated reinforcement plus prompting as treatment for off-task behavior in children with attention deficit hyperactivity disorder. *Journal of Applied Behavior Analysis, 35,* 199–204.

Hains, A. H., & Baer, D. M. (1989). Interaction effects in multielement designs: Inevitable, desirable, and ignorable. *Journal of Applied Behavior Analysis, 22,* 57–69.

Hersen, M., & Barlow, D. H. (1976). *Single case experimental* designs: Strategies for studying behavior change. Pergamon Press.

Iwata, B. A., Dorsey, M. F., Slifer, K. J., Bauman, K. E., & Richman, G. S. (1994). Toward a functional analysis of self-injury. *Journal of Applied Behavior Analysis, 27*, 197–209. (Reprinted from Analysis and Intervention in Developmental Disabilities, 1982, Vol. 2, pp. 3–20.)

Johnston, J. M., Pennypacker, H. S., & Green, G. (2020). *Strategies and tactics of behavioral research and practice* (4th ed.). Routledge.

Kazdin, A. E. (1982). *Single-case research designs: Methods for clinical and applied settings*. Oxford University Press.

Kazdin, A. E. (2020). *Single-case research designs: Methods for clinical and applied settings* (3rd ed.). Oxford University Press.

Kazdin, A. E., & Geesey, S. (1977). Simultaneous-treatment design comparisons of the effects of earning reinforcers for one's peers versus oneself. *Behavior Therapy, 8*, 682–693.

Kennedy, C. H., & Souza, G. (1995). Functional analysis and treatment of eye poking. *Journal of Applied Behavior Analysis, 28*(1), 27–37.

Laraway, S., Snycerski, S., Michael, J., & Poling, A. (2003). Motivating operations and terms to describe them: Some further refinements. *Journal of Applied Behavior Analysis, 36*, 407–414.

Ledford, J. R., & Gast, D. L (Eds.). (2018). *Single case research methodology*. Routledge.

Leitenberg, H. (1973). The use of single-case methodology in psychotherapy research. *Journal of Abnormal Psychology, 82*, 87–101.

Masson, D. (n.d.). *Balanced Latin square generator*. https://damienmasson.com/tools/latin_square/

McGill, P. (1999). Establishing operations: Implications for the assessment, treatment, and prevention of problem behavior. *Journal of Applied Behavior Analysis, 32*, 393–418.

McGonigle, J. J., Rojahn, J., Dixon, J., & Strain, P. S. (1987). Multiple treatment interference in the alternating treatments design as a function of the intercomponent interval length. *Journal of Applied Behavior Analysis, 20*, 171–178.

Podlesnik, C. A., Jimenez-Gomez, C., & Kelley, M. E. (2021). Matching and behavioral momentum: Quantifying choice and persistence. In W. W. Fisher, C. C. Piazza, & H. S. Roane (Eds.), *Handbook of applied behavior analysis* (2nd ed., pp. 94–114). Guilford Press.

Shadish, W. R., Cook, T. D., & Campbell, D. T. (2002). *Experimental and quasi-experimental designs for generalized causal inference*. Houghton Mifflin.

Shapiro, E. S., Kazdin, A. E., & McGonigle, J. J. (1982). Multiple-treatment interference in the simultaneous- or alternating-treatments design. *Behavioral Assessment, 4*, 105–115.

Sidman, M. (1960). *Tactics of scientific research*. Basic Books.

Stevens, M. A., & Burns, M. K. (2021). Practicing keywords to increase reading performance of students with intellectual disability. *American Journal on Intellectual and Developmental Disabilities, 126*(3), 230–248.

Taylor, L. K., Alber, S. R., & Walker, D. W. (2002). The comparative effects of a modified self-questioning strategy and story mapping on the reading comprehension of elementary students with learning disabilities. *Journal of Behavioral Education, 11*, 69–87.

Trump, C. E., Herrod, J. L., Ayres, K. M., Ringdahl, J. E., & Best, L. (2021). Behavior momentum theory and humans: A review of the literature. *The Psychological Record, 71*(1), 71–83.

Ulman, J. D., & Sulzer-Azaroff, B. (1975). Multielement baseline design in educational research. In E. Ramp & G. Semb (Eds.), *Behavior analysis: Areas of research and application* (pp. 377–391). Prentice-Hall.

Wunderlich, K. L., Vollmer, T. R., Mehrkam, L. R., Feuerbacher, E. N., Slocum, S. K., Kronfli, F. R., & Pizarro, E. (2020). The stability of function of automatically reinforced vocal stereotypy over time. *Journal of Applied Behavior Analysis, 53*(2), 678–689.

CHAPTER 12

Baer, D. M., Wolf, M. M., & Risley, T. R. (1968). Some current dimensions of applied behavior analysis. *Journal of Applied Behavior Analysis, 1*(1), 91–101.

Barlow, D. H., Hayes, S. C., & Nelson, R. O. (1984). *The scientist practitioner: Research and accountability in clinical and educational settings*. Pergamon Press.

Barton, E. E. (2015). Teaching generalized pretend play and related behaviors to young children with disabilities. *Exceptional Children, 81*(4), 489–506.

Carnett, A., Sigafoos, J., & Neely, L. (2022). Programming for generalization and maintenance. In J. L. Matson, & Sturmey, P. (Ed.), *Handbook of autism and pervasive developmental disorder. Autism and Child Psychopathology Series*. Springer.

Chen, C. H., Lee, I. J., & Lin, L. Y. (2015). Augmented reality-based self-facial modeling to promote the emotional expression and social skills of adolescents with autism spectrum disorders. *Research in Developmental Disabilities, 36*, 396–403.

Clark, N. M., Cushing, L. S., & Kennedy, C. H. (2004). An intensive onsite technical assistance model to promote inclusive educational practices for students with disabilities in middle school and high school. *Research and Practice for Persons With Severe Disabilities, 29*(4), 253–262.

Coon, J. C., & Rapp, J. T. (2018). Application of multiple baseline designs in behavior analytic research: Evidence for the influence of new guidelines. *Behavioral Interventions, 33*(2), 160–172.

Fisher, W. W., Piazza, C. C., & Roane, H. S. (2002). Sleep and cyclical variables related to self-injurious and other

destructive behaviors. In S. Schroeder, M. L. Oster-Granite, & T. Thompson (Eds.), *Self-injurious behavior: Gene-brain-behavior relationships* (pp. 205–202). American Psychological Association.

Harvey, M. T., May, M. E., & Kennedy, C. H. (2004). Nonconcurrent multiple baseline designs and the evaluation of educational systems. *Journal of Behavioral Education, 13*(4), 267–276.

Hayes, S. C. (1981). Single case experimental design and empirical clinical practice. *Journal of Consulting and Clinical Psychology, 49*(2), 193–211.

Hinton, V. M., & Flores, M. M. (2019). The effects of the concrete-representational-abstract sequence for students at risk for mathematics failure. *Journal of Behavioral Education, 28*(4), 493–516.

Horner, R. D., & Baer, D. M. (1978). Multiple-probe technique: A variation of the multiple baseline. *Journal of Applied Behavior Analysis, 11*, 189–196.

Kennedy, C. H. (2022). The nonconcurrent multiple-baseline design: It is what it is and not something else. *Perspectives on Behavior Science, 45*(3), 647–650.

Kennedy, C. H., Cushing, L., & Itkonen, T. (1997). General education participation increases the social contacts and friendship networks of students with severe disabilities. *Journal of Behavioral Education, 7*, 167–189.

Rincón, C. L., Muñoz-Martínez, A. M., Hoeflein, B., & Skinta, M. D. (2023). Enhancing interpersonal intimacy in Colombian gay men using functional analytic psychotherapy: An

experimental nonconcurrent multiple baseline design. *Cognitive and Behavioral Practice, 30*(1), 82–95.

Slocum, T. A., Pinkelman, S. E., Joslyn, P. R., & Nichols, B. (2022). Threats to internal validity in multiple-baseline design variations. *Perspectives on Behavior Science, 45*(3), 619–638.

Smith, S. W., Kronfli, F. R., & Vollmer, T. R. (2022). Commentary on Slocum et al. (2022): Additional considerations for evaluating experimental control. *Perspectives on Behavior Science, 45*(3), 667–679.

Stokes, T. F., & Baer, D. M. (1977). An implicit technology of generalization 1. *Journal of Applied Behavior Analysis, 10*(2), 349–367.

Tawney, J. W., & Gast, D. L. (1984). *Single-subject research in special education*. Merrill.

Watson, P. J., & Workman, E. A. (1981). The non-concurrent multiple baseline across-individuals design: An extension of the traditional multiple baseline design. *Journal of Behavior Therapy and Experimental Psychiatry, 12*, 257–259.

CHAPTER 13

Boren, J. J. (1963). The repeated acquisition of new behavioral chains. *American Psychologist, 18*, 421.

Boren, J. J., & Devine, D. D. (1968). The repeated acquisition of behavioral chains. *Journal of the Experimental Analysis of Behavior, 11*, 651–660.

Carroll, R. A., Joachim, B. T., St. Peter, C. C., & Robinson, N. (2015). A comparison of error-correction procedures on skill acquisition during discrete-trial instruction. *Journal of Applied Behavior Analysis, 48*(2), 257–273.

Danforth, J. S., Chase, P. N., Dolan, M., & Joyce, J. H. (1990). The establishment of stimulus control by instructions and by differential reinforcement. *Journal of the Experimental Analysis of Behavior, 54*, 97–112.

Dennis, L. R., & Whalon, K. J. (2021). Effects of teacher- versus application-delivered instruction on the expressive vocabulary of at-risk preschool children. *Remedial and Special Education, 42*(4), 195–206.

Hains, A. H., & Baer, D. M. (1989). Interaction effects in multielement designs: Inevitable, desirable, and ignorable. *Journal of Applied Behavior Analysis, 22*(1), 57–69.

Higgins, S. T., Woodward, B. M., & Henningfield, J. E. (1989). Effects of atropine on the repeated acquisition and performance of response sequences in humans. *Journal of the Experimental Analysis of Behavior, 51*, 5–15.

Kennedy, C. H., Caruso, M., & Thompson, T. (2001). Experimental analyses of gene–brain–behavior relations: Some notes on their application. *Journal of Applied Behavior Analysis, 34*, 539–549.

Kirby, M. S., Spencer, T. D., & Ferron, J. (2021). How to be RAD: Repeated acquisition design features that enhance internal and external validity.

Perspectives on Behavior Science, 44(2–3), 389–416.

Tanious, R., & Onghena, P. (2021). A systematic review of applied single-case research published between 2016 and 2018: Study designs, randomization, data aspects, and data analysis. *Behavior Research Methods, 53*, 1371–1384.

CHAPTER 14

Baer, D. M., Wolf, M. M., & Risley, T. R. (1987). Some still-current dimensions of applied behavior analysis. *Journal of Applied Behavior Analysis, 20*, 313–327.

Bartlett, S. M., Rapp, J. T., & Henrickson, M. L. (2011). Detecting false positives in multielement designs: Implications for brief assessments. *Behavior Modification, 35*(6), 531–552.

Boyajian, A. E., DuPaul, G. J., Handler, M. W., Eckert, T. L., & McGoey, K. E. (2001). The use of classroom-based brief functional analyses with preschoolers at-risk for attention deficit hyperactivity disorder. *School Psychology Review, 30*, 278–293.

Cooper, L. J., Wacker, D. P., Sasso, G. M., Reimers, T. M., & Donn, L. K. (1990). Using parents as therapists to evaluate appropriate behavior of their children: Application to a tertiary diagnostic clinic. *Journal of Applied Behavior Analysis, 23*, 285–296.

Eckert, T. L., Ardoin, S. P., Daly, E. J., III, & Martens, B. K. (2002). Improving oral reading fluency: A brief experimental

analysis of combining an antecedent intervention with consequences. *Journal of Applied Behavior Analysis, 35*, 271–281.

Henry, J. E., Kelley, M. E., LaRue, R. H., Kettering, T. L., Gadaire, D. M., & Sloman, K. N. (2021). Integration of experimental functional analysis procedural advancements: Progressing from brief to extended experimental analyses. *Journal of Applied Behavior Analysis, 54*(3), 1045–1061.

Iwata, B. A., Dorsey, M. F., Slifer, K. J., Bauman, K. E., & Richman, G. S. (1982). Toward a functional analysis of self-injury. *Analysis and Intervention in Developmental Disabilities, 2*, 3–20.

Richman, D. M., Wacker, D. P., Brown, L. J. C., Kayser, K., Crosland, K., Stephens, T. J., & Asmus, J. (2001). Stimulus characteristics within directives: Effects on accuracy of task completion. *Journal of Applied Behavior Analysis, 34*, 289–312.

Wacker, D., Berg, W., Harding, J., & Cooper-Brown, L. (2004). Use of brief experimental analyses in outpatient clinic and home settings. *Journal of Behavioral Education, 13*, 213–226.

Wallace, M. D., & Iwata, B. A. (1999). Effects of session duration on functional analysis outcomes. *Journal of Applied Behavior Analysis, 32*, 175–183.

CHAPTER 15

Baer, D. M., Wolf, M. M., & Risley, T. R. (1987). Some still-current dimensions of applied behavior analysis. *Journal of Applied Behavior Analysis, 20,* 313–327.

Barlow, D. H., & Hersen, M. (1984). *Single case experimental designs: Strategies for studying behavior change* (2nd ed.). Pergamon.

Carr, E. G., & Durand, V. M. (1985). Reducing behavior problems through functional communication training. *Journal of Applied Behavior Analysis, 18,* 111–126.

Epstein, L. H., & Dallery, J. (2022). The family of single-case experimental designs. *Harvard Data Science Review, 3,* 1–21.

Fisher, W. W., & Mazur, J. E. (1997). Basic and applied research on choice responding. *Journal of Applied Behavior Analysis, 30*(3), 387–410.

Herrnstein, R. J. (1970). On the law of effect. *Journal of the Experimental Analysis of Behavior, 13,* 243–266.

Kazdin, A. E. (1982). *Single-case research designs: Methods for clinical and applied settings.* Oxford University Press.

Kelley, M. E., Lerman, D. C., & Van Camp, C. M. (2002). The effects of competing reinforcement schedules on the acquisition of functional communication. *Journal of Applied Behavior Analysis, 35,* 59–63.

Kennedy, C. H., Caruso, M., & Thompson, T. (2001). Experimental analyses of gene-brain-behavior relations: Some notes on their application. *Journal of Applied Behavior Analysis, 34*(4), 539–549.

Kennedy, C. H., Meyer, K. A., Knowles, T., & Shukla, S. (2000). Analyzing the multiple functions of stereotypical behavior for students with autism: Implications for assessment and treatment. *Journal of Applied Behavior Analysis, 33,* 559–571.

Lattal, K. A. (2008). JEAB at 50: Coevolution of research and technology. *Journal of the Experimental Analysis of Behavior, 89*(1), 129–135.

Lee, R., McComas, J. J., & Jawor, J. (2002). The effects of differential and lag reinforcement schedules on varied verbal responding by individuals with autism. *Journal of Applied Behavior Analysis, 35,* 391–402.

Mace, F. C. (1994). Basic research needed for stimulating the development of behavioral technologies. *Journal of the Experimental Analysis of Behavior, 61,* 529–550.

Martens, B. K., Ardoin, S. P., Hilt, A. M., Lannie, A. L., Panahon, C. J., & Wolfe, L. A. (2002). Sensitivity of children's behavior to probabilistic reward: Effects of a decreasing-ratio lottery system on math performance. *Journal of Applied Behavior Analysis, 35,* 403–406.

McDowell, J. J. (2013). On the theoretical and empirical status of the matching law and matching theory. *Psychological Bulletin, 139*(5), 1000–1028.

Neuringer, A. (2002). Operant variability: Evidence, functions, and theory. *Psychonomic Bulletin and Review, 9,* 672–705.

Poling, A., Edwards, T. L., Weeden, M., & Foster, T. M. (2011). The matching law. *The Psychological Record, 61,* 313–322.

Richman, D. M., Wacker, D. P., & Winborn, L. (2001).

Response efficiency during functional communication training: Effects of effort on response allocation. *Journal of Applied Behavior Analysis, 34,* 73–76.

Ringdahl, J. E., Winborn, L. C., Andelman, M. S., & Kitsukawa, K. (2002). The effects of non-contingently available alternative stimuli on functional analysis outcomes. *Journal of Applied Behavior Analysis, 35,* 407–410.

Smith, J. D. (2012). Single-case experimental designs: A systematic review of published research and current standards. *Psychological Methods, 17*(4), 1–69.

Tang, J.-C., Patterson, T. G., & Kennedy, C. H. (2003). Identifying specific sensory modalities maintaining the stereotypy of students with multiple profound disabilities. *Research in Developmental Disabilities, 24,* 433–451.

Tiger, J. H., Hanley, G. P., & Bruzek, J. (2008). Functional communication training: A review and practical guide. *Behavior Analysis in Practice, 31,* 16–23.

CHAPTER 16

Beavers, G. A., Iwata, B. A., & Lerman, D. C. (2013). Thirty years of research on the functional analysis of problem behavior. *Journal of Applied Behavior Analysis, 46*(1), 1–21.

Binder, C., & Watkins, C. L. (2013). Precision teaching and direct instruction: Measurably superior instructional technology in schools.

Performance Improvement Quarterly, 26(2), 73–115.

Carr, E. G., Newsom, C. D., & Binkoff, J. A. (1980). Escape as a factor in the aggressive behavior of two retarded children. *Journal of Applied Behavior Analysis, 13*, 101–117.

Catania, A. C. (1988). The behavior of organisms as work in progress. *Journal of the Experimental Analysis of Behavior, 50*, 277–281.

Catania, A. C. (2013a). *Learning* (5th ed.). Sloan Publishing.

Catania, A. C. (2013b). A natural science of behavior. *Review of General Psychology, 17*(2), 133–139.

Cook, T. D., Campbell, D. T., & Shadish, W. (2002). *Experimental and quasi-experimental designs for generalized causal inference*. Houghton Mifflin.

Coopmans, C., Vertesi, J., Lynch, M. E., & Woolgar, S (Eds.). (2014). *Representation in scientific practice revisited*. MIT Press.

Cushing, L. S., & Kennedy., C. H. (1997). Academic effects of providing peer support in general education classrooms on students without disabilities. *Journal of Applied Behavior Analysis, 30*, 139–150.

DeProspero, A., & Cohen, S. (1979). Inconsistent visual analyses of intrasubject data. *Journal of Applied Behavior Analysis, 12*, 573–579.

DeRosa, N. M., Sullivan, W. E., Roane, H. S., Craig, A. R., & Kadey, H. J. (2021). *Single-case experimental designs*. In W. W. Fisher, C. C. Piazza, & H. S. Roane (Eds.), *Handbook of applied behavior analysis* (2nd

ed., pp. 155–172). Guilford Press.

Diller, J. W., Barry, R. J., & Gelino, B. W. (2016). Visual analysis of data in a multielement design. *Journal of Applied Behavior Analysis, 49*(4), 980–985.

Fisch, G. S. (2001). Evaluating data from behavioral analysis: Visual inspection or statistical models? *Behavioural Processes, 54*, 137–154.

Fisher, W. W., Kelley, M. E., & Lomas, J. E. (2003). Visual aids and structured criteria for improving visual inspection and interpretation of single-case designs. *Journal of Applied Behavior Analysis, 36*, 387–406.

Furlong, M. J., & Wampold, B. E. (1982). Intervention effects and relative variation as dimensions in experts' use of visual inference. *Journal of Applied Behavior Analysis, 15*, 415–421.

Gold, M. W. (1976). Task analysis of a complex assembly task by retarded children. *Exceptional Children, 43*, 78–85.

Hacking, I. (1983). *Representing and intervening*. Cambridge University Press.

Haring, T. G., & Kennedy., C. H. (1988). Units of analysis in task-analytic research. *Journal of Applied Behavior Analysis, 21*, 207–216.

Holzinger, A. (2014). Visual insights: A practical guide to making sense of data. *Online Information Review, 38*(7), 994–995.

Iversen, I. H. (1988). Tactics of graphic design: A review of Tufte's The visual display of

quantitative information. *Journal of the Experimental Analysis of Behavior, 49*, 171–189.

Jones, R. R., Weinrott, M. R., & Vaught, R. S. (1978). Effects of serial dependency on the agreement between visual and statistical inference. *Journal of Applied Behavior Analysis, 11*, 277–283.

Kahng, S. W., Chung, K. M., Gutshall, K., Pitts, S. C., Kao, J., & Girolami, K. (2010). Consistent visual analyses of intrasubject data. *Journal of Applied Behavior Analysis, 43*(1), 35–45.

Kazdin, A. E. (1982). *Single-case research designs*. Oxford University Press.

Lane, J. D., & Gast, D. L. (2014). Visual analysis in single case experimental design studies: Brief review and guidelines. *Neuropsychological Rehabilitation, 24*(3–4), 445–463.

Latour, B., & Woolgar, S. (2013). *Laboratory life: The construction of scientific facts*. Princeton University Press.

McConomy, M. A., Root, J., & Wade, T. (2022). Using task analysis to support inclusion and assessment in the classroom. *TEACHING Exceptional Children, 54*(6), 414–422.

McInerny, G. (2013). Embedding visual communication into scientific practice. *Trends in Ecology & Evolution, 28*(1), 13–14.

Parsonson, B. S., & Baer, D. M. (2015). The visual analysis of data, and current research into the stimuli controlling it. In T. R. Kratochwill & J. R. Levin (Eds.), *Single-case research design and analysis: New directions for psychology and education* (pp. 15–40). Taylor & Francis.

Shavelson, R. J., & Towne, L. (2002). *Scientific research in education*. National Academies Press.

Sidman, M. (1960). Normal sources of pathological behavior. *Science, 132*, 61–68.

Skinner, B. F. (1938). *The behavior of organisms: An experimental analysis*. Copley.

Smith, L. D., Best, L. A., Stubbs, D. A., Archibald, A. B., & Roberson-Nay, R. (2002). Constructing knowledge: The role of graphs and tables in hard and soft psychology. *American Psychologist, 57*, 749–761.

Smith, R. G., & Churchill, R. M. (2002). Identification of environmental determinants of behavior disorders through functional analysis of precursor behaviors. *Journal of Applied Behavior Analysis, 35*, 125–136.

Tufte, E. R. (1983). *The visual display of quantitative information*. Graphics Press.

Tufte, E. R. (1997). *Visual explanations: Images and quantities, evidence and narrative*. Graphics Press.

Vollmer, T. R., Ringdahl, J. E., Roane, H. S., & Marcus, B. A. (1997). Negative side effects of noncontingent reinforcement. *Journal of Applied Behavior Analysis, 30*, 161–164.

White, O. R. (1971). *A pragmatic approach to the description of progress in the single case* [Unpublished doctoral dissertation]. University of Oregon.

CHAPTER 17

Barlow, D. H., & Nock, M. K. (2009). Why can't we be more idiographic in our research? *Perspectives on Psychological Science, 4*(1), 19–21.

Barton, E. E., Lloyd, B. P., Spriggs, A. D., & Gast, D. L. (2018). Visual analysis of graphic data. In J. R. Ledford & D. L. Gast (Eds.), *Single case research methodology: Applications in special education and behavioral sciences* (pp. 179–214). Routledge.

Becraft, J. L., Borrero, J. C., Sun, S., & McKenzie, A. A. (2020). A primer for using multilevel models to meta-analyze single case design data with AB phases. *Journal of Applied Behavior Analysis, 53*(3), 1799–1821.

Birnbrauer, J. S. (1981). External validity and experimental investigation of individual behaviour. *Analysis and Intervention in Developmental Disabilities, 1*(2), 117–132.

Busk, P. L., & Marascuilo, L. A. (1988). Autocorrelation in single-subject research: A counterargument to the myth of no autocorrelation. *Behavioral Assessment, 10*(3), 229–242.

Campbell, D. T. (1988). *Methodology and epistemology for social sciences: Selected papers*. University of Chicago Press.

Cohen, J. (1977). *Statistical power analysis for the behavioral sciences*. Academic Press.

Common, E. A., Lane, K. L., Pustejovsky, J. E., Johnson, A. H., & Johl, L. E. (2017).

Functional assessment–based interventions for students with or at-risk for high-incidence disabilities: Field testing single-case synthesis methods. *Remedial and Special Education, 38*(6), 331–352.

Dowdy, A., Peltier, C., Tincani, M., Schneider, W. J., Hantula, D. A., & Travers, J. C. (2021). Meta-analyses and effect sizes in applied behavior analysis: A review and discussion. *Journal of Applied Behavior Analysis, 54*(4), 1317–1340.

Edgington, E. S. (1969). Approximate randomization tests. *Journal of Psychology, 72*(2), 143–149.

Edgington, E. S. (1980). Validity of randomization tests for one-subject experiments. *Journal of Educational Statistics, 5*(3), 235–251.

Ferron, J. M., & Levin, J. R. (2014). Single-case permutation and randomization statistical tests: Present status, promising new developments. In T. R. Kratochwill & J. R. Levin (Eds.), *Single-case intervention research: Methodological and statistical advances* (pp. 153–183). American Psychological Association.

Gast, D. L., & Spriggs, A. D. (2010). Visual analysis of graphic data. In D. L. Gast (Ed.), *Single subject research methodology in behavioral sciences* (pp. 199–233). Routledge.

Gettinger, M., Kratochwill, T. R., Eubanks, A., Foy, A., & Levin, J. R. (2021). Academic and behavior combined support: Evaluation of an integrated supplemental intervention for early elementary students. *Journal of School Psychology, 89*, 1–19.

Glass, G. V. (1976). Primary, secondary, and meta-analysis of research. *Educational Researcher, 5*(10), 3–8.

Glass, G. V., Wilson, V. L., & Gottman, J. M. (1975). *Design and analysis of time-series experiments*. Colorado Associated University Press.

Gottman, J. M., Glass, G. V., & Kratochwill, T. R. (1978). Analysis of interrupted time-series experiments. In T. R. Kratochwill (Ed.), *Single subject research: Strategies for evaluating change* (pp. 197–234). Academic Press.

Hedges, L. V. (1982). Estimation of effect size from a series of independent experiments. *Psychological Bulletin, 92*(2), 490–499.

Hedges, L. V., Pustejovsky, J. E., & Shadish, W. R. (2012). A standardized mean difference effect size for single case designs. *Research Synthesis Methods, 3*(3), 224–239.

Hedges, L. V., Pustejovsky, J. E., & Shadish, W. R. (2013). A standardized mean difference effect size for multiple baseline designs across individuals. *Research Synthesis Methods, 4*(4), 324–341.

Johnston, J. M., Pennypacker, H. S., & Green, G. (2020). *Strategies and tactics of behavioral research and practice* (4th ed.). Routledge.

Keren, G. (2014). Between-or within-subjects design: A methodological dilemma. In G. Keren & C. Lewis (Eds.), *A handbook for data analysis in the behavioral sciences:*

Methodological issues (Vol. 1, pp. 257–275). Psychology Press.

Killeen, P. R. (1978). Stability criteria. *Journal of the Experimental Analysis of Behavior, 29*(1), 17–25.

Kratochwill, T. R. (1978). *Single subject research: Strategies for evaluating change*. Academic Press.

Kratochwill, T. R., Horner, R. H., Levin, J. R., Machalicek, W., Ferron, J., & Johnson, A. (2023). Single-case intervention research design standards: Additional proposed upgrades and future directions. *Journal of School Psychology, 97*, 192–216.

Kratochwill, T. R., & Levin, J. R. (2014). *Single-case intervention research: Methodological and statistical advances*. American Psychological Association.

Lane, J. D., & Gast, D. L. (2014). Visual analysis in single case experimental design studies: Brief review and guidelines. *Neuropsychological Rehabilitation, 24*(3–4), 445–463.

Levin, J. R., Ferron, J. M., & Gafurov, B. S. (2018). Comparison of randomization-test procedures for single-case multiple-baseline designs. *Developmental Neurorehabilitation, 21*(5), 290–311.

Lieberman, R. G., Yoder, P. J., Reichow, B., & Wolery, M. (2010). Visual analysis of multiple baseline across participants graphs when change is delayed. *School Psychology Quarterly, 25*(1), 28–44.

Lipsey, M. W., & Wilson, D. B. (2000). *Practical meta-analysis*. Sage.

Lord, F. M., & Novick, M. R. (1968). *Statistical theories of mental test scores*. Addison-Wesley.

Ma, H. H. (2006). An alternative method for quantitative synthesis of single-subject researches: Percentage of data points exceeding the median. *Behavior Modification, 30*(5), 598–617.

Maggin, D. M., & Odom, S. L. (2014). Evaluating single-case research data for systematic review: A commentary for the special issue. *Journal of School Psychology, 52*(2), 237–241.

Manolov, R., & Solanas, A. (2009). Percentage of non-overlapping corrected data. *Behavior Research Methods, 41*(4), 1262–1271.

Molenaar, P. C. (2004). A manifesto on psychology as idiographic science: Bringing the person back into scientific psychology, this time forever. *Measurement, 2*(4), 201–218.

Molenaar, P. C. (2008). On the implications of the classical ergodic theorems: Analysis of developmental processes has to focus on intra-individual variation. *Developmental Psychobiology, 50*(1), 60–69.

Moeyaert, M., Manolov, R., & Rodabaugh, E. (2020). Meta-analysis of single-case research via multilevel models: Fundamental concepts and methodological considerations. *Behavior Modification, 44*(2), 265–295.

Moeyaert, M., Zimmerman, K. N., & Ledford, J. R. (2018). Synthesis and meta-analysis of single case research. In J. R. Ledford & D. L. Gast (Eds.), *Single case research methodology: Applications in special education and behavioral sciences* (3rd ed., pp. 393–416). Routledge.

Nesselroade, K. P., Jr., & Grimm, L. G. (2018). *Statistical applications for the behavioral and social sciences*. John Wiley & Sons.

Parker, R. I., Hagan-Burke, S., & Vannest, K. (2007). Percentage of all non-overlapping data (PAND) an alternative to PND. *Journal of Special Education*, *40*(4), 194–204.

Parker, R. I., & Vannest, K. J. (2012). Bottom-up analysis of single-case research designs. *Journal of Behavioral Education*, *21*, 254–265.

Parker, R. I., Vannest, K. J., Davis, J. L., & Sauber, S. B. (2011). Combining nonoverlap and trend for single-case research: Tau-U. *Behavior Therapy*, *42*(2), 284–299.

Pustejovsky, J. E. (2015). Measurement-comparable effect sizes for single-case studies of free-operant behavior. *Psychological Methods*, *20*(3), 342–359.

Pustejovsky, J. E. (2018). Using response ratios for meta-analyzing single-case designs with behavioral outcomes. *Journal of School Psychology*, *68*, 99–112.

Pustejovsky, J. E. (2019). Procedural sensitivities of effect sizes for single-case designs with directly observed behavioral outcome measures. *Psychological Methods*, *24*(2), 217–235.

Pustejovsky, J. E., & Ferron, J. M. (2017). Research synthesis and meta-analysis of single-case designs. In J. M.

Kaufmann, D. P. Hallahan, & P. C. Pullen (Eds.), *Handbook of Special Education* (2nd ed., pp. 168–186). Routledge.

Raudenbush, S. W., Spybrook, J., Liu, S., & Congdon, R. (2005). *Optimal design for multi-level and longitudinal research*. Version 3.01 [Computer software] www.wtgrantfoundation.org

Revusky, S. H. (1967). Some statistical treatments compatible with individual organism methodology. *Journal of the Experimental Analysis of Behavior*, *10*(3), 319–330.

Richman, D. M., Barnard-Brak, L., Grubb, L., Bosch, A., & Abby, L. (2015). Meta-analysis of noncontingent reinforcement effects on problem behavior. *Journal of Applied Behavior Analysis*, *48*(1), 131–152.

Salzberg, C. L., Strain, P. S., & Baer, D. M. (1987). Meta-analysis for single-subject research: When does it clarify, when does it obscure? *Remedial and Special Education*, *8*(2), 43–48.

Scruggs, T. E., Mastropieri, M. A., & Casto, G. (1987). The quantitative synthesis of single-subject research: Methodology and validation. *Remedial and Special Education*, *8*(2), 24–33.

Shadish, W. R., Hedges, L. V., & Pustejovsky, J. E. (2014). Analysis and meta-analysis of single-case designs with a standardized mean difference statistic: A primer and applications. *Journal of School Psychology*, *52*(2), 123–147.

Shadish, W. R., Kyse, E. N., & Rindskopf, D. M. (2013).

Analyzing data from single-case designs using multilevel models: New applications and some agenda items for future research. *Psychological Methods*, *18*(3), 385–405.

Shadish, W. R., & Rindskopf, D. M. (2007). Methods for evidence-based practice: Quantitative synthesis of single-subject designs. *New Directions for Evaluation*, *2007*(113), 95–109.

Shadish, W. R., Rindskopf, D. M., & Hedges, L. V. (2008). The state of the science in the meta-analysis of single-case experimental designs. *Evidence-Based Communication Assessment and Intervention*, *2*(3), 188–196.

Shadish, W. R., & Sullivan, K. J. (2011). Characteristics of single-case designs used to assess intervention effects in 2008. *Behavior Research Methods*, *43*, 971–980.

Sidman, M. (1960). *Tactics of scientific research*. Basic Books.

Slocum, T. A., Detrich, R., Wilczynski, S. M., Spencer, T. D., Lewis, T., & Wolfe, K. (2014). The evidence-based practice of applied behavior analysis. *Behavior Analyst*, *37*(1), 41–56.

Smith, J. D. (2012). Single-case experimental designs: A systematic review of published research and current standards. *Psychological Methods*, *17*(4), 510–550.

Tarlow, K. R. (2017). An improved rank correlation effect size statistic for single-case designs: Baseline corrected Tau. *Behavior Modification*, *41*(4), 427–467.

Wampold, B. E., & Worsham, N. L. (1986). Randomization tests for multiple-baseline designs. *Behavioral Assessment*, *8*(2), 135–143.

Weaver, E. S., & Lloyd, B. P. (2019). Randomization tests for single case designs with rapidly alternating conditions: An analysis of p-values from published experiments. *Perspectives on Behavior Science*, *42*, 617–645.

White, O. R. (1987). Some comments concerning "The quantitative synthesis of single-subject research." *Remedial and Special Education*, *8*(2), 34–39.

White, O. R. (1971). *The split middle: A quickie method of trend estimation. [Unpublished master's thesis]*. University of Oregon.

White, O. R., & Haring, N. G. (1980). *Exceptional teaching*. Charles E. Merrill.

Wolery, M., Busick, M., Reichow, B., & Barton, E. E. (2010). Comparison of overlap methods for quantitatively synthesizing single-subject data. *Journal of Special Education*, *44*(1), 18–28.

CHAPTER 18

Baer, D. M., Wolf, M. M., & Risley, T. R. (1968). Some current dimensions of applied behavior analysis. *Journal of Applied Behavior Analysis*, *1*, 91–97.

Baer, D. M., Wolf, M. M., & Risley, T. R. (1987). Some still-current dimensions of applied behavior analysis. *Journal of Applied Behavior Analysis*, *20*(4), 313–327.

Brantlinger, E., Jimenez, R., Klingner, J., Pugach, M., & Richardson, V. (2005). Qualitative studies in special education. *Exceptional Children*, *71*(2), 195–207.

Carr, J. E., Austin, J. L., Britton, L. N., Kellum, K. K., & Bailey, J. S. (1999). An assessment of social validity trends in applied behavior analysis. *Behavioral Interventions*, *14*, 223–231.

Cox, J. A., & Kennedy, C. H. (2003). Transitions between school and hospital for students with multiple disabilities: A survey of causes, educational continuity, and parental perceptions. *Research and Practice for People With Severe Disabilities (formerly JASH)*, *28*, 1–6.

Critchfield, T. S. (2011). Translational contributions of the experimental analysis of behavior. *The Behavior Analyst*, *34*, 3–17.

Enright, R. (2018, April 7). Behavior modification and the image of humanity. *Psychology Today*.

Fawcett, S. B. (1991). Social validity: A note on methodology. *Journal of Applied Behavior Analysis*, *24*, 235–239.

Ferguson, J. L., Cihon, J. H., Leaf, J. B., Van Meter, S. M., McEachin, J., & Leaf, R. (2019). Assessment of social validity trends in the journal of applied behavior analysis. *European Journal of Behavior Analysis*, *20*(1), 146–157.

Finn, C. A., & Sladeczek, I. E. (2001). Assessing the social validity of behavioral interventions: A review of treatment acceptability measures.

School Psychology Quarterly, *16*(2), 176.

Foster, S. L., & Mash, E. J. (1999). Assessing social validity in clinical treatment research: Issues and procedures. *Journal of Consulting and Clinical Psychology*, *67*(3), 308–319.

Goldiamond, I. (1976). Protection of human subjects and patients. *Behaviorism*, *4*, 1–42.

Hawkins, R. P. (1991). Is social validity what we are interested in? Argument for a functional approach. *Journal of Applied Behavior Analysis*, *24*, 205–213.

Kazdin, A. E. (1977). Assessing the clinical or applied significance of behavior change through social validation. *Behavior Modification*, *1*, 427–452.

Kazdin, A. E. (1980). Acceptability of alternative treatments for deviant child behavior. *Journal of Applied Behavior Analysis*, *13*, 259–273.

Kennedy, C. H. (1992). Trends in the measurement of social validity. *The Behavior Analyst*, *15*, 147–156.

Kennedy, C. H. (2002). The maintenance of behavior as an indicator of social validity. *Behavior Modification*, *26*, 594–606.

Leko, M. M., Cook, B. G., & Cook, L. (2021). Qualitative methods in special education research. *Learning Disabilities Research and Practice*, *36*(4), 278–286.

Lerman, D. C. (2024). Putting the power of behavior analysis in the hands of nonbehavioral professionals: Toward a blueprint for dissemination.

Journal of Applied Behavior Analysis, 57(1), 39–54.

Luiselli, J. K. (2021). Social validity assessment. In J. K. Luiselli (Ed.), *Applied behavior analysis treatment of violence and aggression in persons with neurodevelopmental disabilities* (pp. 85–103). Springer.

Makeover, H. B. (1950). The quality of medical care. *American Journal of Public Health, 41,* 824–832.

Poling, A., & Edwards, T. L. (2011). Translational research: It's not 1960s behavior analysis. *The Behavior Analyst, 34*(1), 23.

Reid, D. H., Parsons, M. B., & Jensen, J. M. (2017). Maintaining staff performance following a training intervention: Suggestions from a 30-year case example. *Behavior Analysis in Practice, 10*(1), 12–21.

Roethlisberger, F. J., & Dickson, W. J. (1939). *Management and the worker.* Harvard University Press.

Rogers, C. R. (1942). *Counseling and psychotherapy: New concepts in practice.* Houghton Mifflin.

Rusch, F. R., & Kazdin, A. E. (1981). Toward a methodology of withdrawal designs for the assessment of response maintenance. *Journal of Applied Behavior Analysis, 14,* 131–140.

Schwartz, I. S., & Baer, D. M. (1991). Social validity assessments: Is current practice state of the art? *Journal of Applied Behavior Analysis, 24,* 189–204.

Schwartz, I. S., & Kelly, E. M. (2021). Quality of life for people with disabilities: Why applied behavior analysts should consider this a primary dependent variable. *Research and Practice for Persons With Severe Disabilities, 46*(3), 159–172.

Tsami, L., Lerman, D., & Toper-Korkmaz, O. (2019). Effectiveness and acceptability of parent training via telehealth among families around the world. *Journal of Applied Behavior Analysis, 52*(4), 1113–1129.

Van Houten, R. (1979). Social validation: The evolution of standards of competency for target behaviors. *Journal of Applied Behavior Analysis, 12,* 581–591.

Walker, H. M., & Hops, H. (1976). Use of normative peer data as a standard for evaluating classroom treatment effects. *Journal of Applied Behavior Analysis, 9,* 159–168.

Wolf, M. M. (1978). Social validity: The case for subjective measurement or How applied behavior analysis is finding its heart. *Journal of Applied Behavior Analysis, 11,* 203–214.

Wolraich, M. L. (1997). Addressing behavior problems among school-aged children: Traditional and controversial approaches. *Pediatrics in Review, 18*(8), 266–270.

INDEX